ABBREVIATIONS COMMONLY USED IN ORTHOPEDIC NURSING

ADL	Activities of daily living
AKA	Above-the-knee amputation
AS	Ankylosing spondylitis
BKA	Below-the-knee amputation
CHD	Congenital hip dysplasia or dislocation
CPM	Continuous passive motion or movement
CT	Computed tomography
CTS	Carpal tunnel syndrome
DJD	Degenerative joint disease
EFD	External fixation device
EMG	Electromyogram
MRI	Magnetic resonance imaging
OA	Osteoarthritis
ORIF	Open reduction with internal fixation
OT	Occupational therapy
PT	Physical therapy
RA	Rheumatoid arthritis
RICE	Rest, ice, compression, elevation
ROM	Range of motion
SLR	Straight leg raises
THR	Total hip replacement
TKR	Total knee replacement
TSR	Total shoulder replacement

ORTHOPEDIC DISORDERS

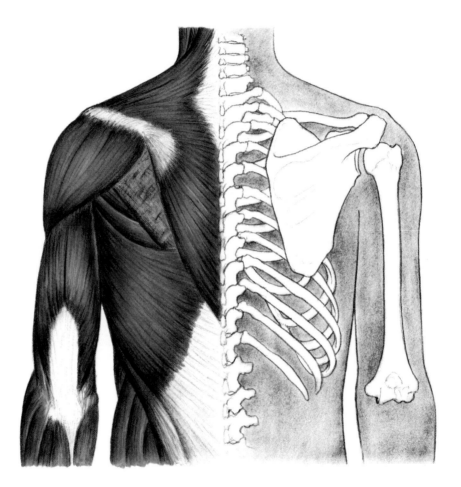

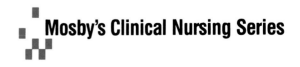
Mosby's Clinical Nursing Series

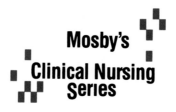

Mosby's Clinical Nursing Series

Cardiovascular Disorders

by Mary Canobbio

Respiratory Disorders

by Susan Wilson and June Thompson

Infectious Diseases

by Deanna Grimes

Orthopedic Disorders

by Leona Mourad

Renal Disorders

by Dorothy Brundage

Neurologic Disorders

by Esther Chipps, Norma Clanin, and Victor Campbell

Immunologic Disorders

by Christine Mudge-Grout

Cancer

by Anne Belcher

Gastrointestinal Disorders

by Dorothy Doughty and Debra Broadwell

Genitourinary Disorders

by Mikel Gray

ORTHOPEDIC DISORDERS

LEONA A. MOURAD, M.S., R.N., O.N.C.

Associate Professor Emeritus
The Ohio State University
College of Nursing
Columbus, Ohio;
Nursing Consultant,
Mourad Consultant Associates
Columbus, Ohio

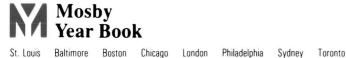

Mosby
Year Book

St. Louis   Baltimore   Boston   Chicago   London   Philadelphia   Sydney   Toronto

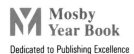

Executive Editor: Don Ladig
Managing Editor: Sally Adkisson
Project Manager: Mark Spann
Designer: Liz Fett

The author wishes to acknowledge the contributions of the
Departments of Orthopedics, Radiology, and Physical Medicine at
The Ohio State University, Columbus, Ohio.

Mosby–Year Book, Inc.
11830 Westline Industrial Drive, St. Louis, Missouri 63146

Library of Congress Cataloging-in-Publication Data

Mourad, Leona A.
    Orthopedic disorders / Leona A. Mourad
        p.   cm. — (Mosby's clinical nursing series)
    ISBN 0-8016-3438-5
    1. Orthopedic nursing.   2. Orthopedics.   3. Bones—Diseases.
    I. Title.   II. Series.
    [DNLM: 1. Bone Diseases—nursing.   2. Muscular Diseases—nursing.
    3. Orthopedics—nursing.   WY   157.6 M929o]
    RD753.M69   1991
    610.73′677—dc20
    DNLM/DLC
    for Library of Congress   91-19569
                                                                CIP

C/CD/VH   9   8   7   6   5   4   3   2

Chapter 15 *"Musculoskeletal Drugs,"* contributed by
Mark Hamelink, MSN, CRNA
Nurse Anesthetist
Morpheus Anesthesia Services, P.C.
South Haven, Michigan

Original illustrations prepared by
George J. Wassilchenko
Tulsa, Oklahoma
and
Donald P. O'Connor
St. Peters, Missouri

Photography by
Patrick Watson
Poughkeepsie, New York

PREFACE

Orthopedic Disorders is the fourth volume in Mosby's Clinical Nursing series, a new kind of resource for practicing nurses.

The *Series* is the result of the most elaborate market research ever undertaken by Mosby–Year Book. We first surveyed hundreds of working nurses to determine what kind of resources practicing nurses want in order to meet their advanced information needs. We then approached clinical specialists—proven authors and experts in 10 practice areas, from cardiovascular to immunology—and asked them to develop a common format that would meet the needs of nurses in practice, as specified by the survey respondents. This plan was then presented to 9 focus groups composed of working nurses over a period of 18 months. The plan was refined between each group, and in the later stages we published a 32-page full-color sample so that detailed changes could be made to improve the physical layout and appearance of the book, section by section and page by page. The result is a new genre of professional books for nursing professionals.

Orthopedic Disorders begins with an innovative color atlas of musculoskeletal structure and function. This review of the anatomy and physiology contains numerous detailed full-color drawings designed to depict normal structure and function.

Chapter 2 includes a discussion of the health history with a focus on musculoskeletal data, physical examination, and assessments of musculoskeletal tissues. Clear full-color photographs show normal musculoskeletal functions and proper positions for assessments. Special assessment techniques are included in an appendix.

Chapter 3 presents detailed information and full-color photographs of diagnostic tests. A consistent format for each diagnostic procedure provides information about the purpose of the test, indications and contraindications, and the associated nursing care, including patient teaching.

Chapter 4 is a discussion of the various types of injuries to musculoskeletal tissues. This chapter includes first aid measures for frequently encountered injuries, principles of trauma management, and definitive treatments for these injuries. Highlights of the chapter are two comprehensive, illustrated tables of fractures. The illustrations can be used for self-learning or for teaching purposes. The nursing process format provides detailed assessments and findings, nursing diagnoses, patient goals, nursing interventions with rationales, expected outcomes, and patient teaching.

Chapters 5 and 6 present the nursing care of patients with inflammatory and degenerative conditions of musculoskeletal tissues. Each disease or condition has its pathophysiologic basis presented. Possible complications are highlighted in boxes so the nurse can be responsive to changes in the patient's condition.

Chapter 7 discusses infectious musculoskeletal conditions, primarily focusing on osteomyelitis with its associated treatments and nursing care.

Chapter 8 discusses metabolic conditions of musculoskeletal tissues, with osteoporosis foremost in the content discussion. Complications, treatments, and nursing care are incorporated throughout.

Chapter 9 discusses spinal curvatures, current treatment regimens, and corresponding nursing care.

Chapter 10 discusses benign and malignant tumors of musculoskeletal tissues with correlations of the various tumors' characteristics, degree of malignancy, and treatment options included. Recent limb salvage procedures are discussed and nursing care is presented positively related to the specific type of tumor.

Chapter 11 focuses on the treatments and nursing care for frequently occurring congenital anomalies, congenital hip dysplasia or dislocation and club foot.

Chapter 12 presents care of patients in casts, traction, and external fixation devices. Information on the types of casts, skin, and skeletal tractions is presented along with indications for use of each. Complete nursing care is presented, including care after removal of the cast or traction. This chapter has detailed information related to potentially severe complications of patients in casts.

Chapter 13 discusses the many different types of surgical procedures for musculoskeletal conditions. Included is discussion of surgical treatment for rotator cuff tears, frequent shoulder dislocations, meniscal and ligament tears, chemonucleolysis for ruptured disks, and the Ilizarov procedure for treating bone nonunions, bone infections, or for limb lengthening.

Chapter 14 presents Patient Teaching Guides for many of the conditions, treatments, or self-care activities associated with orthopedic diseases or trauma. The guides are designed to be copied and handed out for individual patient teaching and learning.

Chapter 15 has excellent content on the many pharmaceutical agents used for patients with musculoskeletal disorders. Many tables are included, listing drugs with similar actions, their trade and generic names, and common dosages.

It is hoped that this book will be used by nurses as they provide care for and with orthopedic patients and their families. It was prepared with thoughtfulness and sensitivity to be a ready and handy resource.

Contents

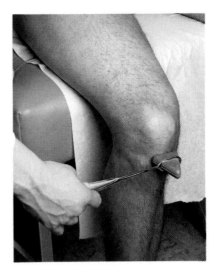

1 COLOR ATLAS OF THE MUSCULOSKELETAL SYSTEM, 1

2 ASSESSMENT, 17

3 DIAGNOSTIC PROCEDURES, 36

X-ray examination, 36
Magnetic resonance imaging (MRI), 37
Computed tomography (CT scan), 38
Bone scintigraphy (bone scans), 38
Arthroscopy, 39
Electromyography, 40
Myelography, 40
Arthrography, 42
Discography, 42
Biopsy of bone, muscle, and synovium, 43
Normal laboratory data, 43

4 MUSCULOSKELETAL TRAUMA, 46

5 INFLAMMATORY MUSCULOSKELETAL CONDITIONS, 63

Rheumatoid arthritis, 63
Ankylosing spondylitis, 74
Epicondylitis and tendinitis (tenosynovitis), 82
Bursitis, 87
Lyme disease, 91

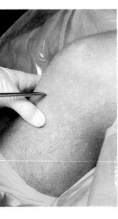

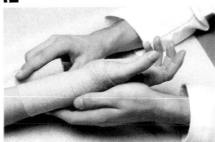

6 DEGENERATIVE MUSCULOSKELETAL CONDITIONS, 97

Osteoarthritis, 97
Carpal tunnel syndrome, 104
Sciatic nerve injury, 110
Hallux valgus, 115

7 INFECTIOUS MUSCULOSKELETAL CONDITIONS, 120

Osteomyelitis, 120
Wound infections, 128

8 METABOLIC MUSCULOSKELETAL CONDITIONS, 129

Osteoporosis, 129
Gout, 136
Osteomalacia, 140

9 CURVATURES OF THE SPINE, 145

Kyphosis, 145
Scoliosis, 150
Lordosis, 155

10 MUSCULOSKELETAL TUMORS, 156

11 CONGENITAL MUSCULOSKELETAL CONDITIONS, 172

Congenital hip dysplasia, 172
Talipes equinovarus, 175

12 CASTS, TRACTION, AND EXTERNAL FIXATION DEVICES, 179

13 SURGERY FOR MUSCULOSKELETAL CONDITIONS, 205

Amputation, 205
Meniscectomy, 211
Open reduction with internal fixation, 218

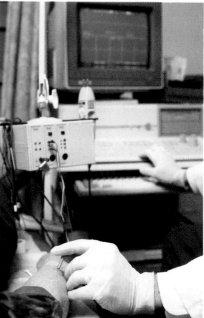

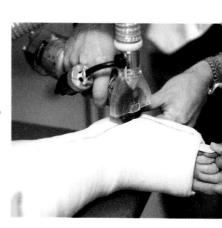

Total hip replacement (THR), 220
Total knee replacement (TKR), 222
Total shoulder replacement (TSR), 224
Total joint replacements for wrist, elbow, or ankle, 225
Endoprosthetic replacement of femoral head, 226
Osteotomy, 228
Spinal fusion with bone grafts or metallic rods, 228
Rotator cuff tears, 230
Recurrent shoulder dislocations, 232
Synovectomy, 232
Chemonucleolysis, 243
Ilizarov method for treatment of bone defects, 248
Rehabilitation, 255

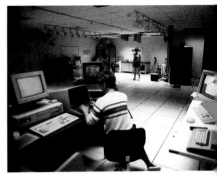

14 PATIENT TEACHING GUIDES

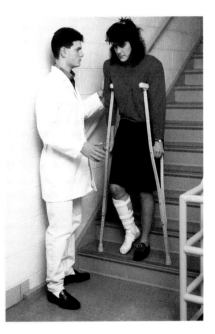

Strains and sprains, 260
Arthritis, 261
What is osteoporosis?, 263
Treatment of osteoporosis, 264
Scoliosis, 265
Low back pain, 266
Ruptured disks, 268
Preventing future back problems, 269
Transcutaneous electrical
    nerve stimulation (TENS), 270
Casts, 271
Home cast care, 272
Traction, 273
Crutch walking, 274
Total hip replacement, 275
Recovery after total hip replacement, 276
Total knee replacement, 277
Recovery after total knee replacement, 278
Total shoulder replacement, 279

15 MUSCULOSKELETAL DRUGS

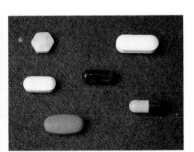

Antiinflammatory medications, 280
Muscle-relaxant medications, 284
Antigout medications, 286
Antirheumatic medications, 287
Antiulcer medications, 290

Appendix: Special assessment techniques for
    musculoskeletal tissues, 292

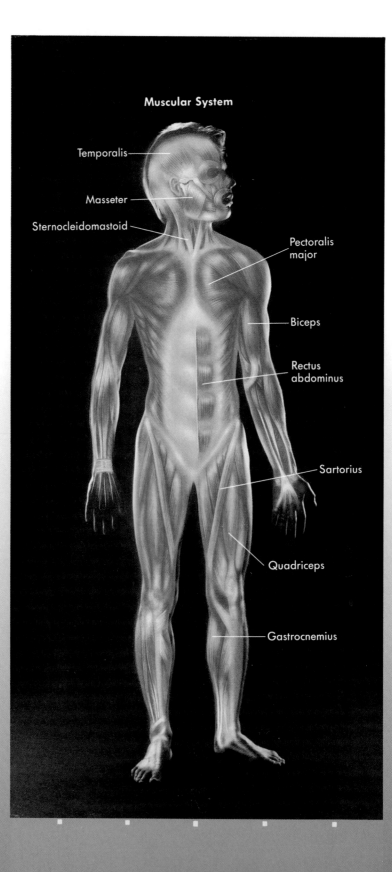

Muscular System

Temporalis

Masseter

Sternocleidomastoid

Pectoralis major

Biceps

Rectus abdominus

Sartorius

Quadriceps

Gastrocnemius

CHAPTER 1

Color Atlas of the Musculoskeletal System

The structures of the musculoskeletal system provide the framework for movement from place to place and for protection of internal organs. Musculoskeletal tissues may be bones, which make up the skeleton of the body, or they may be muscles, ligaments, tendons, cartilage, or joints. These tissues give shape to the body, protect internal organs and tissues, store minerals, serve as sites for hematopoiesis, and help prevent injury to specific musculoskeletal structures or to other organs and tissues.

When the musculoskeletal tissues are unable to perform their usual functions, the affected tissue (or tissues) influence a person's mobility, support, protection, and ability to carry on usual activities. Trauma is a major cause of musculoskeletal disorders, and automobile accidents and injuries are the leading causes of immobility and death. Injuries from sports and physical fitness activities are major factors affecting the health of youngsters or young to middle-aged adults. Middle-aged and older adults are affected by rheumatic, inflammatory, and degenerative conditions of the musculoskeletal tissues. Young children and adolescents also may be affected by rheumatic and inflammatory conditions but to a lesser extent than older persons.

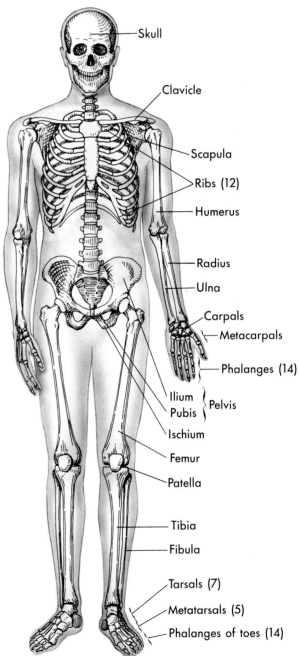

Skull
Clavicle
Scapula
Ribs (12)
Humerus
Radius
Ulna
Carpals
Metacarpals
Phalanges (14)
Ilium
Pubis } Pelvis
Ischium
Femur
Patella
Tibia
Fibula
Tarsals (7)
Metatarsals (5)
Phalanges of toes (14)

SKELETON

The human skeleton is composed of 206 bones which, following Wolff's law, are shaped according to their function. Thus bones may be long, as in the arms and legs; short, as in the ankles and wrists; flat, as in the sternum and scapulae; irregular, as in the vertebrae; or round, as in the patellae. The bones of the arms, legs, shoulders, and pelvis make up the appendicular skeleton; the bones of the skull and face and the auditory ossicles, vertebrae, ribs, sternum, and hyoid bone make up the axial skeleton (Figures 1-1 to 1-3).

FUNCTIONS OF BONES

Support the body, enabling a person to stand erect
Protect internal organs and tissues
Assist movement in coordination with muscles and joints
Provide storage areas or reservoirs for minerals
Serve as sites for formation of blood cells in the bone marrow (hematopoiesis)

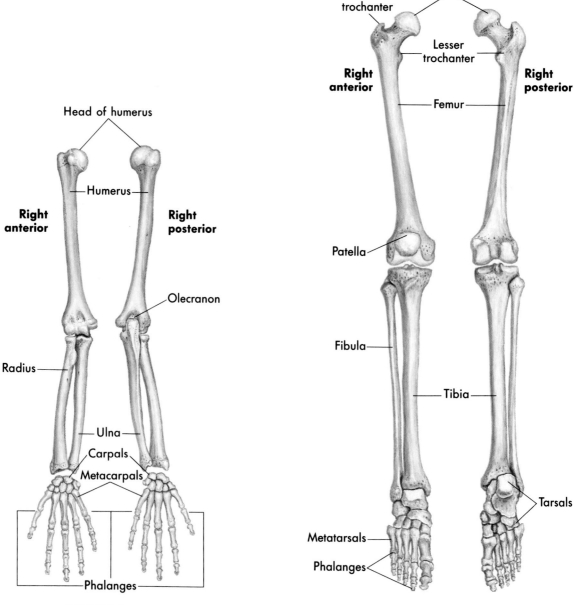

FIGURE 1-1
Bones of the arm.

FIGURE 1-2
Bones of the leg.

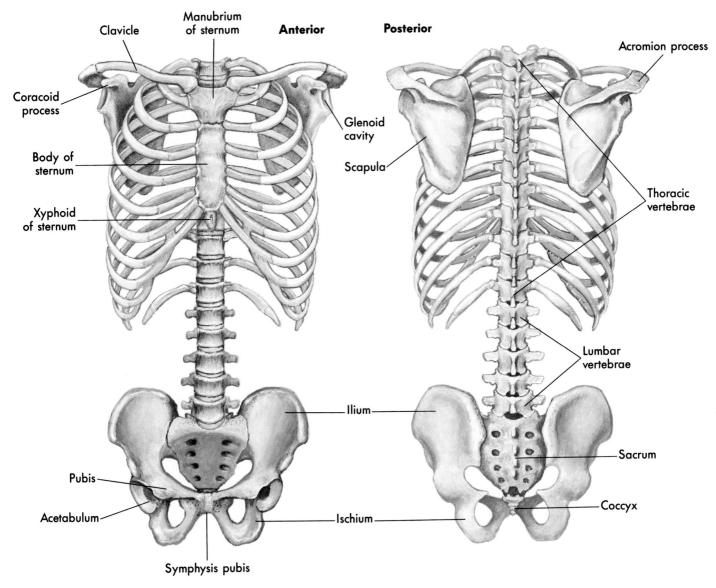

FIGURE 1-3
Bones of the trunk and pelvis.

SKELETAL GROWTH

The skeleton begins to develop prenatally through a process called *osteogenesis*. The skeleton is completely formed by the end of the third prenatal month. After birth secondary centers develop in the epiphyseal regions, and bone growth proceeds from the end toward the center. When the bone has reached its final size and growth ceases, the epiphyseal growth centers are replaced by bone cells. While bones are growing, they lengthen and the outer diameter increases slightly. New bone is continuously deposited on the outer surfaces while the inner surfaces are reabsorbed, until the bone achieves its final shape. These formation-resorption processes help remodel or shape the bone to maximize its load-bearing ability while minimizing its mass or weight. Bone growth and ossification usually continue longitudinally in girls until 15 years of age and in boys until age 16. However, bone maturation and shaping continue until 21 years of age in both sexes with such regularity that a person's age can be fairly closely determined by x-ray examination of bones.

STRUCTURE OF BONE TISSUES

Figure 1-4 shows the gross structure and individual parts of a long bone. The long shaft of the bone is the diaphysis, and the ends are the epiphyses. The epiphyses are covered by cartilage, which cushions them and provides protection during weight bearing and movement. The shaft is separated from the epiphysis by the growth plate and by nutrient arteries of the metaphysis. The shaft of the bone is composed of hard, dense bone cells called compact bone, whereas the ends of bones are made up of soft, spongy bone cells called cancellous bone. Cancellous bone cells in the crests of the iliac bones and in the tibiae, sternum, and ends of long bones contain red bone marrow for hemopoiesis. The shafts of long bones contain yellow marrow composed primarily of fat cells, whose function is to replenish red marrow cells when necessary.

The surface of a bone has many prominences (Figure 1-5), which serve both as attachments for ligaments and tendons and to protect nerves and blood vessels. Prominences may be rounded, knucklelike protuberances (condyles); small, round projections (tubercles); large, irregular processes (trochanters); or narrow ridges or crests (frontal bone and iliac crests). Projections may be transverse (transverse processes of vertebrae and ears), or they may extend posteriorly (posterior spinous processes) or anteriorly, as in the nasal cartilages. Bones also contain alveoli (sockets), fossae (depressions), fissures (narrow slits), foramina (openings for nerves, muscles, and blood vessels), sinuses (cavities), and sulci (grooves).

The tough outer covering of bones (periosteum) contains nutrient arteries to nourish the bone cells. Fibers in the periosteum, called Sharpey's fibers, penetrate the bone to help hold the periosteum to the bone. The periosteal blood vessels communicate with vessels in the central canal of the haversian system, which is the microscopic structural unit of compact bone.

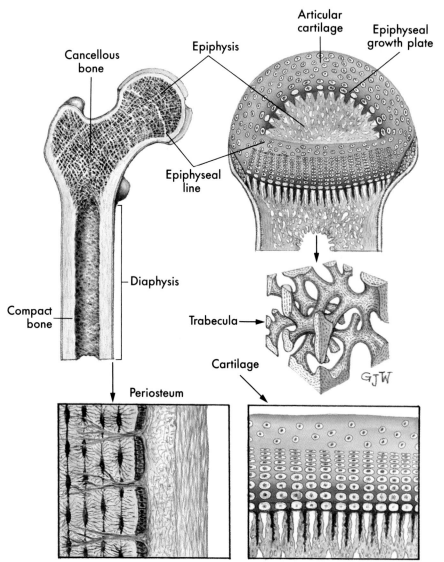

FIGURE 1-4
Gross structure of a long bone.

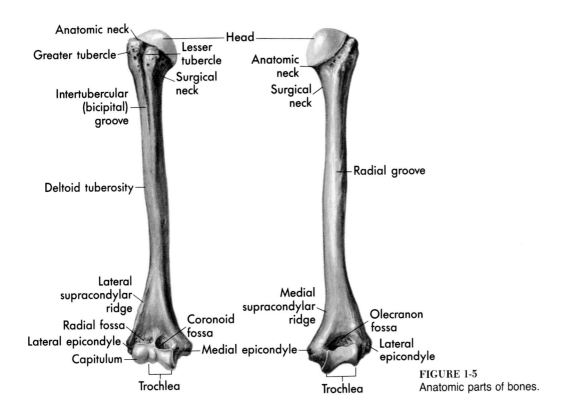

FIGURE 1-5
Anatomic parts of bones.

THE HAVERSIAN SYSTEM

The haversian system is composed of four parts (Figure 1-6):

- Lamellae—concentric layers of cylindrical, calcified matrix cells aligned parallel to the shaft of the bone
- Lacunae—small cavities or spaces in lamellae filled with tissue fluids and bone cells (osteocytes)
- Canaliculi—very small canals that connect with larger canals, called haversian canals
- Haversian canal—a channel extending lengthwise through the center of each haversian system; it contains blood vessels to provide nutrients and to remove wastes produced by bone growth and resorption

Compact bone contains thousands of haversian systems held together by interstitial and circumferential lamellae.

Cancellous, or spongy, bone tissues do not have haversian systems. Instead, cancellous tissues are made up of weblike formations of spaces filled with red marrow; the spaces are separated by bony projections called trabeculae. Trabeculae are arranged along the lines of stress, an arrangement that gives bones their strength.

BONE FORMATION AND RESORPTION

Bones are living structures that are continuously in the process of bone formation counterbalanced by bone resorption. Formation and resorption are subject to the actions of osteocytes, the major bone-forming cells, and osteoclasts, the cells responsible for bone resorption. Osteocytes mature from osteoblasts, spindle-shaped cells found in the endosteum and beneath the periosteum of bones. Osteoblasts remain dormant until needed for bone growth, when they mature into osteocytes.

The processes of formation and resorption prevent bones from becoming excessively thick or thin. These processes are related to the metabolism and to the levels of calcium and phosphate in the body. Approximately 98% of the body's extracellular calcium is contained in bones. Blood serum concentrations of calcium and phosphate are regulated by hormonal secretions of the parathyroid glands, by absorption in the intestines, and by retention or excretion through the kidneys, so that relatively stable concentrations are maintained for homeostasis. Low calcium levels stimulate production of parathyroid hormone (PTH), which stimulates osteoclasts to break down bone structure; this frees calcium phosphate crystals to increase serum calcium concentrations. Additionally, the intestinal ion

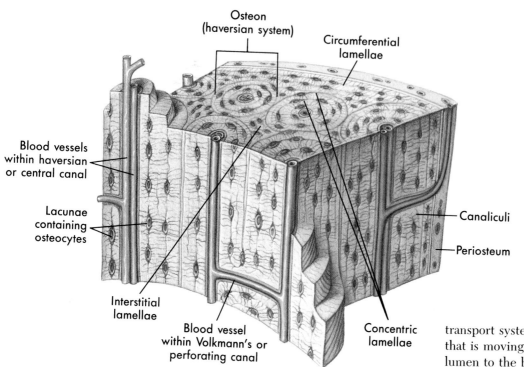

FIGURE 1-6
Cross-section of compact bone, including the haversian system.

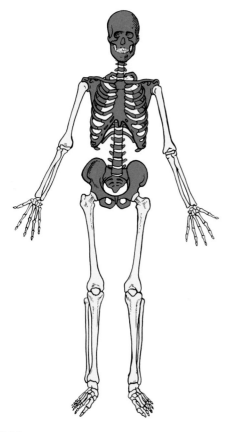

FIGURE 1-7
Distribution of red and yellow bone marrow.

transport system absorbs calcium that is moving the ion from the gut lumen to the blood. Calcium retention increases in the renal tubules, raising serum calcium levels and thereby concurrently reducing the retention or resorption of phosphate. Through these processes calcium levels remain relatively constant, and bones remain strong with a relatively stable calcium content.

Bone strength, formation, and resorption are also affected by the amount and metabolism of vitamin D, which facilitates the absorption of calcium and phosphorus from the intestine. A deficiency of either vitamin D or sunshine (needed to activate sterol precursors to vitamin D in the skin) causes bone changes, a condition known in children as rickets and in adults as osteomalacia.

HEMATOPOIESIS

Along with helping to maintain body posture and protecting organs, bones function as organs for hematopoiesis (or hemopoiesis). Hematopoiesis is the process of producing and developing blood cells, and it takes place in the marrow of the bones. The two types of bone marrow are red and yellow (Figure 1-7). Red marrow in the cancellous areas of bones, particularly the sternum, iliac crests, and tibiae, produces red blood cells, white blood cells, and megakaryocytes, the "mother cells" of platelets. Each of these blood cells develops from primitive "stem" cells, the cells from which the individual cells then differentiate into the specific blood cells in the red marrow. Hematopoiesis requires hemopoietin, which is produced in the kidneys, as a catalyst to stimulate cell production. The only function for yellow marrow occurs in times of stress, when it can be transformed into red marrow to assist with hematopoiesis.

MUSCLES

Muscles are masses of tissues that cover bones and provide bulk to the body, help hold body parts together, and help move one or more parts from place to place. Muscles interact with nerves, minerals, skin, and other connective tissues to bring about muscle contraction for movement in space. There are three types of muscles—skeletal, smooth, and cardiac—but the following discussion concerns only skeletal muscles.

Individual skeletal muscles may be short or long, depending on their position or placement on specific bones. Muscles vary in diameter and length; some are more than 30 cm long and 10 to 60 μm in diameter.

STRUCTURE OF SKELETAL MUSCLES

Skeletal muscles make up 40% to 45% of the body's weight (Figures 1-8 to 1-10). They contain muscle tissue plus nerves, blood vessels, and connective tissue elements. They vary in size from very small to large muscle masses, such as the thigh muscles. Skeletal muscles may be short and blunt, long and narrow, triangular, quadrilateral, flat, bulky, or irregu-

---

NAMES OF MUSCLES

Muscles are given Latin names according to their actions, as in flexor and adductor; for their location, as in femoris and pectoralis; for their shape, as in deltoid (triangular) or quadratus (square); for the direction of their fibers, as in transversus or rectus; for the number of divisions composing the muscle, as in biceps (two heads), triceps (three heads), and quadriceps (four heads); and for their points of attachment, as in carpi (wrist) and abdominis (abdomen). Thus the quadriceps femoris muscle is the four-headed or four-sectioned muscle made up of the vastus lateralis, rectus femoris, vastus medialis, and vastus intermedius of the thigh.

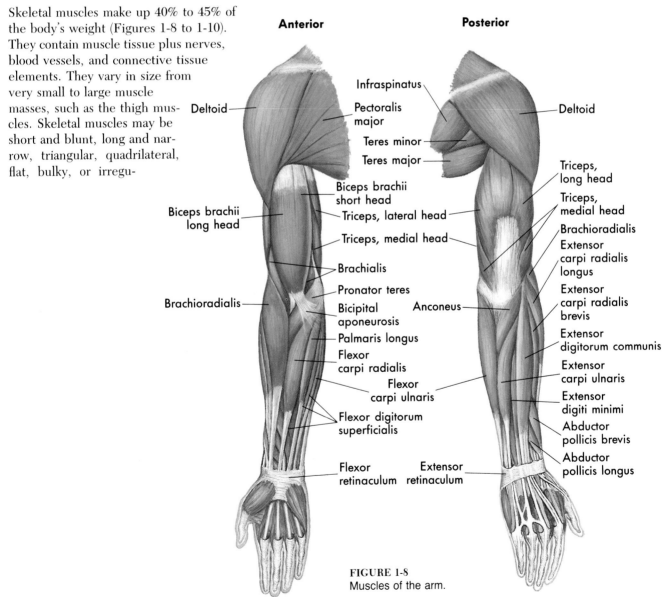

FIGURE 1-8
Muscles of the arm.

lar. Skeletal muscle fibers may be arranged parallel to the long axis of the bone to which they are attached, or they may be obliquely attached, curved as in sphincters, pennate (like feathers in a plume), or bipennate (double feathered), as shown in Figure 1-9. The arrangement of the fibers in specific muscles aids in producing the optimum contraction of the particular muscle.

Muscles are attached at each end to a bone, ligament, tendon, or fascia. One end of the muscle, the more fixed end, is called the origin; the more movable end is the muscle insertion.

Skeletal muscles may be red or white. Red muscles get their color from the pigment myoglobin. Closely related to hemoglobin, myoglobin acts as a temporary oxygen store for the muscle. White muscle fibers contain less myoglobin. White muscles react rapidly when stimulated, whereas red muscles carry out slower, sustained movements.

Normally, muscles are full-bellied and supple. With aging, they lose some fibers through degeneration, and these fibers may be replaced with fibrous connective tissue. Loss of muscle fiber and an increase in connective tissue cause loss of full muscle strength, which is noticeable in older persons.

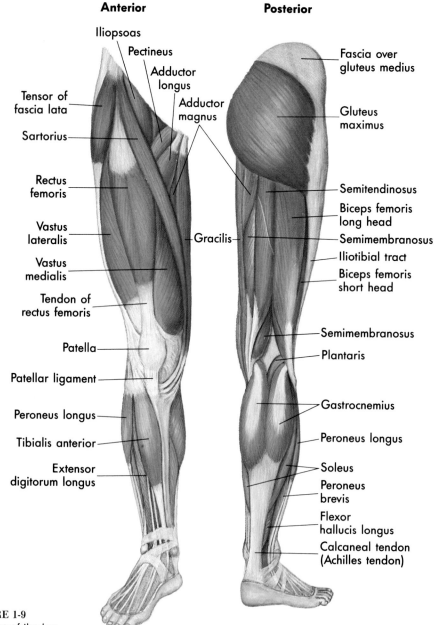

FIGURE 1-9
Muscles of the leg.

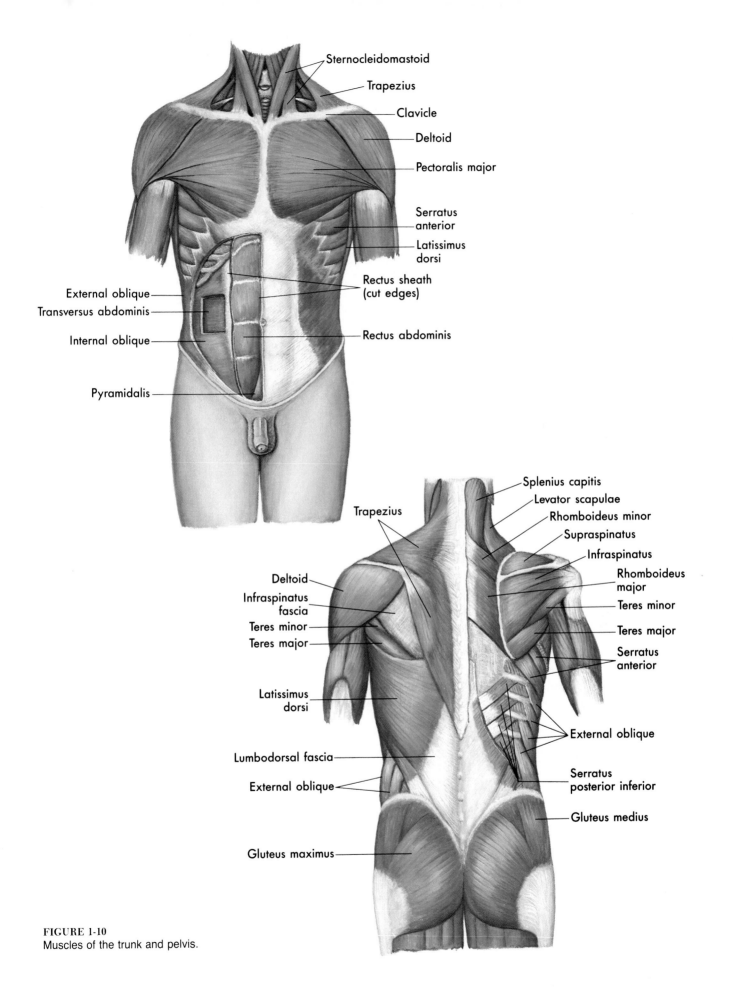

Sternocleidomastoid

Trapezius

Clavicle

Deltoid

Pectoralis major

Serratus anterior

Latissimus dorsi

Rectus sheath (cut edges)

External oblique

Transversus abdominis

Internal oblique

Rectus abdominis

Pyramidalis

Trapezius

Splenius capitis

Levator scapulae

Rhomboideus minor

Supraspinatus

Infraspinatus

Rhomboideus major

Deltoid

Infraspinatus fascia

Teres minor

Teres major

Teres minor

Teres major

Serratus anterior

Latissimus dorsi

External oblique

Lumbodorsal fascia

External oblique

Serratus posterior inferior

Gluteus medius

Gluteus maximus

FIGURE 1-10
Muscles of the trunk and pelvis.

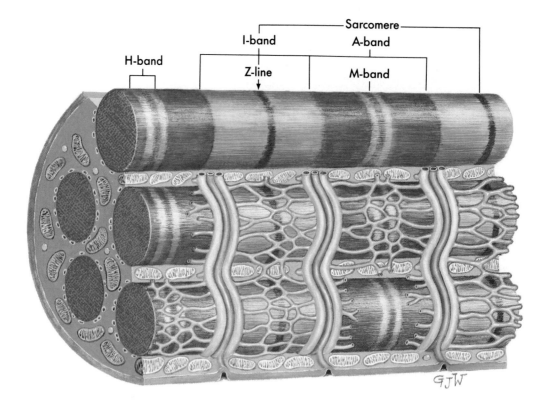

FIGURE 1-11
Lines and bands in striated muscle.

MUSCLE FIBERS

All muscles are composed of the basic cellular unit, called the muscle fiber, which is a cell containing many internal structures. The outer covering of the muscle fiber, or cell, is called the sarcolemma, and the interior cytoplasm is called sarcoplasm.

Skeletal muscles are composed of many cells, or fibers. Some muscle fibers are elongated cells that may extend the entire length of the particular muscle. Bundles of muscle fibers are called fasciculi, and each fasciculus is surrounded by a connective tissue called the endomysium. The endomysium connects with connective tissue partitions called perimysia, which in turn are connected to the outer muscle covering called the epimysium. These three connective tissues provide pathways for nerves and blood vessels to pass inward to the muscle cells.

Skeletal muscles are called voluntary muscles because they are controlled or moved voluntarily. They are also described as striated, because alternating light and dark bands, or striations, can be seen when muscle tissue is viewed under a light microscope. The light bands are known as I bands and the dark ones as A bands (Figure 1-11). As viewed through an electron microscope, each I band is crossed by a dark area, known as the Z line, and each A band has a lighter

area within it, called the H band. Each H band has a dark streak, called the M line (see Figure 1-11). The area of a muscle fiber between two Z lines is called a sarcomere.

MUSCLE CONTRACTION AND RELAXATION

Contraction of the muscle takes place in the sarcomere. During contractions, the sarcomere shortens and the I and H bands shorten and disappear; the A band retains its length but abuts the two Z bands. Contraction is effected by the muscle filaments (myofibrils), as the A bands, which contain the proteins myosin and actin, interact with the I band, which contains only actin filaments in the cross-bridge area where contraction occurs (see Fig 1-13). The interaction (contraction) occurs after an impulse is transmitted along a motor nerve to the sarcolemma of the muscle and is transmitted to the sarcomere through the T tubules to the motor endplate (Figure 1-12). Release of calcium ions into the sarcoplasm is triggered where the sarcoplasm is bound with troponin in the thin filaments of the myofibrils. The calcium-troponin molecules permit myosin to interact with actin, enabling the muscle sarcomeres to contract. When myosin interacts with actin, it pulls the thin filaments toward the center of each sarcomere, shortening the muscle fibers; this shortening is

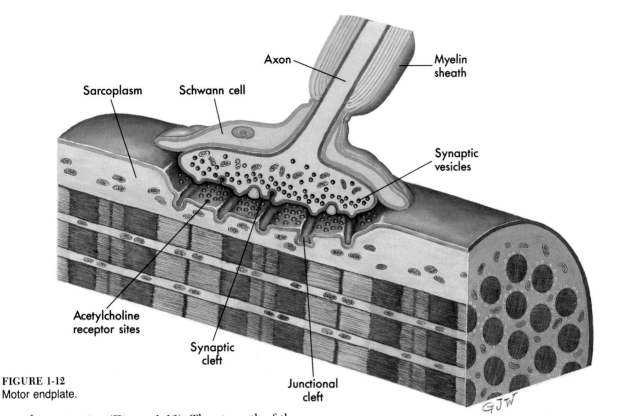

FIGURE 1-12
Motor endplate.

muscle contraction (Figure 1-13). The strength of the contraction is determined by the number of motor units contracting the sarcomeres and by the number of times per second that each motor unit is stimulated. Muscle cells respond either entirely or not at all to the stimulus—that is, they follow the all-or-none law as they contract. A stimulus strong enough to bring about contraction is called a liminal stimulus; a less intense stimulus is called subliminal. Treppe is a phenomenon that occurs when a second stimulus takes place at the apex of a preceding one. The additive effects of the rapid subliminal stimuli increase the strength of the contraction.

The muscle must be able to relax as well as contract. Muscle relaxation is currently thought to be brought about by separation of the calcium-troponin combination, with the calcium ions reentering the muscle sarcoplasm, and the troponin inhibiting the interaction of myosin and actin. The sarcoplasmic cells are sometimes referred to as the relaxing factor of muscle cells. The sarcoplasm may produce a substance, currently called relaxin, that keeps the muscle relaxed between stimuli.

The energy for muscle contraction comes from the hydrolysis of adenosine triphosphate (ATP) into adenosine 5′-diphosphate (ADP) + phosphate + energy.

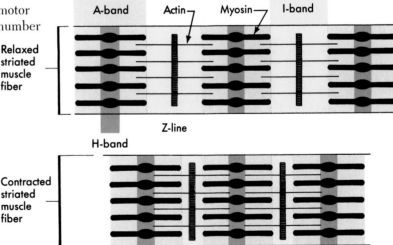

FIGURE 1-13
Relaxation and contraction of muscle fibers.

Breaking the high-energy bands in ATP provides the energy to support muscle contraction. Additional energy sources are phosphocreatine, a protein energy source found only in muscle tissues, and oxygen, which aids contraction by oxidizing the lactic acid that results from the anaerobic hydrolysis of the high-energy ATP bands.

MUSCLE SPASM VS MUSCLE TWITCH

A muscle spasm results from involuntary contraction of a muscle or group of muscles; it is caused by repetitive activation of entire motor units, which in turn is caused by the repetitive firing of a motor nerve. Tetanus is a sustained contraction caused by a repetitive series of stimuli conducted along the sarcolemmal membrane.

A muscle twitch occurs when a liminal stimulus is attained. All muscle fibers associated with the stimulated nerve contract and then relax.

An **isotonic twitch** causes the muscle to change length when constant tension is applied throughout its contraction. An isometric twitch is one in which the muscle remains or retains a constant length, even with a sudden increase in muscle tension.

Muscle Tone

Tone in muscles provides assistance to passive elongation or stretch and ensures a rapid reaction to an external stimulus. It results from a continuous flow of stimuli from the spinal cord to each motor unit. Muscle tone can be increased or decreased, depending on the activity within the nervous system. Tone is increased in anxiety states and decreased during restful periods.

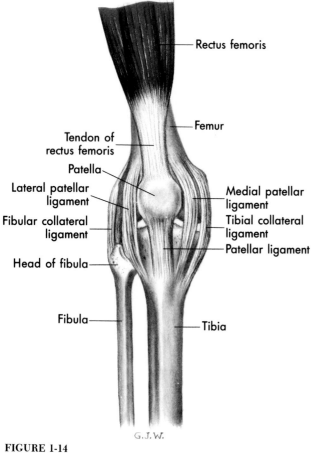

Rectus femoris

Femur

Tendon of rectus femoris

Patella

Lateral patellar ligament

Fibular collateral ligament

Head of fibula

Fibula

Tibia

Medial patellar ligament

Tibial collateral ligament

Patellar ligament

G.J.W.

FIGURE 1-14
Ligaments and tendons of the knee joint.

LIGAMENTS

Ligaments are tough, relatively long bands of dense, connective tissues that hold bones to bones. They are composed of type I collagen fibers (see page 13) arranged in parallel bundles, which gives them great strength with limited extensibility. Ligaments may encircle a joint to add strength and stability, as they do around the hip joint, or they may hold obliquely or parallel to the ends of bones across the joint, as they do in and around the knee joint (Figure 1-14).

Ligaments provide the greatest stability to the joint when they are taut. They allow movement in some directions while restricting movement in other directions. Ligaments may be injured by partial tears, called sprains, or they may be torn loose from their attachment to the bones, called an avulsion.

TENDONS

Tendons are very strong, tough, long strands or cords of dense connective tissues that form at the ends of muscles (see Figure 1-14). The fibers of tendons are arranged in longitudinal and parallel rows into nonelastic cords with high tensile strength. Tendons can transmit great forces from contractile muscles to bone or cartilage tissues while remaining undamaged themselves. Tendons are composed of type I collagen fibers, which give them their strength. The Achilles tendon of the posterior heel area is the longest and largest tendon in the body, being 10 to 14 cm long. Other tendons may be only 2 to 3 cm in length.

CARTILAGE

Cartilage is a semismooth layer of elastic, resilient supporting tissue found at the ends of bones (see Figure 1-15, page 14). Cartilage forms a cap over the bone end to provide protection and support to the bone for its weight-bearing activities.

Adult cartilage is made up of cells called chondrocytes, which are usually arranged in clusters. Between the clusters of chondrocytes are "ground substances" of complex protein-carbohydrate molecules that give cartilage its elasticity and moldability. Cartilage absorbs weight and also shock, stress, and strain to prevent injury to itself, to other joint tissues, and to bones. The outer surfaces of cartilage are undulating, with small depressions and valleys. The area of cartilage nearest the bone end is called the perichondrium; it has blood vessels to bring nutrients to the cartilage and to remove wastes. The thickness of cartilage layers varies from 2 to 4 cm, and thickness may vary from one area to another within a specific joint or from joint to joint. The color of cartilage varies from shades of white to yellow.

The outer cartilage layers have no blood vessels of their own; they receive their nourishment from synovial fluids forced into the elastic, spongy cartilage layers during weight bearing and other joint movements.

Cartilage **must** have joint movement and weight bearing to remain healthy. It will shrink and atrophy if the joint is not used, since the cells would not be replenished with nutrients from the synovial fluid. Cartilage may also wear unevenly and may fray if joints are not stable, anatomically correct, or normally shaped. When cartilage cells are moderately or severely dam-

TYPES OF CARTILAGE

1. **Hyaline**—Hyaline cartilage is bluish white and translucent. The collagen fibers in it are arranged in an interlacing network with large water content between the cells. In adult hyaline cartilage, water constitutes about 70% to 80% of the net weight, giving this type of cartilage great elasticity, sponginess, and moldability. Hyaline cartilage is found over the ends of bones of synovial joints, in the walls of the trachea, in the larynx and nasal septum, and over the ends of the ribs.
2. **Fibrous** (also called fibrocartilage)—Fibrous cartilage is white and is made up of thick bundles of collagen fibers, which give it great strength to act as a shock absorber. Fibrocartilage is found in the symphysis pubis and between each vertebra, as well as in tendons and ligaments of synovial joints.
3. **Yellow**—Yellow cartilage has a dense network of collagen fibers, giving it great flexibility and strength. It is easily bent but returns to its original shape. Yellow cartilage is found in the outer ear, epiglottis, and eustachian tube.

aged and die, they are replaced with new cells if the area is small, or they may be replaced with fibrous tissue and become scars. Scarred cartilage is no longer spongy or resilient and therefore is less able to withstand loading, stress, or strain than healthy cartilage. Weight bearing and joint movements keep cartilage from becoming thin, unhealthy, or damaged, conditions that eventually could lead to degenerative joint disease.

COLLAGEN

Collagen is the major supporting element in connective tissues, making up approximately half of the total body protein in adults. It is made up of three individual strands that are coiled tightly throughout the collagen fiber and stabilized by interchain hydrogen bonds. This coiling gives the connective tissues flexibility and resilience.

Collagen is referred to as type I, type II, or type III. Type I collagen is found in all major connective tissues such as bones and tendons, in the fibrocartilaginous tissues of the symphysis pubis, between vertebrae, and in the dentin of the teeth. Because type I collagen shows very little distensibility under mechanical stress, it gives strength to tendons and ligaments in and around joints. Type II collagen fibers are found in

hyaline cartilage, where they lend their special properties of moldability, flexibility, and sponginess to the strength of the cartilage. Type III collagen fibers are the most distensible and are found in blood vessel walls, skin tissues, and the uterine wall, as well as in several other organs that need distensibility to function normally.

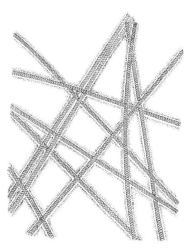

SYNOVIUM

Synovium is a layer of cells that form a membrane to line the inner surfaces of synovial joints (Figure 1-15). Synovium forms from cells within the inner layer of a joint capsule. It has numerous villous folds that contain blood vessels and lymphatic channels. The cells that form the synovial membrane are made up primarily of type I collagen. The blood vessels in the synovial folds are derived from type III collagen, which gives them distensibility.

The villous folds in the synovial membrane are filled with synovial fluid secreted from the membrane. The synovial fluid bathes and lubricates the joint and articular cartilage, aids in joint movements, provides nutrients and oxygen to the joint tissues, and carries out phagocytic and other immunologic functions within the joint.

FIGURE 1-15
Structures of a synovial joint (the knee).

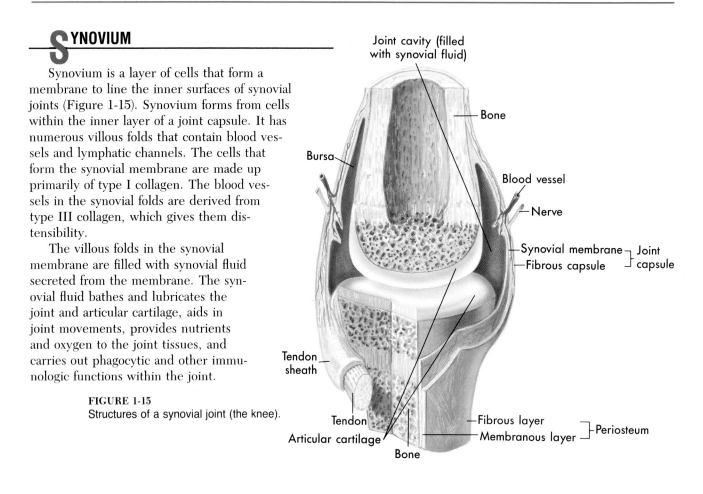

JOINTS

Joints are articulations where bones are joined to one another, or where two surfaces of bones come together. Joints help hold the bones firmly together while permitting movement between them. Joints may be classified by the type of material between the bones and by their degree of movement.

Joints that are classified by the material between them are called fibrous, cartilaginous, or synovial joints. Joints classified according to movement are called immovable (synarthrotic), slightly movable (amphiarthrotic), or freely movable (diarthrotic).

Most joints are freely movable, or diarthrotic. They are also known as synovial joints, because they are lined with the synovial membrane. Also found in freely movable joints are bones, cartilage covering the ends of bones, ligaments that hold the bones together,

synovial fluid, blood vessels, lymphatics, and nerves. Some synovial joints, such as the knee, also have a disk, called the meniscus, which is a pad of cartilage that cushions the joint (see Figure 1-15). Synovial joints have a casing or covering surrounding them, called the joint capsule, which is an extension of the periosteum of the articulating bones. Ligaments also encase the capsule to add strength.

Freely movable (diarthrotic) joints are classified by their types of movements. Slightly movable (amphiarthrotic) joints are connected by cartilage, which permits slight movement between them. Some examples of such joints are the symphysis pubis, the manubriosternal joint (the attachments of the sternum to the first 10 ribs), and the intervertebral joints. Immovable joints are connected by sutures or fibrous tissues between the bones; this arrangement holds the bones so tightly together that no movement occurs between them.

The degree of movement of a joint is called its range of motion (ROM). Only diarthrotic, or freely movable, joints have one or more ranges of motion (Figure 1-16). The types of movement, with examples of each, are as follows:

Angular   Movements that change the size of the angle between articulating bones
- Flexion—Bending forward, which shortens or decreases the angle between the bones
- Extension—Bending backward, which lengthens or increases the angle between the bones
- Abduction—Moving a part away from the midline of the body
- Adduction—Moving a part toward the midline of the body
- Plantar flexion—Stretching the foot and toes down and back, which increases the angle between the top of the foot and the front of the leg
- Dorsiflexion—Flexing or tilting the foot and toes upward toward the leg, which decreases the angle between the foot and the front of the leg
- Hyperextension—Stretching an extended part beyond its normal anatomic position

Circular   Movement around an axis
- Rotation—Moving or pivoting a bone on its own axis, as in side-to-side movement of the head
- Circumduction—Moving a part so that its distal end forms a circular movement while the rest of the movement forms a cone, as in "winding up" to throw a ball
- Supination—Turning the palm upward while rotating the forearm outward
- Pronation—Turning the palm downward while rotating the forearm inward

Gliding   Movement of one joint surface barely over another without any circular or angular movement

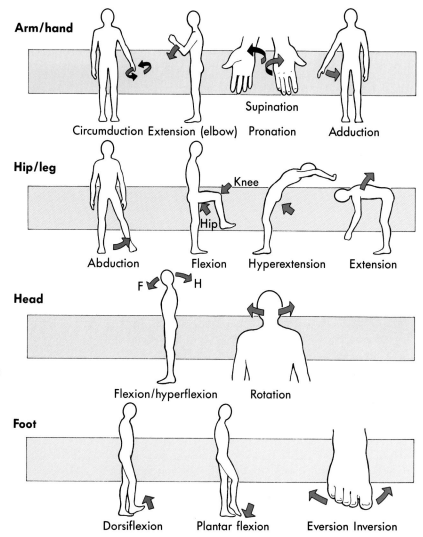

FIGURE 1-16
Body movements provided by synovial (diarthrodial) joints.

Special movements
- Elevation—Moving a part upward, or lifting
- Depression—Moving a part downward, or lowering
- Inversion—Turning the sole of the foot inward
- Eversion—Turning the sole of the foot outward
- Protraction—Moving a part forward
- Retraction—Moving a part backward
- Opposition—Moving parts together, as in bringing the thumb to touch each finger

TYPES OF JOINTS

Freely movable (diarthrotic) joints
Uniaxial: Permits movement in one axis and in only one plane
Hinge
  Permits back and forth extension and flexion. Examples: Knee, elbow, and finger joints.
Pivot
  Permits movement of one bone articulating with a ring or notch of another bone. Examples: Projection of the second cervical vertebra articulating with a ring-shaped portion of the first cervical vertebra; the head of the radius, which articulates with the radial notch of the ulna.

Biaxial: Permits movement around two perpendicular axes in two perpendicular planes
Saddle
  Saddle-shaped bone ends articulate with each other. Example: Found only in the base of each thumb.
Condyloid or ellipsoidal
  The condyle of one bone fits into the elliptically shaped portion of its articulating bone. Examples: Distal end of radius, which articulates with three wrist bones; the condyles of the occipital bone, which fit into elliptical depressions in the atlas.

Multiaxial: Permits movement in three or more planes and around three or more axes
Ball and socket
  Spheroid or ball-shaped bone fits into a concave curved area of its articulating bone. Example: Hip and shoulder joints.

Gliding
  Permits movement along various axes through relatively flat articulating surfaces. Examples: Joints between two vertebrae.

Slightly movable (amphiarthrotic) joints
Symphysis
  Permits limited movement between bones. Examples: Symphysis pubis, intervertebral joints, and manubriosternal joint.

Immovable (synarthrotic) joints
Sutures
  Fibrous tissue projections interlock between articulating bones with only a thin layer of fibrous tissue separating them. Examples: The bones of the skull are held together by suture-type joints.
Syndesmoses
  Ligaments connect the two articulating bones. Examples: Between distal ends of the radius and ulna; between distal ends of the tibia and fibula.
Gomphoses
  A fibrous membrane holds the root of a tooth in the alveolar process of the maxilla or mandible forming the joint.

BURSAE

Bursae are sacs or cavities lined with synovial membrane that contain synovial fluid; they serve as cushioning areas between tendons and bones, tendons and ligaments, or between other tissues where friction occurs. Synovial fluid from a bursa acts as a lubricant between contiguous tissues. Anatomically, bursae are part of the musculoskeletal tissues, but a new bursa can develop from pressure or friction over a prominent part; as, for example, the bursa that forms over a bunion in a hallux valgus deformity of the metatarsophalangeal joint. (Figure 1-15 shows a bursa around the knee joint.)

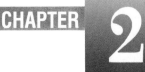

CHAPTER 2

Assessment

Thorough assessment of the musculoskeletal tissues is a vital part of medical and nursing care. Physicians examine the patient to gain a clearer understanding of his condition, which aids in determining a medical diagnosis. Nurses assess patients to determine their health status in light of the medical diagnosis. Both assessments gather information that guides the efforts of all health team members in providing the specific kinds of care the patient needs to regain mobility and health.

PATIENT CONSIDERATIONS

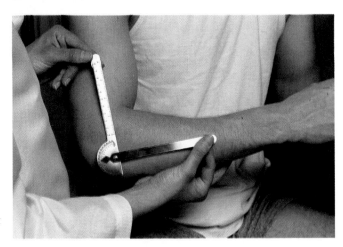

Before beginning the interview, health history, and physical assessment, the nurse should make every effort to establish a milieu to ensure the patient's comfort and cooperation. The patient should be positioned as comfortably as possible with regard to any musculoskeletal injury or condition that might be present or that might be the purpose of the examination. Thus the patient may need to lie down on the examining table from the beginning of the examination, or may be more comfortable sitting in a chair. The nurse should help the patient arrange injured or diseased parts in the most comfortable position, using pillows or blankets for support and warmth if needed. The temperature of the examining area should be comfortable for all participants, there should be no glare from the lights, and the room or cubicle should be private, with doors closed or curtains drawn. The nurse should see that those accompanying the patient are comfortable and available if needed. The interview and examination should proceed sequentially.

HEALTH HISTORY

The health history may be obtained by one of two methods if the patient comes to the examiner with a specific complaint or concern. In this situation, the examiner may need to deal with an injured, deformed, or bleeding tissue to prevent additional injury or pain. The examination thus might occur while the health history is obtained. First, the onset of the symptoms or the source of the injury is determined, and then the site is inspected for gross bleeding, deformity, pain or discomfort, or other symptoms. Emergency care may then be given, before a complete health history is obtained.

The health history may also be obtained as part of the overall picture on a patient's office visit or hospital admission. The health history must be thorough to ensure the most accurate assessment and evaluation of the patient's current condition. Areas other than physical assessment must be included, such as age, sex, weight, height, employment, activities of daily living, nutritional status, medications (especially information about antiinflammatory drugs, muscle relaxants, and steroids), hobbies, family health history, past illnesses and surgical procedures, and current health status.

When taking the health history, the nurse should observe the patient while he is responding to the questions. The nurse should note (1) the patient's affect (whether it is appropriate to what the patient is saying), (2) the position the patient maintains (shifting or moving as if to find a more comfortable position if he states that he is in pain, (3) facial expressions (appearance of tiredness, wrinkling or frowning, or worried expressions), and (4) ability to stay on the subject without drifting to other topics. The nurse should also note the patient's interactions with family members, if present.

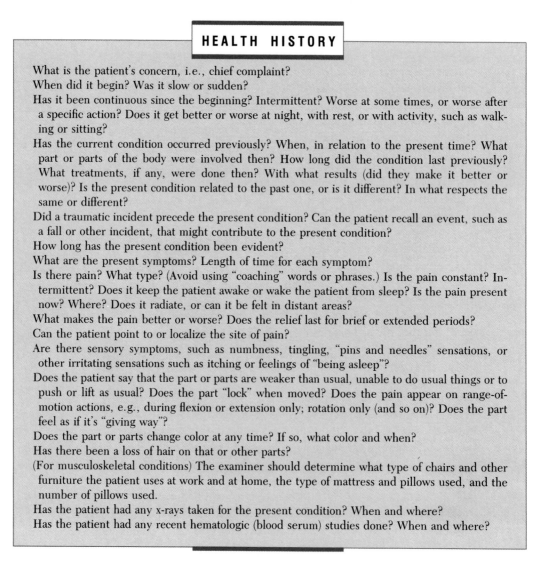

HEALTH HISTORY

What is the patient's concern, i.e., chief complaint?

When did it begin? Was it slow or sudden?

Has it been continuous since the beginning? Intermittent? Worse at some times, or worse after a specific action? Does it get better or worse at night, with rest, or with activity, such as walking or sitting?

Has the current condition occurred previously? When, in relation to the present time? What part or parts of the body were involved then? How long did the condition last previously? What treatments, if any, were done then? With what results (did they make it better or worse)? Is the present condition related to the past one, or is it different? In what respects the same or different?

Did a traumatic incident precede the present condition? Can the patient recall an event, such as a fall or other incident, that might contribute to the present condition?

How long has the present condition been evident?

What are the present symptoms? Length of time for each symptom?

Is there pain? What type? (Avoid using "coaching" words or phrases.) Is the pain constant? Intermittent? Does it keep the patient awake or wake the patient from sleep? Is the pain present now? Where? Does it radiate, or can it be felt in distant areas?

What makes the pain better or worse? Does the relief last for brief or extended periods?

Can the patient point to or localize the site of pain?

Are there sensory symptoms, such as numbness, tingling, "pins and needles" sensations, or other irritating sensations such as itching or feelings of "being asleep"?

Does the patient say that the part or parts are weaker than usual, unable to do usual things or to push or lift as usual? Does the part "lock" when moved? Does the pain appear on range-of-motion actions, e.g., during flexion or extension only; rotation only (and so on)? Does the part feel as if it's "giving way"?

Does the part or parts change color at any time? If so, what color and when?

Has there been a loss of hair on that or other parts?

(For musculoskeletal conditions) The examiner should determine what type of chairs and other furniture the patient uses at work and at home, the type of mattress and pillows used, and the number of pillows used.

Has the patient had any x-rays taken for the present condition? When and where?

Has the patient had any recent hematologic (blood serum) studies done? When and where?

PHYSICAL ASSESSMENT

The equipment needed for examining musculoskeletal and other tissues is shown in Figure 2-1. It includes a stethoscope, sphygmomanometer, thermometer, scale, percussion hammer, goniometer, pin and cotton (for sensory discrimination), tape measure, and tourniquet (for checking capillary fragility, if needed, and for checking Trousseau's sign for tetany).

The following principles should be observed when performing the physical examination:

- **Normal (uninvolved) tissues are examined before injured, inflamed, or otherwise involved tissues.**
- Bilateral observations must always be made for comparison.
- Local (site-specific) signs and symptoms are compared with systemic findings.
- Palpation is done gently, while observing facial and other responses to note sensitivity or tenderness within tissues.
- Movements are assessed within norms for ranges of movements, with bilateral comparisons.
- Bilateral comparisons are made with the parts in the same position while being examined.
- Inspection (observation) *always* includes looking at both sides of the patient for: (1) shape, contour, size, and symmetry; (2) signs of inflammation (heat or hot areas, color changes, edema or swelling, pain, tenderness, or soreness); (3) bruises or ecchymotic or discolored areas; (4) muscle fullness, hypertrophy, or atrophy; (5) deformity or excess or missing members, toes, or fingers.

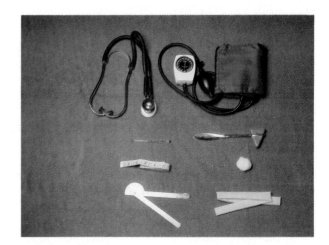

FIGURE 2-1
Equipment for musculoskeletal assessment.

- The steps for musculoskeletal examination follow this pattern:
  1. Inspection
  2. Auscultation
  3. Palpation
  4. Range-of-motion measurements (active movements are done before passive) and joint play
  5. Muscle strength measurements
  6. Reflex testing

The findings should be documented completely after the examination.

PHYSICAL EXAMINATION

POSTURE

The patient can be examined while standing, sitting, or lying (if that is the only pain-free position) (Figure 2-2). First, observe body alignment and stature. Then observe for the following: obvious deformities, spinal curvatures, and hypertrophied or atrophied limbs; size of body and stature related to age and sex; and scars, marks, masses, and skin openings or drainage (if visible while clothed). Note: Initial observations of gait, posture, stature, and gross abnormalities may be made as the patient enters the examining room while clothed. For the rest of the examination, the patient should be positioned with the joints in the position of greatest stability for comfort.

Normal findings. Posture is upright and erect. Head is in midline and perpendicular to shoulders and spinal column. Shoulders and pelvis are aligned. Arms hang freely from shoulders. Feet are planted firmly on floor with toes pointing straight ahead. There is a concave curve to the cervical and lumbar spines and a convex curve to the thoracic spine. *Stature*—Normal for age and sex according to actuarial tables. *Symmetry*—Two sides appear equal but may have slight differences because of handedness. *Gait*—Easy and rhythmic; steps are about 12 to 18 inches in length with normal heel-toe placement; stride is without "hitch," lurch, sway, or tilt. Arms swing freely, and patient is balanced and erect through each phase of walking away, turning, and returning. As patient turns, the head and face turn before the rest of the body. *Older adult:* Posture is less upright and erect. Head and neck may be more forward. Shoulders may be rolled or hunched forward. Feet may be closer together or farther apart (especially in women), with angle of feet and legs decreased at hip

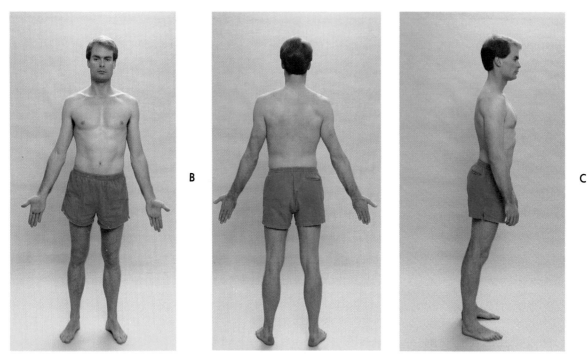

FIGURE 2-2
Inspection of body posture. **A,** Anterior view. **B,** Posterior view. **C,** Lateral view. (From Seidel.[91])

area, leading to varus placement of legs and feet. Upper extremities appear longer and out of proportion to rest of body. *Gait*—Patient is slower to initiate and stop; may have shuffle at times, with less ankle and knee lifting. Steps are shorter, more rapid, and less rhythmic.

Variations. Head and neck are in front of shoulders. Lumbar lordotic curve is flatter as a result of lumbar disk disease. *Stature*—Patient may be shorter or taller than average. *Gait*—Patient may have abnormal gait, such as steppage, ataxic, or quadriceps gait. *Older adult:* Posture is slightly (or more) "bent over" with pronounced thoracic curve (dowager's hump) as a result of osteoporosis or osteoarthritis; may have loss of height from osteoporosis. Body contour is less "fleshed out" because of loss of subcutaneous fat. *Gait*—Patient may have one or more gait disturbances such as festinating, ataxic, arthrogenic, or steppage gait (see SA).

HEAD AND FACE

Inspect the following: size and shape of head, ears, jawline, and chin; hair distribution, color, and thickness; and neck (front and back, noting alignment of head and shoulders). Note symmetry of skin folds, wrinkles, muscles, and layers of fatty tissues. Palpate hair and scalp for bumps or masses (wens); feel texture

of hair; feel ear pinnae for tophi or other lesions.

Normal findings. Shape of head is symmetric (occasionally slightly asymmetric). Ears are positioned in midtemporal area of skull; pinnae of ears are near skull. Jawline recedes or juts forward in a pronounced manner. No tophi, lumps, or bumps are felt when palpating skull or ear pinnae. Hair is evenly distributed with full thickness; texture may be fine, medium-fine, or coarse, curly or straight (natural or permanent wave). Skin folds or wrinkles are symmetric. *Older adult:* Patient may be partly or completely bald, or hair may be thinner and straighter than in younger adult. Layers of fat under chin may obscure neck structures.

Variations. Tumors may make face or neck appear asymmetric. Layers of fat (double chin) may obscure neck and chin structures. Tophi related to gout may be present on ear pinnae (tophi would be noted in both pinnae). Baldness may be related to endocrine disease or medications (steroids cause hair loss and changes in hair texture). Wens (small sebaceous cysts that occur in the epithelium of hair follicles) are frequently numerous when present.

TEMPOROMANDIBULAR JOINT

Palpate just anterior to tragus of each ear with finger to locate temporomandibular joint (TMJ); feel joint movements as patient opens and closes mouth. Have patient slide lower jaw side to side, move it forward (protract), and then move it back to original position (retract). Ask patient to clench teeth as you palpate and press firmly on contracted muscles.

Normal findings. A space of 3 to 6 cm is present between teeth as patient opens mouth. No soreness, pain, or tenderness is noted, and patient does not complain of headaches. No crepitus is felt (some patients normally may have some slight clicking or snapping in TMJ area). Mandible can move laterally 1 to 2 cm in either direction; patient can move lower jaw forward slightly and retract it easily. Clenching teeth produces no pain or muscle spasm.

Variations. Patient may have difficulty opening mouth as a result of injury or arthritic changes. TMJ may be painful because of arthritic changes or malocclusion of teeth. Muscle spasms may be secondary to trigeminal neuralgia. *Older adult:* Patient may have difficulty keeping mouth closed because of muscle weakness or secondary to cerebrovascular accident. Both upper and lower jaws may show recession as a result of loss of teeth without replacement with dentures. TMJ may be painful because of arthritic changes. Muscle spasms may be secondary to trigeminal neuralgia.

CERVICAL SPINE AND NECK
Range of Motion and Joint Play

Ask patient to perform the following maneuvers (Figure 2-3):

- Bend head forward to put chin to chest (to check flexion)
- Bend head backward as far as possible, chin toward ceiling (to check hyperextension)
- Bend head to each side, putting ear to shoulder without hunching shoulder (to check lateral bending)
- Turn head side to side, putting chin to shoulder (to check rotation)

To assess strength of trapezius and sternocleidomastoid muscles: Apply opposing force while patient does each movement. To assess joint looseness or play: Put joint in resting position (position in which joint is under least stress); assess *passively.* Temporomandibular joint: Have mouth slightly open. Facet of cervical spine: midway between flexion and extension

Normal findings. Flexion to 45 degrees; lateral bending to 40 degrees; rotation to 70 degrees. *Older adult:* Patient may have slightly less degree of hyperextension and rotation. Joint play for all ages is less than 4 mm in any direction.

Variations. Hyperextension and flexion are markedly limited because of cervical vertebral disk or osteoarthritic changes. Joint play of more than 4 mm indicates ligament laxity; less than 3 mm indicates "freezing" of joint from injury or arthritic changes.

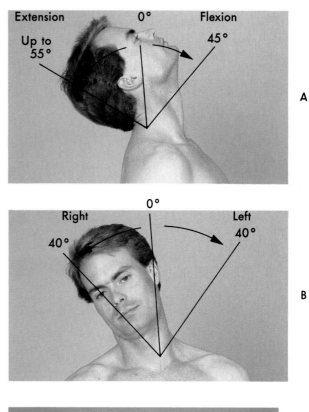

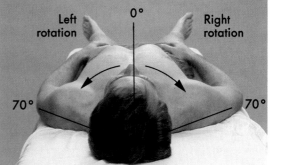

FIGURE 2-3
Range of motion of the cervical spine. **A,** Flexion and hyperextension. **B,** Lateral bending. **C,** Rotation. (From Seidel.[91])

NECK
Palpation

Palpate neck, front and back, for amount of tissue tension or differences in tension, tissue thickness, variations in temperature, locations of any masses, enlarged lymph nodes (anterior and posterior cervical chains, scalene, or supraclavicular, occipital, submandibular, submental, preauricular or postauricular nodes), skin moisture, and changes in sensations.

Normal findings. Neck is soft and firm, and tissues are easily movable. Temperature is same as in face and head. Lymph nodes in all areas are not palpable; no

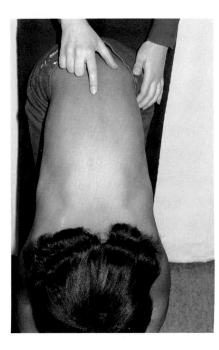

FIGURE 2-4
Inspection of spine for lateral curvature and lumbar convexity. (From Seidel.[91])

masses are noted. There are no sensations of numbness, tingling, spasms, or anesthesia. *Older adult:* Neck is soft and fairly firm, yet feels less soft than in younger adult because of some loss of subcutaneous fatty tissue. Veins may be more easily visible or prominent. Temperature is same as in face. No lymph nodes are enlarged. There are no sensory changes.

Variations. Mass may be present in or around lymph nodes as a result of Hodgkin's disease, non-Hodgkin's lymphoma, leukemia, or other cancer. Numbness or tingling may be present because of cervical radiculopathy. *Older adult:* Sensory changes may be present as a result of cervical radiculopathy. Cervical and supraclavicular lymph nodes may be enlarged because of head, neck, or lung malignancies.

THORACIC AND LUMBAR SPINE

Patient should be standing, if possible, with back to you and with back fully exposed. Inspect back from shoulders to buttocks. Note position of back of head and neck in relation to spinal column. Assess equality of height of shoulders. Assess each vertebral spinous process in relation to ones above and below. Note curvatures of spinal column by having patient turn to side. Note equality of height of iliac crests. Have patient bend forward to touch toes; inspect spinal curvatures (Figure 2-4) (put skin dot with water-soluble pen or pencil over each spinous process for easier visibility). Note position of legs, feet, and toes when patient is

standing erect and when bending forward. Assess muscles along both sides of vertebral column when patient is standing erect and when bending forward. Inspect for dimpling, hairy patch of skin or nevus in sacral or coccygeal area of vertebrae. Observe for spinal opening of skin along vertebral column.

Normal findings. Head rests centrally over vertebral column. Vertebrae are in straight line when viewed from behind. Spinal curves are concave of cervical and lumbar spines and convex of thoracic and sacral vertebrae. Iliac crest heights are even; no laterality is noted when patient is bending forward. Legs and feet are in alignment with trunk when patient is standing or bending forward. Muscles along vertebral column are symmetric in size, shape, and contour. Skin areas of back and vertebral column show no openings, hairy patches, or dimpling.

Variations. Patient may have lateral curvature (scoliosis), excessive thoracic curvature (kyphosis), or flattened or excessive lordosis. Iliac crests may be unequal. Paraspinal muscles may be asymmetric in muscle mass (one side may seem more prominent) or may be positioned higher on one side. One shoulder may appear higher than other. Normal lordotic curve may be lost in obese patients or because of herniated disk in lumbar vertebrae or sacroiliac condition. Young adult (20 to 30 years of age) may have more rigid spine with head flexed forward related to beginning or severity of ankylosing spondylitis. There may also be associated low back pain with ankylosing spondylitis. *Older adult:* Head may list to side because of osteoarthritic changes in cervical vertebrae. Excessive thoracic curvature (called senile kyphosis or dorsum rotundum) may be related to osteoporosis. Normal lordotic curve may be lost because of osteoarthritic or disk disease and osteoporosis or obesity.

Palpation

Palpate spinal column, pressing on each spinous process and into each laminar and intervertebral area. Press thumbs into paraspinal muscles along transverse processes of vertebrae. Percuss for tenderness over spinous process with thumbs or fingers along each spinous process, lightly tapping each spinous process with ulnar aspect of fist.

Normal findings. No tenderness or soreness is noted in patient of any age. No muscle tenderness or spasm is evident.

Variations. Patient may have tenderness or pain when tapped because of diskitis or herniation of disk. *Young adult:* Patient may have pain and tenderness with muscle spasms because of diskitis, ankylosing spondylitis, or herniated disk. Osteomyelitis also must be ruled out in spinal tenderness, as must spinal involvement from tuberculosis. Gibbus may be noted in patients 10 years of age or older. (Gibbus is a sharp, angular deformity associated with spinal deformity, thoracic vertebral fracture or, in an older adult, osteoporosis.)

Range of Motion (Figure 2-5)

Ask patient to perform the following maneuvers:

- Bend forward at waist to touch toes (to check flexion)
- Bend backward from waist as far as possible (to check hyperextension)
- Bend to each side as far as possible (to check lateral bending)
- Swing upper trunk from waist in a circular movement, front to side to back to side, while examiner stabilizes pelvis (to check rotation)

Normal findings. Flexion of 75 to 90 degrees; hyperextension of 30 degrees; bilateral/lateral bending of 35 degrees; rotation of upper trunk to 30 degrees forward and backward. *Older adult:* Movements may be limited in degree, especially hyperextention and rotation.

Variations. Muscle movements may be rigid because of ankylosing spondylitis, disk herniation, or arthritic or osteoporotic changes.

Joint Play

To assess: Place vertebral column in resting position (patient should be lying prone or in side-lying position). Gently try to move adjacent vertebrae passively, while patient breathes through mouth to avoid contracting muscles.

Normal findings. Slight joint play to 4 mm with joints resting midway between flexion and extension.

Variations. Excessive tightness or play may be associated with neuromuscular diseases such as cerebral palsy or muscular dystrophy.

SHOULDERS

Patient should be standing, with his back to you. Inspect equality of height of shoulders, contour and shape of

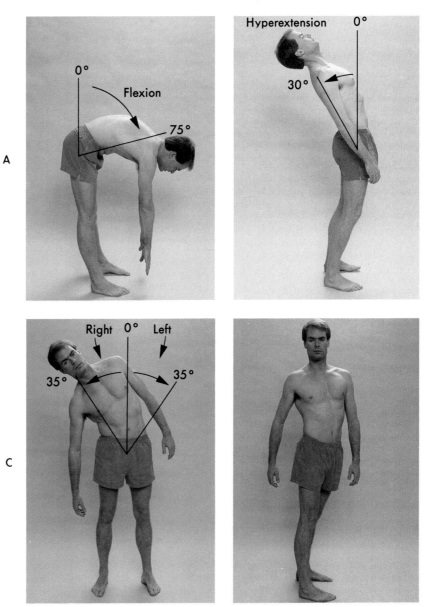

FIGURE 2-5
Range of motion of thoracic and lumbar spines. **A,** Flexion. **B,** Hyperextension. **C,** Lateral bending. **D,** Rotation of the upper trunk. (From Seidel.[91])

shoulders, and bony prominences at shoulder joints. Inspect shoulder girdle, both scapulae, and clavicles. Inspect scapulae for size and equality of height. Observe size and shape of trapezius muscles and whether they pull neck and shoulders together or laterally unevenly. Inspect and palpate clavicles with patient facing you.

Normal findings. Shoulders are somewhat rounded and firm, with smooth contours and no bony projections. Each scapula is smooth, with dorsal projection equal bilaterally. Each shoulder is equidistant from the vertebral column and located over thoracic ribs two through seven. Clavicles cross chest from sternal manubrium to shoulder joint. Each clavicle is continuous and smooth, without bumps or curves. Trapezius muscles are firm, full, and supple and do not pull scapulae and neck together or have lateral tightness. Deltoid, triceps, and biceps muscles may be slightly hypertrophied from "handedness" activities, e.g., tennis, baseball, handball, or other sports in which one hand predominates.

Variations. Shoulder joint may have some deformity as a result of trauma or arthritic changes. Patient may have pain and functional changes with sensory loss because of cervical arthropathy or secondary to cerebrovascular accident. Clavicle (one or both) may be irregular from healed fracture. Scapula may be "winged" (noted by an outward prominence when hands are pushed against a wall). *Young adult:* Patient may have step deformity of shoulder as a result of dislocation of acromioclavicular joint.

Palpation

Palpate shoulder with each hand, coming down to each scapula to palpate its surfaces and edges. Palpate trapezius muscles for shape, firmness, and equality bilaterally. Assess for "winging" of scapulae by having patient stand close to a wall and push against it with the hands. Inspect triceps, biceps, and deltoid muscles for firmness, fullness, and suppleness and for masses or bulges. Palpate for pain in or around shoulder joint, clavicles, and scapulae, noting tender, hot pressure, or "trigger" points, changes in sensations, and numbness or tingling.

Normal findings. *Older adult:* One or both shoulder joints may have bony projections along acromioclavicular joints, with associated loss of roundedness and smooth contour. Clavicles are straight and smooth. Scapulae are smooth equidistant from vertebral column without "winging." Trapezius muscles may show less fullness, suppleness, and strength. Deltoid, biceps, and triceps muscles may show some atrophy, sagging, or loss of firmness. Patient may complain of mild tenderness or soreness in one or both shoulder joints, often associated with weather changes.

Variations. *Older adult:* Patient may have arthritic changes in shoulder or deformity resulting from trauma or cerebrovascular accident, accompanied by loss of function of shoulder and extremity with associated muscle atrophy. Patient may have numbness or tingling associated with cervical or shoulder arthritic changes.

Range of Motion (Figure 2-6)

Ask patient to perform the following maneuvers:

- Shrug shoulders (to check symmetry)
- Raise both arms forward and then straight up above head (to check flexion)
- Extend and stretch both arms behind back (to check hyperextension)
- Lift both arms laterally and straight up above head (to check abduction)
- Swing each arm across front of body (to check adduction)
- Place both arms behind hips with elbows out (to check internal rotation)
- Place both arms behind head with elbows out (to check external rotation)

Normal findings. Shoulders rise symmetrically; forward flexion of 180 degrees; hyperextension of 50 degrees; shoulder abduction of 180 degrees; shoulder adduction of 50 degrees; internal rotation of 90 degrees; external rotation of 90 degrees. *Older adult:* Range of motion for each area may be 5 to 10 degrees less than average.

Variations. One shoulder may be lower than other as a result of trauma. Range of motion may be limited because of trauma or surgery or secondary to neuromuscular condition. *Older adult:* As above, plus changes caused by arthritic condition or sedentary lifestyle and lack of exercise.

Muscle Strength

To assess strength of trapezius, deltoid, biceps, and triceps muscles: Have patient shrug shoulders while you try to press each shoulder down (tests trapezius and deltoid muscles). Have patient flex and extend arm while you exert opposing force (tests biceps and triceps muscles).

Normal findings. Patient can resist force for each muscle tested. *Older adult:* Patient can resist force for brief periods.

Variations. Range of motion in each age group may be limited because of conditions listed previously.

Rotator Cuff

To assess anterior portion of rotator cuff muscles: Stand behind patient and place fingers of one hand in acromioclavicular joint; grasp arm with other hand just above elbow and gently pull arm back, palpating acromioclavicular joint area in notch formed by acromion spine of scapula and clavicle. To assess posterior portion: Have patient adduct arm across chest and place hand on opposite shoulder; stand in front of patient and palpate posterior surface of head of humerus by placing thumb on anterior surface and fingers on posterior aspect of shoulder; posterior portion of rotator cuff is now beneath your fingers.

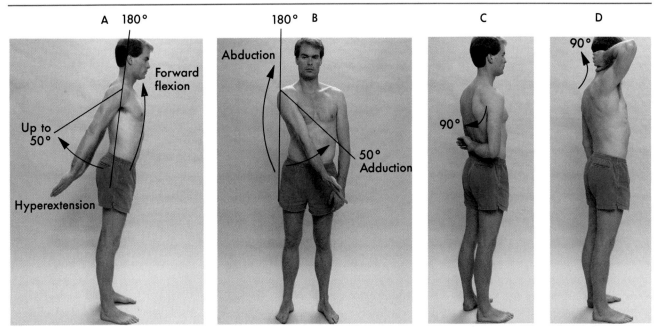

FIGURE 2-6
Range of motion of the shoulder. **A,** Forward flexion and hyperextension. **B,** Abduction and adduction. **C,** Internal rotation. **D,** External rotation. **E,** Shrugged shoulders. (From Seidel.[91])

Normal findings. No soreness, tenderness, or pain with palpation is noted in any age group. No swelling, masses, or gaps (tears) are felt in the cuff.

Variations. Torn tendons of the rotator cuff muscles (supraspinatus, infraspinatus, teres minor, and subscapularis) most commonly occur in sports injuries to pitchers, quarterbacks, or others who use a constant throwing motion.

Joint Play

To assess glenohumeral joint: Place arm in 55 degrees abduction, 30 degrees horizontal adduction. To assess acromioclavicular joint: Arm should be resting in normal physiologic position at side. To assess sternoclavicular joint: Have patient rest arm at side in normal physiologic position; passively (no active movement from patient) move joint backward, then forward, then laterally with fingers of one hand in each joint area. (Sternoclavicular joint play is checked with fingers of both hands.)

Normal findings. Joint play is approximately 4 mm with arm passively moved for patient of any age.

Variations. Joints may be tighter with little play because of surgical scarring or arthritic changes or because of repetitive trauma and scarring.

ELBOWS

Inspect skin areas of upper arm around elbow on all sides and front and back; then inspect forearm skin around elbow. Place arm in flexed and extended positions; assess for roundness and firmness of elbow in flexion and for any masses, edema, or bogginess in joint area. Assess supracondylar area (just above epicondyles) for supracondylar lymph nodes.

Normal findings. Skin of elbow is more rounded with elbow in flexion. No masses, bogginess, or tenderness is noted along medial or lateral condyles of humerus, along grooves of olecranon process and epicondyles, or along extensor surface of ulna. Supracondylar lymph nodes are not palpable.

Variations. Subcutaneous nodules just inferior to olecranon process (elbow joint) may indicate rheumatoid arthritis. Tenderness or increased pain with pronation and supination of elbow and forearm, accompanied by point tenderness in lateral epicondyle, may indicate tendinitis or epicondylitis (tennis elbow); pain with point tenderness in medial epicondyle may indicate golfer's elbow.

Carrying Angle of Arm

The carrying angle is the angle formed by the elbow between the arm and forearm. To assess: Have arm in

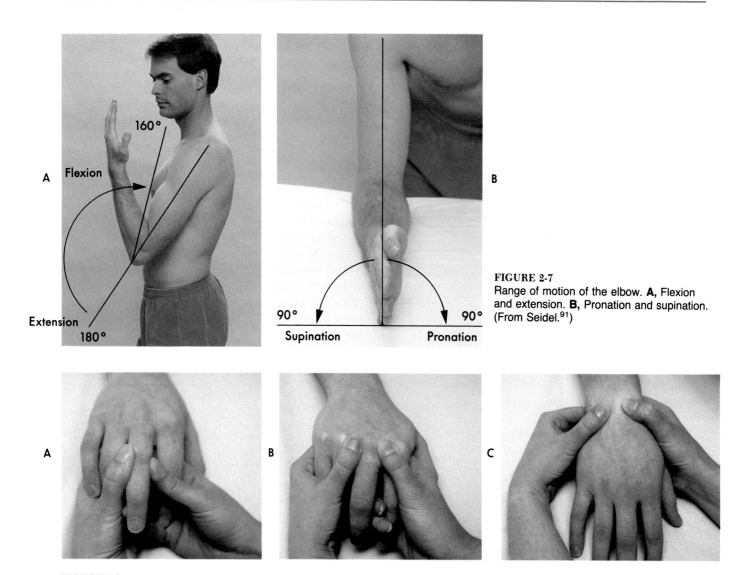

FIGURE 2-7
Range of motion of the elbow. **A,** Flexion and extension. **B,** Pronation and supination. (From Seidel.[91])

FIGURE 2-8
Palpation of the joints of the hand and wrist. **A,** Interphalangeal joints. **B,** Metacarpophalangeal joints. **C,** Radiocarpal groove and wrist. (From Seidel.[91])

passive extension; check for dislocation or partial dislocation (subluxation) of elbow by noting carrying angle, discomfort or pain, partially flexed elbow, pronated forearm, and refusal to use arm.

Normal findings. Carrying angle at elbow is between 5 and 15 degrees in adults.

Variations. Cubitus valgus (forearm farther outward than arm) and cubitus varus (forearm carried more inward) can occur in any patient of any age because of acute injury, posttraumatic arthritis, and other arthritides. Dislocation or subluxation may occur at any age as a result of acute trauma.

Range of Motion and Muscle Strength (Figure 2-7)

Ask patient to perform the following maneuvers:

- Bend and straighten elbow
- Flex elbow at right angle, then rotate hand from palm side down to palm side up
- Maintain flexion and then extension while you apply opposing force

Normal findings. Flexion of 160 degrees; extension of 180 degrees; pronation and supination of 90 degrees each. Patient can maintain flexion or extension against force.

Variations. Loss of full amounts of flexion and extension, pronation or supination may be secondary to posttraumatic arthritis, rheumatoid arthritis, osteoarthritis or postcerebrovascular accident atrophy. Loss of full muscle strength may be secondary to neuromuscular conditions, cerebral palsy, or muscular dystrophy.

WRISTS, HANDS, AND FINGERS
Inspection

Inspect and palpate all skin areas in each structure for smoothness, contour, position, symmetry, firmness, tenderness, edema, deformity, atrophy or hypertrophy of palmar muscles, increased size of hands and fingers, and short, thick, fat hands or fingers or very long, slender fingers (Figure 2-8). Inspect for radial or ulnar deviation of hand at wrist. Inspect finger (interphalangeal) joints and wrist-finger (metacarpophalangeal) joints for excess flexion or hyperextension. Count number of digits, completeness, and symmetry; inspect straightness of fingers. Check each joint separately for enlargement, tenderness, edema, pain, nodules, bogginess, color changes, and tenseness of joint. Inspect palm for muscle fullness or atrophy and for webbing at metacarpophalangeal joint. Inspect dorsal surface of hand for skin contours, blood vessels, and tendon ridges and swelling along tendon. Inspect palm for ridges, creases, and central depression.

Normal findings. Skin surfaces are smooth, warm, firm, symmetric (handedness may make one hand slightly larger with more muscular development). Hand is aligned with wrist, and fingers are aligned with wrist and forearm. No edema, soreness, tenderness, deformity, or sensory changes are noted. Thenar surface below thumb on palmar surface is more prominent than hypothenar surface near little finger. Size of hands and fingers is in relation to other body structures. Metacarpophalangeal and interphalangeal joints are not tender, swollen, boggy, hot, malformed, or tense. Fingers are not webbed. Tendon ridges and blood vessels are visible on dorsum of hand. Palm has central depression between thenar ridges. (Creases may run at angles superficially through portions of palm but not completely across palm.) All 10 digits are complete and tapered to nail ends; third finger is longer than other fingers. *Older adult:* Contours of wrist, hands, and fingers are somewhat less smooth and firm. Palm has less muscle fullness. Blood vessels on dorsum of hand may be more prominent and appear smaller and more tortuous. Less subcutaneous fat may be noted on wrists, hands, and fingers. Sensations may be slightly decreased yet within normal limits.

Variations. *Adult and older adult:* Wrists may have bony projections and deformity, with radial or ulnar deviation of hands at wrists because of arthritic changes. Joints of wrist and interphalangeal joints may be hot, tender, painful, deformed, edematous, boggy, or tense because of rheumatoid arthritis. Swan neck and bouton-

nière deformities of interphalangeal joints may be related to rheumatoid arthritis. Bouchard or Haygarth nodes in proximal and middle joints are related to rheumatoid arthritis, and Heberden nodes in distal interphalangeal joints are associated with osteoarthritis. Unusually large hands and fingers may be associated with acromegaly; short, thick, fat hands and fingers may be related to cretinism. Circumscribed area of swelling with nodular mass along tendon on dorsum of hand may be a ganglion. Digits may be partly or completely absent from trauma or congenital anomaly. Very long, slender fingers may be related to Marfan's syndrome.

Palpation

Palpate wrist structures and each finger individually after inspection is completed. Palpate for sensations and point discrimination in wrists and each finger individually. Perform Tinel's sign or test (see Appendix). Palpate anatomic snuff box area (locate on radial side of wrist by having patient extend thumb away from fingers); palpate for tenderness.

Normal findings. Sensations are within normal limits in patients of all ages. Tinel's sign is negative, indicating no carpal tunnel syndrome is present. No numbness is noted in any surface in wrist or finger areas. No tenderness is noted in anatomic snuff box.

Variations. Camptodactyly (flexion contracture of proximal interphalangeal joint, usually of little finger) and ectrodactyly (lobster-claw hand) may be noted. Clawed fingers may be a result of trauma.

Range of Motion (Figure 2-9)

Ask patient to perform the following maneuvers:

- Bend fingers forward at metacarpophalangeal joints, then stretch fingers up and back at knuckles
- Touch thumb to each fingertip and to base of little finger
- Make a fist
- Spread fingers apart, then bring them back to touch each other
- Bend hand up and down at wrist
- With palm down, turn each hand to right and left

Joint Play

To assess elbow (ulnohumeral) joint: Have elbow in 70 degrees flexion, 10 degrees supination; passively palpate joint play. To assess radiohumeral joint: Have elbow fully extended and supinated and proximal radioulnar joint: elbow in 70 degrees flexion, 35 degree supination and distal radioulnar joint: elbow in 10 degree supination.

Normal findings. All movements are possible and performed. Metacarpophalangeal flexion of 90 degrees; hyperextension of up to 20 degrees. Hand-wrist flexion

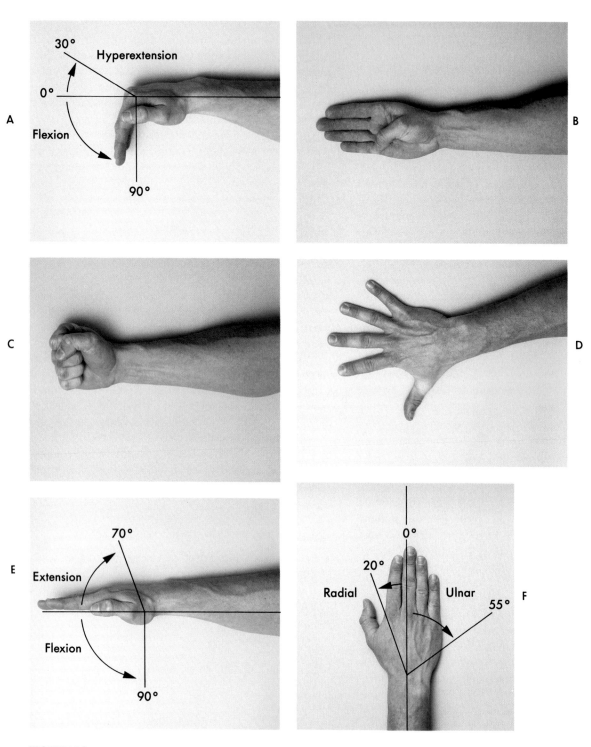

FIGURE 2-9
Range of motion of the hand and wrist. **A,** Metacarpophalangeal flexion and hyperextension.
B, Finger flexion: thumb to each fingertip and to the base of the little finger. **C,** Finger flexion:
fist formation. **D,** Finger abduction. **E,** Wrist flexion and hyperextension. **F,** Wrist radial and
ulnar movement. (From Seidel.[91])

of 90 degrees; hyperextension of 70 degrees. With palms down, hand turns to radial side 20 degrees and to ulnar side 55 degrees. Joint play for each area is 4 mm.

Variations. Ranges of motion for patient of any age may be altered because of trauma, neuromuscular conditions, muscular dystrophy, or arthritic changes. Patient of any age may have joint stiffness secondary to trauma, arthritides, or neuromuscular diseases. Joint laxity may be related to Marfan's syndrome.

Joint Play (Wrists)

Assess joint play of wrist by putting wrist (radiocarpal) joint in neutral position with slight ulnar deviation.

Normal findings. Patient may have less than 4 mm play in wrist.

Variations. Excessive laxity may be related to Marfan's syndrome.

Joint Play (Interphalangeal Joints)

Assess play in each interphalangeal joint by putting joint in slight flexion.

Normal findings. Patient may have less than 4 mm play in each joint.

Variations. Lack of joint play may be result of rheumatoid or osteoarthritic changes.

Palpation (Arteries)

Palpate radial and ulnar arteries to count pulsations.

Normal findings. All pulsations are equal in number and strength in both wrists.

Variations. Ulnar pulsations may be difficult to palpate because of ulnar deviation caused by rheumatoid arthritis.

LOWER EXTREMITIES AND PELVIS
Inspection

Initial inspection of lower extremities can be grossly made as patient walks into examining area while observing patient's gait during each phase. Note components of step. Have patient walk away from and return to same spot. Observe gait while standing in positions anterior, posterior, and lateral to patient. Note contour and shape of extremities (you should be in same place as extremities; seated is best for observing thighs, legs, and feet). Have patient stand still so as to observe characteristics of extremities, including swelling (edema) of knee or ankle area; bulges around knees; and knotty or irregular tracks of veins.

Normal findings. Gait is smooth and coordinated with base width of 2 to 4 inches between heels and step length of 15 to 18 inches (length of step is usually related to person's height). Extremities are symmetric in size. Contour varies with age, size, and weight.

Variations. Gaits vary for patients of different ages.

Inspection (Posterior)

Observe and inspect pelvis from behind patient: Observe sacral triangle; (imaginary) tip of triangle is top of gluteal cleft with base bordered on sides by posterosuperior iliac crests or spines. Dimples, one over each iliac spine, may mark lateral borders of triangle base. Assess plane on which iliac crests, and extend thumbs across back in a straight line from crest. Assess gluteal muscles; observe for roundness and equality of size of each buttock. Observe gluteal cleft (is it in midline?) Observe lower buttock border for gluteal fold. Observe anterior pelvis and lower abdominal areas for symmetry, masses, and pelvic hair distribution over mons pubis. Palpate inguinal lymph nodes.

Normal findings. Base of sacral triangle forms straight line. Plane of iliac crests is level and horizontal. Buttocks and gluteal muscles are symmetric in size, shape, and roundness. Gluteal cleft is in midline below spinal column; gluteal folds are in same horizontal plane.

Variations. Adult and older adult: Tenderness in hip joint may be caused by arthritic changes. Tenderness, especially point tenderness over trochanters (one or both) may be caused by trochanteric bursitis. Unstable pelvis may indicate fractures of pelvis. Tilt of plane may be caused by scoliosis, unequal leg length, or muscle weakness or impairment. Deviation in roundness or symmetry of gluteal structures may be result of atrophy of muscles, trauma, tumor, or unequal leg length.

HIPS
Inspection and Palpation

Inspect each hip area anteriorly and posteriorly with patient standing. Palpate each hip, iliac crest, and trochanteric area for tenderness or instability (patient should be supine for palpation). Palpate pelvis for stability.

Normal findings. Anterior iliac crests are in level, horizontal lines opposite each other. No masses are palpable in groin (no enlarged lymph nodes), and no masses are visible.

Inspection (Posterior)

Posterior iliac crests are in level horizontal line. No tenderness, instability, or crepitus is noted. Pelvis is stable when hands are pressed on iliac crests and hips and when pelvis is squeezed together from sides.

Variations. Uneven iliac crests may be result of trauma or spinal curvatures. Enlargement of lymph nodes may be caused by infection in lower extremity or by malignant disease.

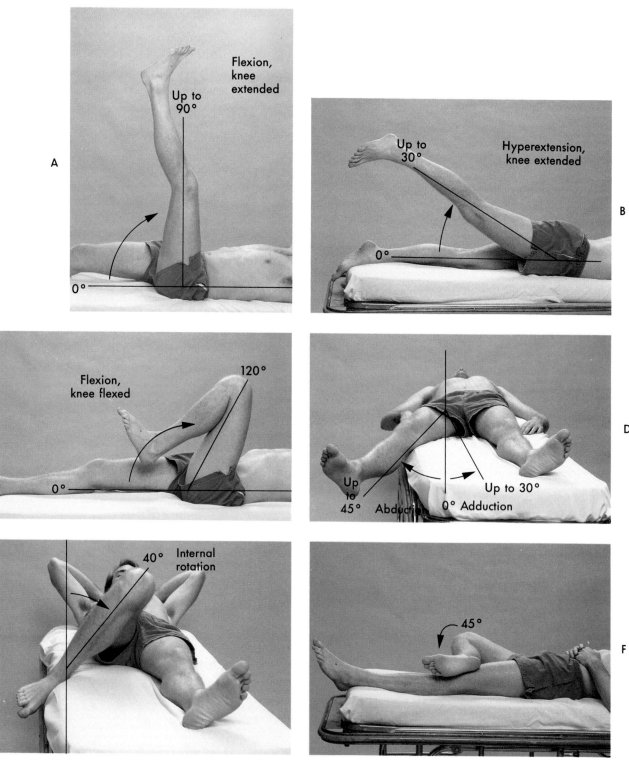

FIGURE 2-10
Range of motion of the hip. **A,** Hip flexion, leg extended. **B,** Hip hyperextension, knee extended. **C,** Hip flexion, knee flexed. **D,** Abduction. **E,** Internal rotation. **F,** External rotation. (From Seidel.[91])

Range of Motion (Figure 2-10)

Ask patient to perform the following maneuvers (assess each hip):

- With patient supine, ask her to raise leg above body with knee extended. (Normal: flexion to 90 degrees
- With patient standing or prone, have her swing each straightened leg behind body. (Normal: Hyperextension of 25 to 30 degrees)
- With patient supine, have her raise one knee to chest while keeping opposite leg straight. (Do on each side.) (Normal: Hip flexion of 120 degrees)
- With patient supine, have her swing leg laterally and medially with knee straight (you should lift opposite leg for medial (adduction) assessment to permit full movement). (Normal: Both abduction and adduction to some degree)
- With patient supine, have her place side of foot on knee of opposite leg; then move flexed knee down toward examining table. (Normal: External rotation of 45 degrees)

Variations. Inability to perform full (normal) hip movements may be result of arthritic, osteoporotic, or low back disorder. Inability to achieve 45 degrees of external rotation may be result of hip or knee arthritides or trauma.

Muscle Strength

Ask patient to perform the following maneuvers:

- With patient sitting with legs dangling over edge of table, have her raise flexed leg; apply force (pressure) on distal thigh above knee.
- With patient prone on table, place forearm over posterior iliac crest on side being tested to stabilize pelvis and ask patient to raise thigh and leg off table while you apply downward force just below gluteal fold.

Normal findings. Patient can resist forcing the leg down and can raise leg against force.

Variations. Inability to resist force may be result of muscle disorder or hip condition.

Trendelenburg's Test

Patient stands with back to you and raises one leg with knee bent.

Normal findings. Pelvis on side opposite raised leg rises.

Variations. Pelvis may stay at same level or drop to lower level in congenital hip dysplasia.

Joint Play

Assess play with hip in 30 degrees flexion, 30 degrees abduction, and slight lateral rotation.

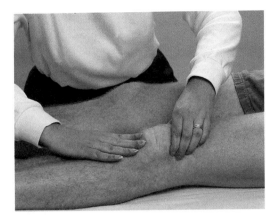

FIGURE 2-11
Procedure for ballottement examination of the knee. (From Seidel.[91])

Normal findings. Joint play is about 4 mm.

Variations. Joint stiffness or tightness may be result of trauma or arthritides.

KNEES

Inspection

Inspect knees for contour and angle of lower leg. Inspect each patella for smoothness, roundness, and position in knee area. Observe for bony growths and edema or swelling around patella or knee contours. Inspect for valleys or hollows around patellae.

Normal findings. Knee joint is fairly smooth and without bony projections, edema, or unequal contour. Patellae are smooth and round in center of knee area. Valleys or hollows are visible around patellae.

Variations. Patellae may be off center or have less smoothness or roundness because of arthritic or traumatic condition. Deviation of angle of lower leg may be present in patients of all ages because of genu valgum (outward deviation of lower leg, or knock-knees) or genu varum (inward deviation of lower leg, or bowleg). Genu recurvatum, or excessive hyperextension of knees with weight bearing, may be result of weak quadriceps muscles.

Palpation

Palpate suprapatellar pouch, lateral and medial hollows, and tibiofemoral joint spaces with thumb and fingers of one or both hands. Also palpate each of above joints while using opposite hand to apply compression over suprapatellar pouch. Palpate for edema or bogginess, fluid movements, or "doughiness." (Figure 2-11). To assess for fluid in knee under patellar area: (1) With patient supine and knee extended, stroke or milk medial side of patella upward (should displace any fluid, if present); or (2) with a single tap, percuss, lateral hollow just adjacent to patella; observe medial side of patella

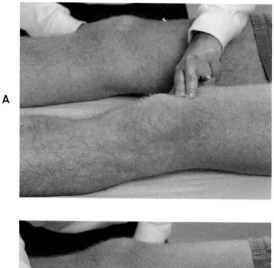

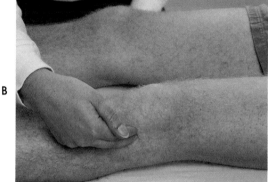

FIGURE 2-12
Testing for the bulge sign in examination of the knee. **A,** Milk the medial aspect of the knee two or three times. **B,** Then tap the lateral side of the patella. (From Seidel.[91])

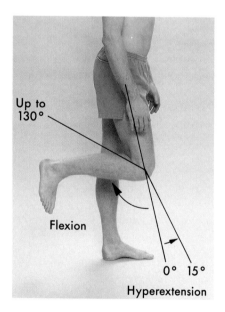

FIGURE 2-13
Range of motion of the knee: flexion and extension. (From Seidel.[91])

for bulging, an indication of fluid displacement (Figure 2-12); or (3) grasp thigh just above knee to displace any fluid in suprapatellar pouch into space between patella and femur; then use second and third fingers of opposite hand to firmly push patella against femur.

Normal findings. No edema, bogginess, or doughiness. No fluid is present in joint area. No sound is noted.

Variations. Edema, bogginess, or doughiness may be result of inflammation or joint effusion. Fluid in joint area may be result of trauma or inflammation in joint. If fluid is present, a palpable tapping or clicking sensation will be noted.

McMurray and Apley's Tests

Special tests for assessment of knee stability include applying lateral pressure to medial aspect of lower leg with one hand while holding head of fibula stable and applying pressure in a medial direction.

Normal findings. No gap or clicking sensation when pressure is applied.

Variations. If collateral ligament is unstable, this maneuver produces palpable gap.

Drawer Test

(The drawer test is used to assess the anterior and posterior cruciate ligaments.) Have patient either supine or sitting with knees flexed at 90-degree angle; hold patient's foot stable between your knees, then grasp knee and draw it forward. Push leg posteriorly for posterior drawer test.

Normal findings. Anterior drawer test may produce minimum forward gliding of knee; no movement of knee is normal for posterior test.

Variations. Anterior: Noticeable forward movement is possible because of weakness or tear in ligament. *Posterior:* Movement is possible because of ligament weakness.

Range of Motion

Ask patient to perform the following maneuvers (Figure 2-13):

- Bend each knee
- Straighten and stretch leg

Normal findings. Flexion to 130 degrees; leg can fully extend; hyperextension to 15 degrees.

Variations. Inability to flex or extend fully may be result of trauma or arthritic condition.

Muscle Strength

Assess strength of knee muscles by applying opposing force with knee in flexion or extension.

Normal findings. Patient can resist force.

Variations. Muscle weakness may be result of neuromuscular or arthritic disorder.

Joint Play

Place knee in 25 degrees of flexion.

Normal findings. Joint play is less than 4 mm.

Variations. Laxity of joint may be result of weakness or tear in ligament. Tightness of joint may be result of trauma or arthritic changes.

THIGHS AND LEGS

Inspection

Inspect thighs and legs for symmetry, contour, and size. Measure circumference of each thigh; if measurement is unequal, measure thigh longitudinally, marking off equal distances on each thigh, then measure each site's circumference. Measure leg lengths (Figure 2-14).

Normal findings. Thighs are symmetric in contour and size; muscles taper from groin to knee, being narrowest at knees. Legs are symmetric in contour and size. Thigh circumferences may differ up to 1 inch related to dominant side. Leg lengths are even, although there may be slight differences.

Variations. Varicose veins may be noted in thighs or legs, being more prominent in posterior thighs and legs.

Palpation

Using both hands, palpate muscles of thigh from groin to knee in a circular manner, simultaneously feeling for muscle masses, consistency of muscle distribution, firmness, and continuity.

Normal findings. Muscles are continuous from groin to knee. No masses, nodules, or gaps are noted. Muscles feel firm and full.

Variations. Soft, flabby muscles with atrophy may be result of neuromuscular condition. Nodular areas on thighs may be result of dystrophic effect from repetitive insulin injections.

ANKLES

Inspection and Palpation

Inspect size, shape, and contour of each ankle. Note contour of medial and lateral malleoli and smoothness or roundness. Palpate around each malleolus for edema, tenderness, or bony growths. Palpate anterior and posterior tibialis arteries in front of and behind each malleolus.

Normal findings. Malleoli are smooth and rounded. Little or no edema is noted around ankles.

Variations. Edema around malleoli may be secondary to cardiovascular or arthritic condition.

Joint Stability

Assess joint stability by stabilizing lower leg with one hand while other hand grasps heel and everts foot.

Normal findings. No gap is present.

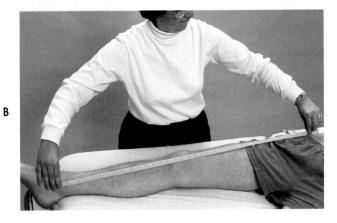

FIGURE 2-14
Measuring leg dimensions. **A,** Leg circumference. **B,** Limb length. (From Seidel.[91])

Variations. Noticeable gap may indicate ligament injury or laxity.

Joint Play

Assess joint play with ankle in 10 degrees plantar flexion midway between inversion and eversion.

Normal findings. Joint play is less than 4 mm.

Variations. Joint stiffness may be result of arthritic changes.

FEET

Inspection

Inspect feet with patient standing; note weight-bearing stance. Observe arch of foot. Observe each toe for size, shape, and contour. Note any corns or calluses. Observe heel prominence and prominences of each metatarsophalangeal joint and of balls of foot (patient may be sitting or supine) on plantar surface. Assess foot color.

Normal findings. Weight bearing occurs on midline of each foot, on imaginary line from heel midline to between second and third toes. Medial longitudinal arches are present; pes cavus (excessively high arch) may be present. Foot is pink in color.

Variations. Pes varus (toeing in) or pes valgus (toeing out) may be present and may be result of tibial torsion. Forefoot may deviate inward (metatarsus varus) or outward (metatarsus valgus). Heel may be off center with weight bearing. Pes cavus or pes planus (absence of arch) may be present, possibly because of degeneration of spinocerebellar pathways. The following conditions may also be present: hallux valgus (lateral deviation of great toe); claw toe (hyperextension of metatarsophalangeal joint with flexion of proximal interphalangeal joint); and hammer toe (hyperextension of metatarsophalangeal joint and distal interphalangeal joint with flexion of proximal interphalangeal joint.

Palpation

Palpate foot for presence of plantar warts (on heel or plantar surface), bunions, and heel spurs. Palpate for soreness or tenderness and warmth and edema around metatarsophalangeal joint of great toe. Palpate each metatarsophalangeal joint. Palpate Achilles tendon area of heels. Palpate dorsalis pedis pulse on dorsal center of metatarsal area of each foot. Palpate for temperature of feet. Perform blanching test of nail beds of toes.

Normal findings. No plantar warts, heel spurs, or bunions are present. No signs of inflammation are present, and no tenderness is noted around metatarsophalangeal joints. Achilles tendon area is smooth and round. Dorsalis pedis pulses are palpable. Feet are warm, and nail beds "pink up" in 2 to 4 seconds.

Variations. Plantar warts cause considerable pain with weight bearing. Bursa may develop at pressure point and form bunion of great toe metatarsophalangeal joint. Gout or gouty arthritis may be present. Absence of dorsalis pedis pulse may be result of arterial disease or trauma. Sluggish "pinking up" (4 to 6 seconds) may indicate arterial disease or may be secondary to beginning compartment syndrome.

Joint Play

Assess joint play with interphalangeal joints in slight flexion.

Normal findings. Joint play is less than 4 mm.

• • •

After completing the physical examination, the examiner auscultates the following:

1. Carotid arteries on each side of neck
2. Apical pulse in fifth intercostal space in left anterior chest
3. Abdominal aorta
4. Breath sounds in apex and lobes of each lung
5. Bowel sounds in four quadrants: right and left upper and lower sides

Normal findings. Pulsations are equal and clearly heard, with no irregular pulsations. Apical pulse is heard in all areas without irregularities or murmurs. The abdominal aorta pulsation is clear without bruits. Breath sounds are heard in all areas, without rales, rhonchi, or wheezes. Bowel sounds are heard in all quadrants (peristalsis usually occurs every 30 seconds).

Variations. Bruits may be heard with atherosclerosis and possibly with abdominal aneurysm. Murmurs may be heard at different stages of heartbeat. Pulse irregularities may be noted. Extra (S_3) heart sound may be heard. Breath sounds may be diminished with emphysema, asthma, pulmonary edema, or pneumonia. Bowel sounds may be decreased with constipation and increased with regional ileitis and ulcerative colitis.

Table 2-1

REFLEXES TESTED DURING PHYSICAL EXAMINATION

Reflex	Site	Normal findings	Abnormal findings
Abdominal	Abdomen around umbilicus	Contraction of umbilicus	No response in upper motor neuron lesions
Achilles or ankle jerk*	Posterior heel	Plantar flexion of foot	Decreased response in ankle in lumbar disk pathology
Anal	Anal skin area	Sphincter contracts	Flaccid sphincter in neurologic conditions
Babinski's	Sole of foot	Absent reflex	Splaying of toes and extension of great toe
Biceps*	Biceps muscle	Flexion of forearm	Partial or no flexion
Brachioradial*	Above wrist on radial surface of forearm	Flexion and supination of forearm	Partial or no flexion
Cervical	Chin (midpoint)	Mouth will close	No response
Chaddock	Lateral outer surface of foot	Flexion of great toe	Extension of great toe
Cremasteric	Proximal inner thigh at groin, only	Scrotal sac pulls up	No pulling up of scrotal sac
Finger flexor*	Finger tips of each finger	Fingers and terminal phalanx of thumb flex	Slow or no flexion
Gag	Lateral posterior wall of oropharynx	Gag initiated; uvula is drawn up and back	No response and no gag evident
Gordon	Lateral midthigh	Flexion of great toe	Extension of great toe
Hamstring	Posterior knee	Leg is drawn backward	Leg remains stationary
Jaw jerk	(same as cervical reflex above)		
Oppenheim	Anterior midcalf tibial surface (crest of tibia)	Flexion of great toe or no reaction	Extension of great toe
Patellar*	Quadriceps tendon below patella (knee is flexed for test)	Leg is drawn forward or extended	Leg remains stationary
Pectoralis major*	Tendon anterior to axilla or chest	Contraction of pectoralis muscle	No contraction
Triceps*	Posterior elbow over triceps aponeurosis	Forearm contracts with extension of forearm	No contraction or extension of forearm

*The most commonly tested reflexes.

GRADING OF REFLEX RESPONSES

0		Absent
1	(+)	Sluggish or diminished
2	(++)	Normal or active
3	(+++)	Increased or slightly hyperactive
4	(++++)	Brisk, may have intermittent clonus
5	(+++++)	Very brisk, sustained clonus

CHAPTER 3

Diagnostic Procedures

X-RAY EXAMINATION

X-rays (also known as radiographs or roentgenograms) are a noninvasive tool used in the diagnosis of orthopedic conditions. Beams of radiation are passed through the body, providing images that visualize bone structure and function and aid in detection of fractures (Figure 3-1). X-rays also show density changes, irregularities in contour, erosion of surfaces, narrowing of joint spaces, spur formation, changes in normal bone or joint shapes, tumors, and the presence of fluid in cavities that should be fluid free. X-rays allow anterior, posterior, lateral, and oblique views of the neck, chest, pelvis, or extremities.

INDICATIONS

To diagnose: Fractures
Degenerative conditions
Impingement
Infection or inflammation
Tumors
To evaluate: Organ size
Skeletal age or maturity

CONTRAINDICATIONS

Pregnancy

NURSING CARE

Have the patient remove jewelry and metal objects. If necessary, the patient may put on a long gown. The patient may be sitting, standing, or lying in a supine, prone, or side-lying position and may require assistance assuming the position. Instruct the patient to hold his breath and to remain still. Several views are usually taken, and the patient is held in the radiology department for a brief time to determine if the films are satisfactory.

PATIENT TEACHING

Explain the purpose of the specific x-ray and the multiple views that may be required. Tell the patient when the examination will be conducted, whether there are intake restrictions, and what amount of time will be needed to complete the study. Tell the patient that the examination is relatively painless, and the results will be known shortly after its completion.

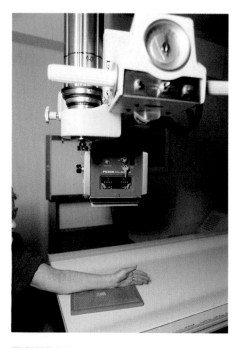

FIGURE 3-1
X-ray of forearm. Height of machine varies from 40 to 72 inches, depending on what is being examined.

MAGNETIC RESONANCE IMAGING (MRI)

Magnetic resonance imaging (MRI) is a diagnostic procedure that produces images of body tissues. It is a noninvasive technique involving the use of electromagnetic (radio) waves to alter the alignment of atoms (hydrogen ions) in the nuclei of cells (Figure 3-2). When the irradiation is stopped, the nuclear atoms return to their original positions, emitting the absorbed energy as signals that are stored by a computer and projected as images. MRI provides excellent soft tissue contrasts for clear evaluation of musculoskeletal conditions and tumors (Figure 3-3).

INDICATIONS

To diagnose: Musculoskeletal trauma
Tumors
Spinal and neurologic conditions
Infection

CONTRAINDICATIONS

Individuals with metallic implants, pacemakers, metallic clips, or staples cannot undergo an MRI study, because these objects would be forcefully drawn to the powerful magnet used for the procedure.

NURSING CARE

Have the patient remove all metallic objects and items that could be damaged by the magnet (e.g., keys and credit cards). Tell the patient to remain as still as possible for the duration of the study. After the procedure, the patient is returned to the nursing unit or discharged if an outpatient.

PATIENT TEACHING

Discuss the purpose of the procedure. Explain that the patient will lie on a table and pass through the center of a magnet. Tell the patient that there will be a steady humming sound during the examination but there should be no pain or discomfort. The examination will take 30 to 60 minutes to complete.

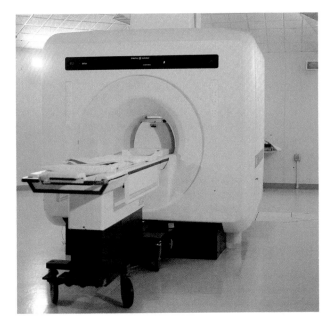
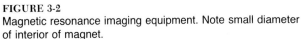

FIGURE 3-2
Magnetic resonance imaging equipment. Note small diameter of interior of magnet.

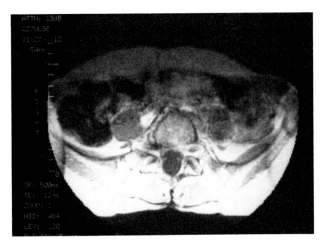

FIGURE 3-3
Printout of magnetic resonance image.

COMPUTED TOMOGRAPHY (CT SCANS)

Tomography is performed to provide a series of radiographic images of bone and tissue. It is a noninvasive examination in which radiographs are taken serially of small "slices" of tissue in cross-sectional, horizontal, and sagittal planes (Figure 3-4). The computer-translated radiographs are displayed on an oscilloscope. Tomographic views are much sharper than conventional x-rays. They more clearly define severe or complicated fractures and outline internal organs or masses more distinctly.

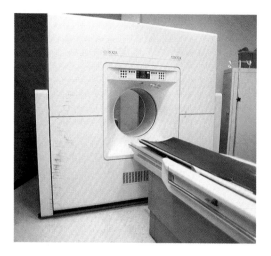

FIGURE 3-4
Set-up for computed tomography. (From Wilson [105a])

INDICATIONS

To diagnose: Musculoskeletal conditions
Spinal and vertebral trauma

CONTRAINDICATIONS

Pregnancy
If a contrast medium is used, precautions must be taken for patients with a history of hypersensitivity.

NURSING CARE

Have the patient remove all jewelry and metal objects. Instruct the patient to remain as motionless as possible during the procedure. Occasionally a sedative may be administered to calm a nervous or restless patient. A radiopaque solution may be given to outline blood vessels more clearly, although most CT scans are done without such an agent. After returning to the nursing unit, the patient can resume usual activities.

PATIENT TEACHING

Discuss the reason for the test. Explain that the patient will lie on a narrow table, which will slowly be advanced into a round opening in the center of the scanner. The scanner will make a clicking sound as it moves around and along the patient's body. The scan will take 10 to 60 minutes to complete, depending on whether portions of the body or the entire body is being examined. If a contrast medium is used, discuss intake restrictions, possible responses to the contrast agent, the method by which the contrast solution will be introduced into the body, and whether it will be removed or absorbed.

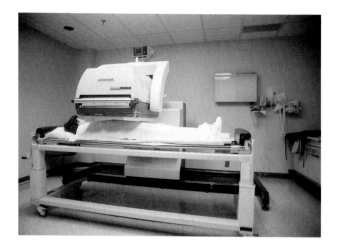

FIGURE 3-5
Patient prepared for bone scan. Patient's feet are tied to help maintain hips in position for maximal scanning uptake.

BONE SCINTIGRAPHY (BONE SCANS)

Bone scintigraphy is the examination of bones through intravenous injection of a radioisotope, usually technetium-99 (^{99}Tc sodium pertechnetate) (Figure 3-5). The radioisotope is scanned by a special camera, which records its distribution throughout the bones in the body and produces an image. The scan reveals increased radioisotope uptake (which shows up as a "hot" spot) if unusual bone reactivity is present.

INDICATIONS

To diagnose: Metastatic lesions
Bone trauma•
Inflammation or infection
To evaluate: Healing progress of bone grafts

CONTRAINDICATIONS

Pregnancy
Lactation

NURSING CARE

Obtain an informed consent. Have the patient remove all metal and jewelry. A sedative may be administered, if necessary. The radioisotope is injected 1 to 3 hours before the bone scan to permit the isotope to circulate to the bone tissue. Have the patient drink one to three glasses of water during the waiting period to aid excretion of radioisotope that is not absorbed in the bones. The patient is transported to the nuclear medicine area and placed on a scanning table. After the procedure, when the patient returns to the nursing unit, check the injection site for edema or redness.

PATIENT TEACHING

Explain the purpose of the procedure. Tell the patient that a scanning camera will move back and forth over her body as the images are recorded. Tell the patient that the procedure takes about 1 hour and is painless.

ARTHROSCOPY

Arthroscopy is the examination of joint tissues with an endoscope (arthroscope), which allows direct visualization of the interior of a joint (Figure 3-6). An arthroscopic study reveals the condition of internal joint tissues, the existence of loose bodies, tears in cartilage or ligaments, or conditions of synovial tissues. Small loose bodies may be removed, torn cartilage may be repaired, and tissues may be biopsied through arthroscopy. Theoretically, arthroscopy may be performed on any joint, but most frequently it is done on the knee, shoulder, and elbow. It is less often performed on the hip and ankle. Complications of arthroscopy include bleeding in the joint, edema, and possible infection.

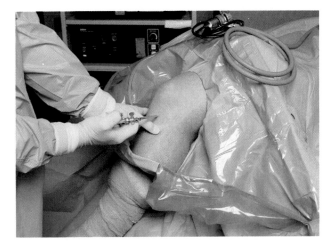

FIGURE 3-6
Patient ready for arthroscopy of knee.

INDICATIONS

To diagnose: Acute and chronic musculoskeletal disorders
The status of ligaments, tendons, cartilage, or synovium inside a joint

CONTRAINDICATIONS

None

NURSING CARE

The patient should have nothing to eat or drink after midnight the day of the procedure. Arthroscopy is performed in the outpatient or inhospital surgical suite; therefore complete a preoperative checklist, and obtain a signed consent. After the procedure, apply a compression dressing and use ice to lessen bleeding and edema. The patient should avoid excessive use of the joint for 24 to 48 hours after the procedure, although walking is permitted after knee arthroscopy. Use of other joints varies with the purpose and extent of the arthroscopic examination or repair. Check all peripheral pulses, and observe for swelling and changes in color or temperature. Assess movement, sensation, and the amount of pain in the surrounding tissue. Administer analgesics as ordered for discomfort or pain.

PATIENT TEACHING

Explain the purpose of the procedure. Discuss the preparatory skin cleansing, administration of a local anesthetic, application of a tourniquet to lessen blood flow, and sterile draping. Tell the patient that the arthroscope may be inserted in more than one area or port to visualize the tissues more thoroughly. The patient should be informed about signs of infection, undue edema or pain, ice applications, restrictions or limitations of joint use and, if discharge is planned, when to return to see the physician.

ELECTROMYOGRAPHY (ELECTROMYOGRAM)

Electromyography is a recording of nerve and muscle responses to electrical stimulation of one or more muscles. The responses are shown on an oscilloscope. A muscle may fail to respond to stimulation or may have a slow or delayed response, depending on the integrity of the nerve and muscle. Electromyography may be performed in conjunction with nerve conduction velocity determination (NCVD), with the nerve responses timed and recorded. The same equipment and procedures are used as for the electromyogram (Figure 3-7).

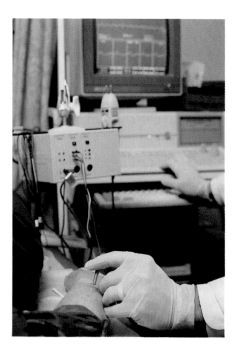

FIGURE 3-7
Patient having electromyogram of forearm. Small needle size makes procedure virtually painless.

INDICATIONS

To diagnose: Muscle conditions (myopathies)
To evaluate: Nerve enervation status

CONTRAINDICATIONS

None

NURSING CARE

There is no specific nursing care. The patient may be required to limit cigarette smoking or caffeine ingestion before the procedure.

PATIENT TEACHING

Explain the procedure and its purpose. Tell the patient that a small, thin needle will be inserted into the muscle or muscles to be tested, and the muscle will be stimulated by an electrical pulsation through the needle. The muscle will twitch or contract, and the results will be recorded on a graph. Tell the patient that he may feel some discomfort as the needle is inserted and the muscle stimulated. Inform him that the procedure takes 10 to 20 minutes and there should be no lasting discomfort.

MYELOGRAPHY (MYELOGRAM)

Myelography uses a radiopaque solution, injected by lumbar or cisternal puncture, to outline the contents of the spinal canal. Radiographic records (myelograms) provide evidence of intervertebral disk integrity or herniation, the presence of tumors, or the existence of developmental or degenerative spinal conditions that could exert pressure on the spinal nerves as they exit the canal. Complications of the procedure include headache, seizures, persistent pain or radiculopathy, arachnoiditis, nausea, and vomiting.

INDICATIONS

To diagnose: Herniations of intervertebral disks
　　　　　　　Tumors
　　　　　　　Developmental or degenerative spinal conditions

CONTRAINDICATIONS

Pregnancy
Allergy to contrast medium
Evidence of increased intracranial pressure

NURSING CARE

Before the procedure the patient is served a clear liquid breakfast; after this, restrict food and fluids. Complete a preoperative checklist, and obtain a signed consent. Ask the patient about sensitivity to the contrast agent. After the myelogram, if iophendylate was used, keep the patient flat in bed, monitor vital signs, and observe the site for edema, bleeding, or spinal fluid leak. Do neurovascular checks (see inside back cover) every 1 to 2 hours, and note complaints of headache. If headache occurs, continue flat bed rest and increase fluid intake to restore spinal fluid; a narcotic analgesic may be administered if ordered. Bed rest is usually required for 8 to 12 hours after the myelogram. Care after a myelogram in which metrizamide was used includes allowing the patient to be up, if desired, because the water-soluble agent has been absorbed into the cerebrospinal fluid and will be eliminated through general circulation. Do laminectomy checks, increase fluid intake, and observe the patient for complaints of headache, nausea, vomiting, or seizures for 4 to 8 hours. If headache occurs, put the patient on flat bed rest. Antiemetics may be administered for nausea or vomiting. Give anticonvulsants if seizures follow the myelogram. If myelography is performed as an outpatient procedure, monitor the patient for 4 to 6 hours before discharge.

PATIENT TEACHING

Explain the purpose of the procedure. The physician will have discussed with the patient whether a contrast agent (metrizamide [Amipaque] or iophendylate [Pantopaque]) or air will be used to visualize the desired area. Discuss the length of the examination and any discomfort the patient may feel. If the patient is discharged, provide instructions about symptoms that could occur at home that would require notifying a physician.

LUMBAR PUNCTURE

Lumbar puncture is a diagnostic procedure that involves inserting a needle into the spinal canal subarachnoid area to collect cerebrospinal fluid for study. Spinal fluid should be clear with no or few white blood cells (0 to 8 cells/mm³) 15 to 45 mg/dl of protein, 45 to 85 mg/dl of glucose, 118 to 130 mEq/L of chloride, and 7 to 15 mg/dl of urea. Spinal fluid pressure should equal 75 to 200 mm water or 8 to 12 mm mercury. Yellowish color of the fluid may indicate the presence of bilirubin or red blood cell pigments. Complications of lumbar puncture include headache, spinal fluid leak from the puncture site, hematoma and, in rare cases, pain radiating to the thigh from nerve root irritation.

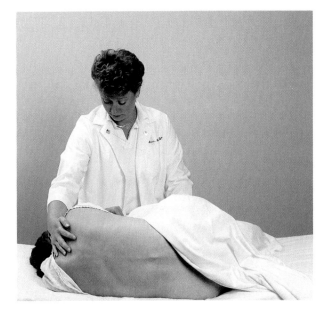

FIGURE 3-8
Positioning of patient for lumbar puncture for myelogram. Patient may also be seated in upright position for lumbar puncture. (From Grimes [39a])

NURSING CARE

Obtain a signed consent before the procedure. Assist the patient into a recumbent side-lying or upright sitting position, according to the physician's request or the purpose of the lumbar puncture (Figure 3-8). Ask the patient to flex the legs and knees to thighs and to bend the head forward, curving the back. Encourage the patient to remain quiet and still. After the lumbar puncture, the patient should lie flat in bed. Monitor vital signs, and check the needle insertion site for edema, soreness, or signs of leakage. Investigate complaints of headache, and place the patient on flat bed rest with fluids forced to replenish spinal fluid, if necessary. Observe the patient for evidence of complications.

PATIENT TEACHING

Explain the need for the procedure, and tell the patient that some pain and discomfort may be felt during the study. Emphasize the need for cooperation and the importance of bed rest after the test. The procedure lasts approximately 10 to 15 minutes.

ARTHROGRAPHY (ARTHROGRAM)

Arthrography is the radiographic study of joint tissues after injection of a contrast solution. Arthrograms show tears of ligaments, tendons, and cartilage and provide information that may not be obtained through arthroscopy. The procedure is commonly done for rotator cuff or meniscal trauma. Complications include edema, bleeding, soreness or pain, and crepitus (noise on joint movement). In rare cases the patient may have an inflammatory or allergic reaction to the contrast agent.

INDICATIONS

To diagnose: Injury to joint ligaments, cartilage, tendons, or muscles

CONTRAINDICATIONS

Joint infection
Active arthritis
Pregnancy
Allergy to contrast medium

NURSING CARE

Ask the patient about sensitivity to the contrast solution, and obtain a signed consent. After the study, apply a compression dressing and ice to lessen edema. Instruct the patient to keep the joint at rest for 12 hours or longer. After that time, use depends on the findings of the arthrogram. Mild analgesics are usually given for pain, which may be related to the original joint condition. Check the joint frequently, noting edema, color changes, heat, and amount of pain.

PATIENT TEACHING

Discuss the purpose of the procedure with the patient. Explain that the involved joint will be thoroughly cleansed and that a local anesthetic will be injected. The radiopaque solution will be injected through a needle inserted into the joint, the needle will be removed, and the site sealed with collodion. Tell the patient that she may feel some discomfort when the contrast dye is injected. Explain that she will be asked to move the joint through its range of motion while x-rays are being taken. The contrast solution will be absorbed into the joint fluids.

DISCOGRAPHY (DISCOGRAM)

Discography is a diagnostic method for studying the intervertebral disk space. A radiopaque solution is injected, and radiographic images are produced. The study should reveal the integrity of the intervertebral disk, show the site or sites of pressure or impingement on contiguous structures, and provide evidence of inflammation or tumor in the disk space. Inflammation (diskitis) is a possible complication of the procedure.

INDICATIONS

To diagnose: Nerve impingement
　　　　　　　Tumors
To evaluate: Condition of the disk space

CONTRAINDICATIONS

Pregnancy
Allergy to contrast agent

NURSING CARE

Ask the patient about sensitivity to the contrast agent and obtain a signed consent. After the procedure, assess the patient's neurologic condition using neurovascular checks (see inside back cover). Observe the injection site for edema, color changes, and bleeding. Administer mild analgesics as ordered for pain or soreness.

PATIENT TEACHING

Explain the reason for the procedure. Tell the patient that a radiopaque solution will be injected into the disk space after the skin is cleansed and a local anesthetic is injected. Use pictures of the spinal column and disk areas to clarify any of the patient's concerns. Discuss the length of the procedure and any discomfort the patient may feel.

BIOPSY OF BONE, MUSCLE, AND SYNOVIUM

Bone, muscle, or synovial biopsy consists of extracting one or more pieces of tissue for microscopic study. Histologic examination may help differentiate a benign tumor from a malignant one, or it may help identify muscle disease and synovial conditions. All biopsies are performed aseptically in the outpatient or inhospital surgical suite. Complications include effusion or hemorrhage into a joint with synovial biopsy, and hematoma or pain with bone or muscle biopsy.

INDICATIONS

To diagnose: Bone tumors
Muscle diseases
Synovial conditions
Arthritis

CONTRAINDICATIONS

None

NURSING CARE

Complete the preoperative checklist, and obtain a signed consent. The patient should have nothing to eat or drink for 1 to 4 hours (or longer) before the procedure. After the biopsy, apply a sterile dressing to the site. Check the site for edema, bleeding, or pain, and change the dressing as warranted. Ice may be ordered to lessen edema or bleeding. A mild analgesic may be ordered to relieve pain.

PATIENT TEACHING

Explain the purpose of the procedure. Teach the patient about the skin cleansing techniques, administration of the local anesthetic, and the use of a needle to obtain the biopsy tissue. Teach the patient about signs of infection and use of the biopsied joint, muscle, or tissue.

NORMAL LABORATORY DATA
BLOOD SERUM VALUES

Test	Normal adult values
Red cell count ($10^6/\mu$L)	Men: 5.11 ± 0.38
	Women: 4.51 ± 0.36
Hemoglobin (g/dl)	Men: 15.5 ± 1.1
	Women: 13.7 ± 1.0
Hematocrit (%)	Men: 46.0 ± 3.1
	Women: 40.9 ± 3
Mean corpuscular volume (MCV)	Men: 90 (80-100) μm^3
	Women: 88 (79-98) μm^3
Mean corpuscular hemoglobin (MCH)	Men: 30 (25.4-34.6) pg
	Women: 30 (25.4-34.6) pg
Mean corpuscular hemoglobin concentration (MCHC)	Men: 34% (31%-37%)
	Women: 33% (30%-36%)
Reticulocyte count (expressed as % of 1000 RBCs)	0.5%-1.5%
Complete white blood count (WBC)	4500-11,000/mm^3
Differential WBC	Expressed as a percent of total WBC
Granulocytes	
Neutrophils	62.0% (range of 60%-70%)
Eosinophils	50-350/mm^3
Basophils	0.4%
Nongranular leukocytes	
Monocytes	5.3%
Lymphocytes	30.0%
Sodium (serum or plasma)	135-145 mEq/L
Potassium (plasma)	3.5-5.0 mEq/L
Chloride (serum)	97-107 mEq/L

Continued.

NORMAL LABORATORY DATA
BLOOD SERUM VALUES—cont'd

Test	Normal adult values
Magnesium (serum)	1.2-1.9 mEq/L
Serum iron	42-135 µg/dl
Serum calcium (ionized)	4.75-5.2 mg/dl
Serum calcium (ionized, calculated, blood)	3.9-4.8 mg/dl
Serum phosphorus	2.5-4.5 mg/dl
Alkaline phosphatase*	3-13 King-Armstrong units or 1.5-4.0 Bodansky units
Acid phosphatase	Method dependent; up to 0.8 IU/L, ACA
Creatinine (24-h urine)	Adult male: 1-2 g/24 h
	Adult female: 0.8-1.8 g/24 h
Creatinine clearance	Adult male: 85-125 ml/min/1.73 m²
	Adult female: 75-115 ml/min/1.73 m²
BUN/creatinine ratio	6-20; mean about 10:1
Creatinine (serum)	Adult males: up to 1.2 mg/dl
	Adult females: up to 1.1 mg/dl
	There are slight differences between the sexes with males higher, since the range relates to the amount of muscle mass present.
Uric acid (serum)	Adult males: 3.4-7.0 mg/dl or slightly more
	Adult females: 2.4-6.0 mg/dl or slightly more
Uric acid (urine)	Approximately 250-750 mg/24 h
Serum glutamic pyruvic transaminase (SGPT)	3-30 IU/L (method dependent)
Serum glutamic oxaloacetic transaminase (SGOT)	8-42 IU/L
Creatinine phosphokinase (CPK)	0-50 IU (method dependent)
Aldolase	1.5-7.2 m/M/min/L
Erythrocyte sedimentation rate (ESR): Westergren method	Males <50 yr: 0-15 mm/h
	Males >50 yr: 0-20 mm/h
	Females <50 yr: 0-25 mm/h
	Females >50 yr: 0-30 mm/h
Zeta sedimentation ratio	<50 yr: <55%
	50-80 yr: 40-60%
Blood platelets	150,000-400,000/mm³
Prothrombin time	10-13 sec
Prothrombin levels	60-140%
O₂ saturation	95-99%
Bleeding time	Ivy: 2-7 min
	Duke: 5 min
CO₂	Arterial: 22-29 mEq/L
	Venous: 23-30 mEq/L
Po₂	80-95 mm Hg
Pco₂	35-45 mm Hg
Serum pH	7.35-7.45
Partial thromboplastin time	25-39 sec (usually stated to be within 10 sec of control)
Fibrinogen	Quantitative: 200-400 mg/dl
Lactic acid dehydrogenase (LDH)	18-44 yr: 115-200 IU/L
	44 yr and up: 115-225 IU/L
Serum albumin	1-31 yr: 3.5-5.0 g/dl with A/G ratio >1.0; after 40 yr, normal range gradually decreases

*In nonpregnant subjects, percent residual activity >25% favors hepatic origin; <10% favors bone origin.

NORMAL LABORATORY DATA
BLOOD SERUM VALUES—cont'd

Test	Normal adult values
Serum proteins	
Immunoglobulins	
IgG	1140 mg/dl (75% of total; range of 564-1765 mg/dl)
IgA	214 mg/dl (10%-15% of total; range of 85-385 mg/dl)
IgM	168 mg/dl (7-10% of total; range of 40-120 mg/dl)
IgD	0.5-3 mg/dl (<1% of total)
IgE	0.01-0.04 mg/dl (<1% of total)
Blood urea nitrogen (BUN)	1-40 year: 5-20 mg/dl; slight increase may occur gradually
Fibrin split products	<10 µg/ml
Serum complement C$_3$	900-2000 µg/ml
Direct bilirubin	up to 0.4 mg/dl
Total bilirubin	0.3-1.0 mg/dl
Coagulation factors	
V	60%-140%
VII	70%-130%
VIII	50%-200%
IX	60%-140%

URINE VALUES (FROM URINALYSIS)

Laboratory test	Normal adult values
Urinalysis	
Albumin	<20 mg/dl
Bilirubin	Negative
Color	Clear, golden yellow
Glucose	Negative
Hemoglobin	Negative
Ketones	Negative
Microscopic urinalysis	
Bacteria	Negative
Casts	0-4 hyaline casts per low-power field
Crystals	Interpreted by physician
Mucous threads	Negative
Red blood cells	0-5 per high-power field
Squamous epithelial cells	Seen on voided specimen in females; negative on voided specimen in males; negative for catheterized specimens
White blood cells	0-5 per high-power field
Uric acid (urine)	250-750 mg/24 h
Sodium (urine)	27-287 mEq/24 h (varies with dietary intake)
Oxalate	Up to 40 mg/24 h
Cystine	Random sample negative
Calculated ionized calcium	Varies with diet; based on average calcium intake of 600-800 mg/24 h, excretion may be 100-250 mg/24
Inorganic phosphorus	0.9-1.3 g/24 h
Creatinine	
Urine	Male: 1-2 g/24 h
	Female: 0.8-1.8 g/24 h
Urine specific gravity	1.001-1.035

CHAPTER 4

Musculoskeletal Trauma

Trauma is the most common cause of death between the ages of 1 and 40 years; it is the third most common cause in the 35 to 54 age group.[71] Each year more than 150,000 people die from trauma, and 3.6 million are admitted to hospitals for injuries.[62] In economic terms, these injuries and deaths cost $100 billion to $140 billion annually.[71] Furthermore, thousands of productive years of life are lost—a consequence that has a major impact on the economy. The loss of these human and economic resources affects each of us, either directly, from loss of a family member or friend, or indirectly, through increased insurance and health care costs.

Head injuries are a common cause of death, but nonfatal injuries such as multiple fractures and soft tissue trauma are also common. Injuries can occur in nearly any activity, even walking, but many are related to sports, running, jogging, accidents at work, or pedestrian mishaps.

Table 4-1 lists the common types of injuries for various age groups and the sources of those injuries. Some injuries may be minor, such as a strain or sprain, but many may be more severe, life threatening, or even fatal.

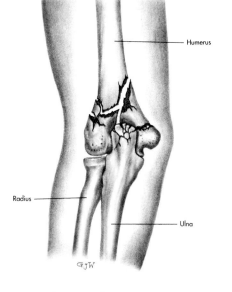

Comminuted Fracture

Humerus

Radius

Ulna

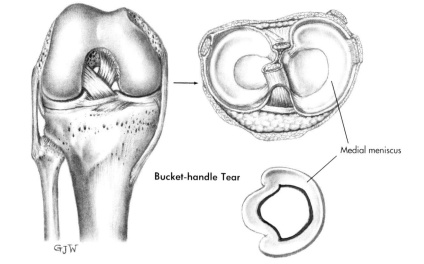

Bucket-handle Tear

Medial meniscus

Table 4-1 _____

AGE-RELATED INJURIES AND THEIR CAUSES

Age (yr)	Types of injuries	Causes of injuries
1-4	Head/neck injuries Lacerations/contusions Fractures Strains/sprains	Play equipment at home, climbing equipment, recreational games or settings, unknown causes
5-10	Lacerations/contusions Fractures Head/neck injuries Strains/sprains	Same causes as above, also running into traffic from sidewalks or yard
10-20	Dislocations Fractured hip, elbow, skull and other bones and others Muscle/tendon strains Joint/ligament strains Concussions Inflammation (bursitis, tendonitis, apophysitis)	High energy trauma (auto accidents, falls), motorcycles, bicycles, low energy falls (downhill accidents, gliding injuries), sports injuries (stretched muscles, twisting, overuse, jumping, football, baseball, etc.)
20-50	Fractures/dislocations Head injuries/concussions Inflammation (as above) Lacerations/contusions Sites: knee, hip, ankle, foot, spine, wrist, hand, elbow, shoulder	Sports injuries (stretched muscles, twisting), stress injuries (fractures), overuse, recreational sports, tennis, swimming, jogging, basketball, football, etc. Auto accidents, pedestrian injuries, boxing
50-65	Same injuries as for 20-50 yrs Inflammation (as above) Degenerative joint disease	Traffic and auto accidents, falls, recreational sports, pathologic fractures
65 or over	Fractured hip or femur, tibia, fibula, pelvis, radius, ulna, humerus, skull/brain injury	Falls, pedestrian injuries, auto accidents, recreational injuries (e.g., walking, jogging, swimming, hiking), osteoporosis, pathologic fractures

PRINCIPLES OF TRAUMA MANAGEMENT

Much has been written about the management of patients with multiple trauma injuries. More of these patients have survived since the advent of local and regional level I trauma centers. Level I centers have all necessary personnel present as a team, as well as the equipment and facilities, to manage different types of trauma cases, whether they involve multiple or single injuries and one person or many. The members of the trauma team are well versed in their specific responsibilities, and they continually practice their techniques and skills so as to be alert and ready when they are needed. Rescue and emergency medical transport teams are taught which hospitals in their areas are level I trauma centers, to avoid any delay in obtaining care for injured people.

The box on p. 48 lists principles of management for injuries in children and adults. In both cases, the ABCs (*a*irway, *b*reathing, and *c*irculation) are priority assessments, accompanied by care while maintaining the in-

dividual with the head and spinal cord immobilized to prevent initial or additional injury to those areas. Secondary assessments (e.g., neurologic responses, condition of genitourinary system) follow the priority assessments, thus completing the assessment of the patient. Each trauma team member, under the direction of the physician team leader, provides specific care according to practiced roles and responsibilities. Consultants are called in and used as needed. The trauma team's assessment and the severity of the injuries determine whether the patient is transferred to the operating room, the intensive care unit, or the nursing unit. Trauma accounts for one of every 10 admissions to short-stay hospitals,[62] and these patients required significant inpatient and outpatient care in the year after discharge.[62]

DEFINITIVE CARE FOR SPECIFIC INJURIES

Along with initial primary and secondary assessments of an injured person, definitive care is one of the principles of trauma management. Definitive care includes all the activities or treatments provided throughout the period from injury through rehabilitation. It includes all the planning, discussing, and determining of the program for the patient's particular situation. Many treatments for various injuries are identical; e.g., RICE—*rest, ice* applications, *compression* and *elevation*—is used in a number of injuries, although the type or time for rest, the type of compression, and the duration of ice applications or elevation may vary. Many operative treatments and the use of casts, traction, or external fixators follow standard principles and to avoid redundancy are discussed together.

The types of musculoskeletal trauma are defined in the box on page 49. Each type is accompanied by some degree of soft tissue trauma, which may aggravate the extent or severity of the injury.

A *contusion* can occur anywhere in the body and usually is the result of a direct blow or fall on the tissue. The force of the blow or fall disrupts capillaries, causing bleeding into the subcutaneous, muscular, or adipose tissues. The involved area becomes black and blue and may be tender, or it may be more painful if the contusion is in a muscle or an area such as the but-

tocks or coccyx, where sitting or walking could cause pain. Usually applying an ice bag or ice wrapped in cloth to the area lessens the bleeding, edema formation, and pain. The discoloration and soreness resolve in 7 to 10 days, most often without additional treatment.

A *strain* results from excessive stretching of a muscle beyond its functional capacity; this leads to bleeding into the tissues, which causes an inflammatory reaction. Pain is a common symptom; it may be severe in an acute strain or dull, aching, and less severe in chronic strains. The person may limit use of the affected muscles and joints.

Strains (and sprains) are classified according to their severity as first, second, or third degree or as grade 1, 2, or 3. A first-degree strain is treated by applying ice to lessen edema and bleeding, plus initial rest to the part, followed by gradual resumption of activities. Immobilization is not advocated. Pain may be relieved with analgesics. After several days, heat may be applied to hasten resolution of the inflammation and pain. The strain usually heals in 4 to 6 weeks without residual effects.

Second-degree strains are also treated with ice applications and rest and elevation of the part, but in these cases the injured muscle *is* immobilized. Crutches are used for strains of the leg; for strains of

---

PRINCIPLES OF TRAUMA MANAGEMENT

Pediatric patients

Immobilize neck
Remove clothing
Perform 60-sec overall examination
Apply electrocardiogram (ECG) leads
Draw blood for complete blood count (CBC), type and
   cross-match, serum amylase
Administer nasal oxygen
Initiate intravenous therapy via cutdown if necessary
X-rays of cervical vertebrae
Insert urinary catheter and temperature probe
If needed: Insert endotracheal tube
   Insert nasogastric tube
   Do peritoneal lavage
   Insert arterial lines
Dress open wounds
Do complete physical examination
Get full history
Get chest x-ray
Check laboratory findings
Calculate trauma score
List positive findings (type and severity of injuries)

Adult patients

Immobilize head, neck, spine
Provide priority care:
   Airway
   Breathing
   Circulation
Provide secondary assessments and care:
   Neurologic responses
   Gastrointestinal/abdominal system
   Genitourinary system
   Musculoskeletal system
   Endocrine system
Management under each system for adults involves similar
   treatments used for pediatric patients (e.g., oxygen therapy, intravenous (IV) infusions, ventilatory assistance)

the arm, the limb is placed in a sling until the edema and tenderness subside. After the pain has resolved, ambulation or use is begun, with progressive active exercises done to the limit of pain. Heat applications are used in place of ice at this stage. Second-degree strains should heal well; however, if the person (especially an athlete) returns to activity while there is still significant edema or bleeding, fibrosis, with a resultant calcium deposit, may delay healing and recovery.

Third-degree strains are treated with ice applications, elevation of the limb, and immobilization in a splint. The patient should be referred to a specialist, since surgical repair may be indicated, depending on the individual's age, the muscle involved, and the location of the tear or tears.

A *sprain* is a tear in a ligament. A first-degree sprain involves tearing of a few fibers with minimum edema, no functional disability, and normal joint motion. Second-degree sprains vary according to the number of fibers disrupted (from one third to all but a few); they also involve more edema, tenderness, and functional disability than do first-degree sprains, although joint motion is normal. Third-degree sprains involve complete separation of the ligament from the bone, significant edema, functional disability, and abnormal joint motion.

First-degree ligament tears are treated by applying ice, resting the joint, applying compression with an elastic bandage, and resuming use and exercises early. Usually there is no residual damage.

Second-degree sprains are also treated with ice, rest, and compression, but they also call for aspiration of excessive joint fluid, support with a splint or immobilization device (taping), and rehabilitative exercises. Residual damage is uncommon and may be related to failure to differentiate a second-degree sprain from a third-degree sprain.

A third-degree sprain is treated with early surgical intervention to restore continuity to the ligament, which helps restore normal ligament tissues and hastens collagenization. Early repair also lessens scar tissue, and sutured ligaments are stronger than unsutured ones. After an appropriate healing period, rehabilitative exercises are started to strengthen the joint structures and surrounding muscles. Residual damage may be associated with joint instability.

A *subluxation* is an injury in which one of the bones is partly dislocated from the joint. It is caused by direct force on the bones making up the joint or by indirect (sideways) force against one or both bones. There may be some associated edema, pain, and functional changes.

Treatments include manual traction to replace the bone within the joint (reduction), compression, immobilization with a splint, and ice application. If there is no bone damage, such as a bone chip, function is fully restored, and use is encouraged when the edema has resolved. There should be no residual damage.

A *dislocation* involves complete separation of the contact between the two bones of a joint. The injury results from moderate to intense pressure or force that pushes the bone from the joint. There is immediate functional alteration and usually pain. Bleeding and edema are usually minimal. X-rays confirm the diagnosis.

Treatment consists of manual traction to replace the bone within the joint. Anesthesia may or may not be used, depending on the patient's age and emotional condition and the specific joint involved. Following reduction, wrapping or compression may be applied, with the arm held in a sling after a shoulder or elbow reduction. Following a hip reduction, traction may be applied to maintain the reduction. Residual damage may cause posttraumatic arthritis.

TYPES OF MUSCULOSKELETAL TRAUMA

Contusion   A bruise with bleeding into the soft tissues.

Strain   An injury to a muscle, tendon, or ligament caused by excessive pull, use, or forcible stretch. It may be an acute injury or may develop from chronic overuse. Strains are referred to as first, second, or third degree (see Table 4-2).

Sprain   An acute injury of a tendon or ligament around or in a joint, resulting in partial or complete tearing of the fibers from their attachments. Sprains are also referred to as first, second or third degree, as shown in Table 4-2.

Subluxation   A partial separation or incomplete dislocation of a bone from a joint.

Dislocation   A complete disruption or separation of contact between the bones of a joint.

Fracture   A partial or complete break in a bone. Table 4-3 lists the classifications of various types of fractures and the causes of injury. Table 4-4 lists the proper names (eponyms) and descriptions of many fractures and provides illustrations of each.

Table 4-2

CLASSIFICATION AND SYMPTOMS OF STRAINS AND SPRAINS

	Strain	Sprain
Tissue involved	Muscle usually, tendon or ligament at times	Tendon or ligament
Classification		
First degree (grade 1)	Excess pull or stretch	Ligament fibers partly torn
Symptoms	Mild pain; edema with some ecchymosis; muscle spasm at times; tenderness; slight loss of function or strength	Mild pain; slight edema; local tenderness; no joint instability; slight change in function for brief period
Second degree (grade 2)	Tear or disruption of some muscle fibers	Incomplete tear of ligament
Symptoms	More pain and edema than in first-degree strain; inflammatory response with redness, bleeding, change in function, local heat	Moderate edema; local pain and tenderness; moderate joint instability; inability to carry out usual activities
Third degree (grade 3)	Complete disruption of muscle fibers, possibly with rupture of overlying fascia	Full or complete tear of ligament or tendon
Symptoms	Severe pain; muscle spasm; pronounced edema; marked ecchymosis with hematoma formation; marked tenderness; loss of function	Marked pain; edema minimum to marked; marked joint disability; loss of function of joint tissues

A *fracture* is a more severe injury than those previously described. A fracture is a break in one or more cortices of a bone. Fractures may be described according to a number of characteristics such as (1) whether the skin is intact (closed fracture) or broken (open fracture), (2) the line of the fracture (transverse, oblique, spiral, or linear), (3) the force causing the fracture (compression), (4) the number of pieces (comminuted), (5) the anatomic position of the distal fragment (displaced, augulated), and (6) whether the fracture involves the joint (intraarticular or extraarticular).

A fracture of the bone is usually accompanied by soft tissue injury involving muscles, arteries, veins, nerves, other bones, and the skin. The degree of involvement generally correlates to the amount of energy or force that caused the fracture. Thus minor force may cause a break in one cortex (greenstick), but moderate to severe forces cause the bone to break into many pieces (comminuted). Greenstick fractures result in little associated soft tissue trauma, whereas comminuted fractures involve considerable soft tissue trauma.

After a fracture, the site is usually numb for 15 to 20 minutes because of trauma to the nerve or nerves at the site. During this nerve "shock" period, the tissues may be used almost normally. People have walked on frac-

tured legs and used fractured arms and hands. After the numbness wears off, the site becomes tender, sore, or painful, leading to guarding and less willingness to use the injured parts. Guarding usually protects the injured tissues from additional trauma.

The numbness, pain, and functional changes associated with fractures are accompanied by edema, bleeding, pallor, and coolness of the site. These signs or symptoms are indications of inflammatory processes, which are initiated following the trauma. Bone healing and callus (bone) formation transpire through the processes of inflammation.

Fracture Healing

Fractures heal in several phases of inflammatory processes. The *inflammatory phase* is initiated after the bone is fractured with bleeding into the site, which causes a hematoma to form between the fractured bone ends and around the bone surfaces. A clot is formed, and the osteocytes at the bone ends die as they are deprived of nutrition. The presence of the necrotic cells sets up an intense inflammatory response accompanied by vasodilation, edema, and exudation of inflammatory cells into the area. Cells that migrate to the site include fibroblasts, lymphocytes, macrophages, and osteoblasts from the bone itself, all of which begin to form new bone. Fibroblasts form granulation tissue, capillary buds develop and invade the fracture site, collagen is formed and calcium is deposited in the collagen meshwork. As the calcium is deposited, callus is formed during this time, referred to as the *reparative phase.* Osteocytes continue to form bone trabeculae according to lines of force or stress; osteoclasts aid in resorbing poorly formed or superfluous trabeculae during what is referred to as the *remodeling phase.* The hematoma and cell debris are removed from the site by phagocytes and phagocytosis, and the necrotic bone is resorbed by osteoclasts. As the fracture site is calcified, the bone is united, making it difficult to discern the fracture site. These processes of bone healing require several months before full strength for weight bearing and normal use is regained.

Many local and systemic factors influence bone healing, some positively and some negatively. Positive local influences include the actions of phagocytes to keep the injured area free of debris and pathogens, and the efforts of osteoblasts to form new bone as osteoclasts aid in resorbing and reshaping the healing bone. Immobilization is a positive local factor; the bone ends and the muscles are held relatively immobile to permit the bridging and consolidating of the fractured bones, this aiding solid bone union. Electric bone stimulation is a positive local factor that aids bone union. Fractures outside of or not involving a joint heal more soundly and without the complication of posttraumatic arthritis.

Some positive systemic factors include an adequate amount of growth hormone, the absence of systemic infections or diseases such as diabetes or cancer, younger age of the injured person, and moderate activity and exercise, which aid circulation, retention of calcium within the bone, and bone healing.

Some local negative factors that delay or inhibit bone healing include foreign objects in the injured site; open fractures, which permit the entrance of pathogens; separation of the fracture fragments, which delays the bridging and consolidation phases; stress at the fracture site from insufficient immobilization; intraarticular fractures; and older age of the injured person. Systemic disease is a major negative influence that prolongs bone healing.

Diagnosis of Fractures

Fractures are diagnosed through physical examination, history of trauma, and hematologic, radiologic, or other studies. Physical examination may show changes in the normal length or shape of the bone, loss of alignment of fragments, deformity, mobility of the fragments with or without crepitus, muscle spasms and edema around the fracture site, and ecchymosis and evidence of he-

matoma or bleeding. Pain is usually present, and the person declines to use the injured part. Numbness and tingling may also be present. The person may guard or protect the injured tissues by holding the part close to the body or by cradling it to prevent additional trauma. The specific indications of a fracture depend on the site of the fracture, the severity and mechanism of injury, the type of fracture, and the amount of associated trauma to the bone and surrounding tissues. The person may relate a history of a fall, a blow, an accident, or other mechanism of injury followed by acute pain, local tenderness at the site, muscle spasms, increased pain with attempted movement or use (or marked numbness for 15 to 20 minutes), and later numbness, tingling, weakness, or paralysis.

X-rays are used to confirm the presence of a fracture or to detect a fracture in other types of injuries that could, for example, result in a nondisplaced, impacted, or compression fracture. Arthroscopy may be needed for intraarticular fractures, hematologic studies may be done for bone and soft tissue injuries, and bone scans may be done if a pathologic fracture is found.

Treatments for Fractures

The specific treatment or treatments for a fractured bone depend on the patient's age, the type of fracture, the bone or bones involved, and the types of treatments available.

For bones to unite, the fractured ends or fragments must be brought into alignment and approximation and held relatively immobile for the time required to heal the specific bone and type of fracture. *Reduction* is the process of aligning and approximating the fracture fragments. Reduction may be done in a *closed* manner, in which the skin remains intact and manual manipulation is used to bring the fragments into alignment. Traction may be applied to aid or hasten closed reduction. *Open* reduction is reduction performed during a surgical procedure; after reduction the fractured fragments are held by internal fixation devices such as a compression plate with screws, and by pins, intramedullary rods, and wires.

Following closed or open reduction, the fractured bones are held immobile with a cast, splint, elastic bandages, skin or skeletal traction, external fixation devices, or a combination of immobilization techniques; e.g., transverse pins are placed above and below the fracture site, the bones are then aligned and the fracture reduced, and a cast is applied that incorporates the pins to maintain the reduction. A sling may be used for nondisplaced fractures of the humerus, along with a swathe to hold the arm immobilized against the body. The nursing care of patients in casts or of those in traction or external fixation devices is discussed in Chapter

12; care of individuals who underwent surgical repair is discussed in Chapter 13.

Nursing Care of Patients with Fractures

The nursing care of a patient with a fracture depends on the person's age, the exact bone or bones fractured, the type of fracture, and the treatment or treatments involved. Because of their active growth cycles, children tend to heal more rapidly than mature adults; therefore their treatments may be shorter in duration before they regain mobility and the fracture achieves union. However, a child's nursing needs may be more intense and more concentrated in a shorter time frame than are those of an adult with a similar injury. Generally, the nursing needs of patients of any age are quite similar, and use of the nursing process provides a framework for meeting the needs of all patients with orthopedic trauma and fractures. The major nursing diagnoses associated with caring for patients with fractures are outlined below. Additional treatments and nursing diagnoses associated with the individual treatments are incorporated into their specific chapters in this book.

Table 4-3

TYPES AND CAUSES OF FRACTURES

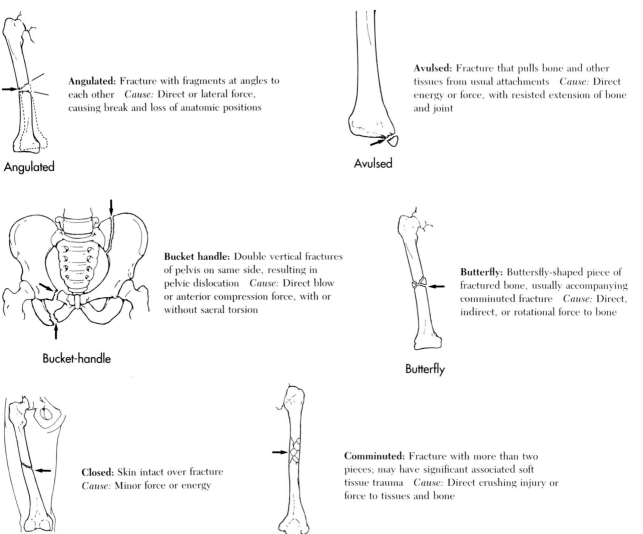

Angulated: Fracture with fragments at angles to each other   *Cause:* Direct or lateral force, causing break and loss of anatomic positions

Angulated

Avulsed: Fracture that pulls bone and other tissues from usual attachments   *Cause:* Direct energy or force, with resisted extension of bone and joint

Avulsed

Bucket handle: Double vertical fractures of pelvis on same side, resulting in pelvic dislocation   *Cause:* Direct blow or anterior compression force, with or without sacral torsion

Bucket-handle

Butterfly: Buttersfly-shaped piece of fractured bone, usually accompanying comminuted fracture   *Cause:* Direct, indirect, or rotational force to bone

Butterfly

Closed: Skin intact over fracture *Cause:* Minor force or energy

Closed

Comminuted: Fracture with more than two pieces; may have significant associated soft tissue trauma   *Cause:* Direct crushing injury or force to tissues and bone

Comminuted

Table 4-3

TYPES AND CAUSES OF FRACTURES—cont'd

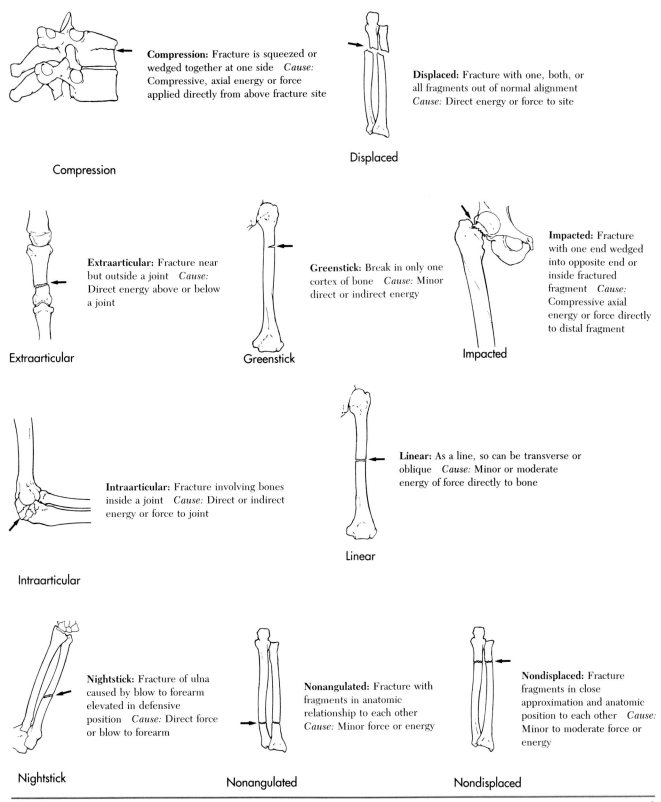

Compression: Fracture is squeezed or wedged together at one side   *Cause:* Compressive, axial energy or force applied directly from above fracture site

Compression

Displaced: Fracture with one, both, or all fragments out of normal alignment   *Cause:* Direct energy or force to site

Displaced

Extraarticular: Fracture near but outside a joint   *Cause:* Direct energy above or below a joint

Extraarticular

Greenstick: Break in only one cortex of bone   *Cause:* Minor direct or indirect energy

Greenstick

Impacted: Fracture with one end wedged into opposite end or inside fractured fragment   *Cause:* Compressive axial energy or force directly to distal fragment

Impacted

Intraarticular: Fracture involving bones inside a joint   *Cause:* Direct or indirect energy or force to joint

Intraarticular

Linear: As a line, so can be transverse or oblique   *Cause:* Minor or moderate energy of force directly to bone

Linear

Nightstick: Fracture of ulna caused by blow to forearm elevated in defensive position   *Cause:* Direct force or blow to forearm

Nightstick

Nonangulated: Fracture with fragments in anatomic relationship to each other   *Cause:* Minor force or energy

Nonangulated

Nondisplaced: Fracture fragments in close approximation and anatomic position to each other   *Cause:* Minor to moderate force or energy

Nondisplaced

Continued.

Table 4-3

TYPES AND CAUSES OF FRACTURES—cont'd

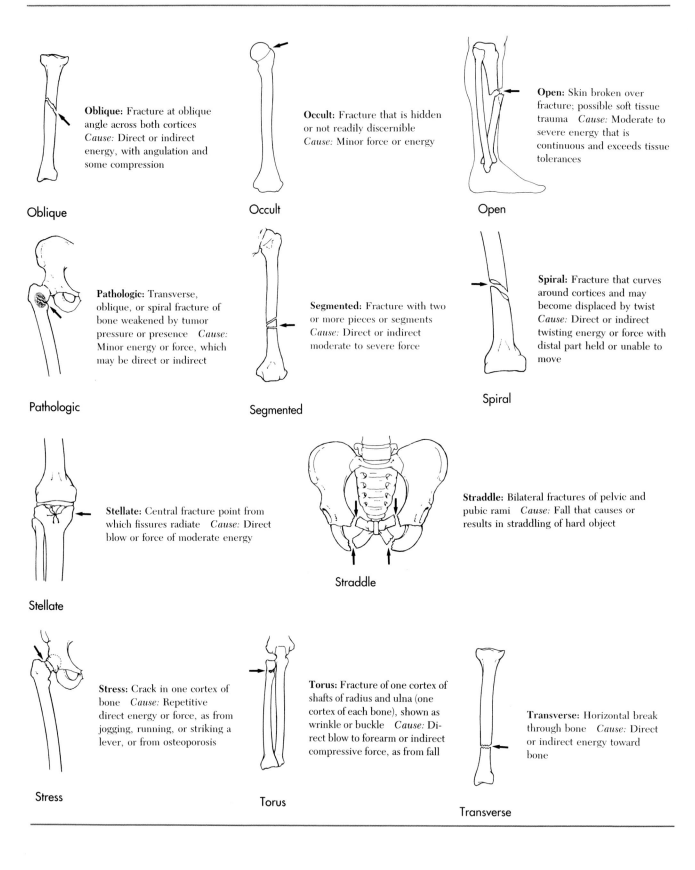

Oblique: Fracture at oblique angle across both cortices *Cause:* Direct or indirect energy, with angulation and some compression

Oblique

Occult: Fracture that is hidden or not readily discernible *Cause:* Minor force or energy

Occult

Open: Skin broken over fracture; possible soft tissue trauma *Cause:* Moderate to severe energy that is continuous and exceeds tissue tolerances

Open

Pathologic: Transverse, oblique, or spiral fracture of bone weakened by tumor pressure or presence *Cause:* Minor energy or force, which may be direct or indirect

Pathologic

Segmented: Fracture with two or more pieces or segments *Cause:* Direct or indirect moderate to severe force

Segmented

Spiral: Fracture that curves around cortices and may become displaced by twist *Cause:* Direct or indirect twisting energy or force with distal part held or unable to move

Spiral

Stellate: Central fracture point from which fissures radiate *Cause:* Direct blow or force of moderate energy

Stellate

Straddle: Bilateral fractures of pelvic and pubic rami *Cause:* Fall that causes or results in straddling of hard object

Straddle

Stress: Crack in one cortex of bone *Cause:* Repetitive direct energy or force, as from jogging, running, or striking a lever, or from osteoporosis

Stress

Torus: Fracture of one cortex of shafts of radius and ulna (one cortex of each bone), shown as wrinkle or buckle *Cause:* Direct blow to forearm or indirect compressive force, as from fall

Torus

Transverse: Horizontal break through bone *Cause:* Direct or indirect energy toward bone

Transverse

Table 4-4

PROPER NAMES (EPONYMS) FOR SPECIFIC FRACTURES

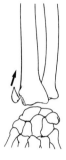

Barton's fracture *Bone involved:* Radius *Description:* Dorsal rim fracture of radius

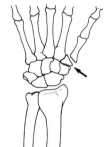

Bennett's fracture *Bone involved:* Base of thumb *Description:* Acute with associated subluxation or dislocation of metacarpal joint of thumb

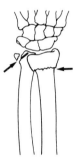

Colles' fracture *Bone involved:* Radius and ulna *Description:* Fractures of distal radius and ulna that may or may not involve wrist joint, cause by extending outstretched hand

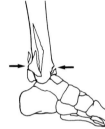

Cotton's fracture *Bone involved:* Ankle *Description:* Trimalleolar fracture of distal tibia (medial, lateral, and posterior articular margin or posterior malleolus of tibia)

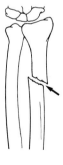

Galeazzi's fracture *Bone involved:* Distal radius *Description:* Fracture of distal third of radius with associated radioulnar dislocation

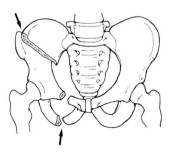

Malgaigne's fracture *Bone involved:* Pelvic ring *Description:* Double fractures in pelvic ring, causing instability in pelvis.

Continued.

Table 4-4

PROPER NAMES (EPONYMS) FOR SPECIFIC FRACTURES—cont'd

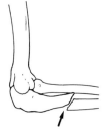

Monteggia's fracture   *Bone involved:* Ulna   *Description:* Fracture of shaft of ulna with displacement of fragments

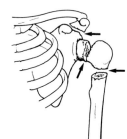

Neer fracture   *Bone involved:* Shoulder and humerus   *Description:* Displaced fracture with three or more pieces

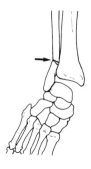

Pott's fracture   *Bone involved:* Malleolus of fibula *Description:* Fracture of fibula, including malleoli of ankle

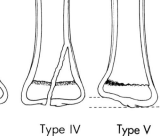

Type I   Type II   Type III   Type IV   Type V

Salter (or Salter-Harris) fracture   *Bone involved:* Epiphyseal area of involved bone   *Description:* Fracture may separate epiphysis from bone; may involve bones above and below epiphysis; may be crush injury to epiphysis

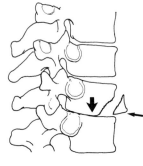

Teardrop fracture   *Bone involved:* Cervical vertebrae   *Description:* Compression fracture of body of a cervical vertebra with separation of a bone fragment

1 ASSESS

ASSESSMENT	OBSERVATIONS
Site of injury	Observe for deformity, edema, ecchymosis, use of injured part, capillary refill, peripheral pulses, color and temperature of tissues, injuries in contiguous or distant tissues Assess for muscle spasms, open areas in skin, hematoma, bleeding areas or clots, dirt or foreign substances in wounds Assess facial expressions or verbal expressions of pain, soreness, numbness, or other complaints; observe attempts to protect tissues by holding, guarding, or avoiding use Assess for presence of dressings, wraps, slings or other protective devices
Presence of pain or discomfort	Observe or ask about pain, its type, amount, severity, or duration Assess or ask about numbness, tingling, "pins and needles," or other sensory complaints Observe for presence of ice bag, hot water bottle, or other heat or cold application Observe for presence of pillows, splints or such Ask about medications that might have been taken or given for pain relief
Tissue perfusion	Assess color, capillary refill, temperature, edema, petechiae, ecchymosis, peripheral pulses Assess vital signs, breath sounds, and rate, depth, and character of pulse and respirations Assess level of consciousness, orientation, anxiety or restlessness Assess skin for dampness or clamminess Assess urinary output Assess appetite, food or fluid intake, weight (if can be moved); diarrhea or constipation, bowel sounds Assess laboratory test results
Stress response	Observe for shivering, nervousness, talkativeness or quietness, pallor, anger, hostility, fear, apathy, crying, chattering teeth Observe for unconsciousness, blood loss, shock, inflammation Observe or listen to concerns about severity of injuries and effects of injuries on self, family, and roles or employment
Pulmonary competence (possible fat embolism)	Observe respiratory rates, depth, character of respirations, dyspnea, shortness of breath, chest pain, changes in color, presence of petechial rash on chest, neck, or conjunctivae, altered consciousness, confusion, restlessness Observe sputum production and color; presence of cough

2 DIAGNOSE

NURSING DIAGNOSIS	SUBJECTIVE FINDINGS	OBJECTIVE FINDINGS
Impaired physical mobility related to bone fracture and soft tissue trauma	Complains of pain, tenderness, and soreness when attempting to move part; "muscles are so sore and can't move part"; feels "slightly numb at times"; states heard bone snap	Marked edema at site, color pale, skin areas ecchymotic and bruised; area of injury cool and deformed and distal part not in usual position, carries injured part protectively without weight or use
Pain related to soft tissue trauma and fracture	Reports sharp, moderate pain at fracture site; pain constant and increases with movement; numbness somewhat less; pain lessened with medication	Marked edema and bruising at site with angulation and deformity; marked reluctance to move or use part; holds it protectively

➔ ➤ ➤

NURSING DIAGNOSIS	SUBJECTIVE FINDINGS	OBJECTIVE FINDINGS
Altered peripheral tissue perfusion (pulmonary) related to fat embolism	States, "I feel strange—like something is wrong"; "I have some chest pain in my left side"; "It's hard to get my breath"	Some difficulty stating day of week, where hospitalized; respirations becoming slightly labored and more rapid; breath sounds decreased in left lower lobe; has petechial rash on chest, neck, and conjunctivae; pulse increased; blood pressure: systolic levels lower than previous readings
Anxiety related to sudden, unexpected injury and loss of mobility	States, "I can't move my leg—it hurts so bad"; "Can't you get the doctor here?"; "I need to go to the bathroom"; "What is going to happen next?"; "Where is my wife?" "I need some medicine for pain"	Very restless with frightened look in eyes and on face; tries to move injured leg; very pale, skin cool and damp; pulse rapid and thready on rare occasions; respirations rapid; systolic blood pressure lower than on admission; urinary output scant compared with IV intake; at times is angry and hostile, at other times tearful
Knowledge deficit related to injury, trauma, and loss of mobility	Asks, "How did the accident happen?"; "Who got hurt?" "Is my leg broken?" "How long will I be here?" "What will be done?" "What did the x-rays show?"	No previous hospitalizations or fractures; questions health team members; repeats some questions as if not hearing answers

3 PLAN

PATIENT GOALS

1. The patient will regain bone union following treatment and healing.
2. The patient will regain mobility with use of sling or ambulatory aid as needed.
3. The patient will experience no neurovascular complications.
4. The patient will regain a pain-free state through bone healing and rehabilitation.
5. The patient will regain circulatory, pulmonary, and peripheral tissue perfusion through recovery.
6. The patient will experience no fat or pulmonary emboli.
7. The patient will experience only mild anxiety.

4 IMPLEMENT

NURSING DIAGNOSIS	NURSING INTERVENTIONS	RATIONALE
Impaired physical mobility related to bone fracture and soft tissue trauma	Assist patient to position of comfort; use care in handling injured tissues, cast, or traction, if used (see Chapter 12).	Helps aid circulation, ease tired muscles, and increase oxygenation to tissues.
	Apply pillows to injured limbs, to back, or under head.	Elevation increases venous return and lessens edema and pain.
	Teach patient to lift self using trapeze or "post position" if possible.	Self-care aids independence and recovery. Post position: bend knee of uninjured leg; place foot securely on bed and lift self while grasping trapeze with all weight on uninjured limb and arms.

NURSING DIAGNOSIS	NURSING INTERVENTIONS	RATIONALE
	Assist patient to be up in chair with injured limb(s) elevated and to ambulate with crutches or walker when permitted; instruct on amount of weight bearing allowed.	Circulation and recovery are aided by being up and ambulating. Weight bearing may be restricted for varying periods according to type of injury and evidence of callus formation.
	Apply ice to area of injury q 4 h.	Ice applications lessen bleeding, decrease edema and pain, and increase comfort.
Pain related to soft tissue trauma and fracture	Assess for type, amount, severity, duration, and continuity of pain; use pain scale (0-10 or other pain scale) to help patient rate pain severity.	Assessment helps determine type of need or intervention required. Edema and trauma to soft tissues are very painful.
	Reposition patient q 2-4 h.	Repositioning eases sore, tired muscles and joints and increases oxygenation and circulation to aid recovery.
	Elevate injured area as ordered; apply ice to site.	Elevation and ice decrease edema and increase oxygenation, thereby lessening pain.
	Ask patient to describe pain; allow patient to describe pain in own words.	"Burning" pain is a sign of pressure on a nerve, or anoxia; "pins and needles" is also a sign of nerve pressure and lessened circulation; throbbing pain is related to edema and tightened compartments (see pages 182-183 for compartment syndrome); limb that feels "asleep" is a sign of nerve pressure.
	Do all eight parts of neurovascular checks (see inside back cover for checks).	Neurovascular status is a critical parameter for circulatory and neurologic function.
	Administer narcotic or nonnarcotic analgesic as ordered q 3-4 h around the clock. (Patient may have patient-controlled analgesia [PCA] pump if condition permits.)	Round-the-clock administration helps maintain therapeutic blood levels for pain relief.
	Monitor for relief of pain after analgesic administration.	Medication type or dosage may need adjustment if analgesia is not adequate. Pain associated with bone fractures is often severe and unrelenting for several days postfracture.
	Administer antiinflammatory medications between narcotic analgesics q 4 h if ordered. (See pages 281 and 282 for analgesics and pages 280-283 for antiinflammatory medications.)	Antiinflammatory medications ease inflammation following trauma and fractures and may be given between narcotics to aid resolution of pain and inflammation.

NURSING DIAGNOSIS	NURSING INTERVENTIONS	RATIONALE
Altered peripheral tissue perfusion (pulmonary) related to fat embolism	Assess for signs of fat embolism: sense of danger or doom, pain in chest, petechial rash over chest from nipple line to neck and on conjunctivae, shock, tachypnea and tachycardia, change in sensorium, confusion or disorientation.	Fat embolism occurs most commonly in long-bone fractures within first 48-72 hr postfracture. Current theories of causes are related to mobilization of fat molecules from bone marrow, chemical changes in blood serum, or other, unknown factors. Fat emboli are serious complications and have a mortality rate of 25%-40%.
	Monitor vital signs q 15 min.	Shock is commonly noted in fat emboli syndromes. Blood pressures drop, tachypnea and tachycardia are common. Temperature may rise to 38.3° C (101° F) or higher over 30 min to 1 hr or longer.
	Listen for breath sounds in all lobes.	Breath sounds may be decreased in affected areas of lungs.
	Assist with chest x-ray if ordered or lung scan if done.	Diagnostic studies may show "snow storm" lung involvement or lack of perfusion in embolized area.
	Administer oxygen per mask or catheter if ordered.	Oxygen may aid respiratory competence and lessen tachypnea or dyspnea.
	Initiate IV therapy as ordered; regulate infusion rates closely.	IV therapy is needed to maintain blood volume and as an avenue for administration of therapeutic fluids such as dextrose. Shock in fat embolism can lead to respiratory distress syndrome, because fat emboli damage lung alveoli, impairing perfusion.
	Assist with blood gas determinations.	Blood gases may show P_{O_2} levels of 50 mm Hg or less.
	Transfer to intensive care unit, if ordered, for mechanical ventilatory assistance if needed.	Mechanical ventilation may be required to raise arterial oxygen to proper levels. Positive end-expiratory pressure may also be used.
	Administer diazepam (Valium) 10-15 mg IV if ordered.	Sedation eases anxiety, lessens tachypnea and tachycardia, and aids muscle relaxation.
	Administer furosemide (Lasix) 40 mg IV if ordered.	Furosemide, a diuretic, lessens pulmonary edema to aid pulmonary perfusion.
	Monitor patient closely for progression or relief of symptoms.	Symptoms should ease if hypovolemic shock is adequately treated, if Pa_{O_2} levels become more normal, and if respiratory distress syndrome is avoided or properly treated.

NURSING DIAGNOSIS	NURSING INTERVENTIONS	RATIONALE
Anxiety related to unexpected injury and loss of mobility	Assess for reactions or responses to injury, treatments, or loss of mobility; may be fearful, angry, hostile, tearful, anxious or withdrawn, depending on associated injuries.	Reactions are usually related to person's perception of threat from injury and/or loss of mobility and are also related to person's usual response(s) to stressors.
	Explain upcoming events, care, or treatments.	Explanations help ease anxiety and increase understanding.
	Discuss inflammatory changes and recovery processes over time; repeat explanations as needed.	Patient may not hear or understand all of initial explanations because of pain, trauma, or unfamiliarity with terms or processes. Repeated explanations may be needed.
	Administer antiinflammatory, muscle relaxant, or analgesic medications q 4 h as needed.	Medications ease muscle spasms and pain or lessen inflammation to lessen stress responses and aid recovery.
	Assist to ambulate or be up in chair as ordered, with or without weight bearing.	Being up or ambulating eases patient's concerns and aids physical mobility to aid recovery.
	Discuss weight loss if or when it occurs.	Weight loss can occur with severe trauma and fractures as a result of catabolism during stress response, lack of physical activity, or lack of adequate intake. Gradual regaining of strength, muscle function, and weight occurs over time.
Knowledge deficit related to injury, trauma and loss of mobility	See Patient Teaching.	

5 EVALUATE

PATIENT OUTCOME	DATA INDICATING THAT OUTCOME IS REACHED
Bone union is progressing.	X-rays show maintenance of reduction and presence of callus bridging fracture site.
Mobility and use of injured tissues are regained.	Patient ambulates with crutches with partial weight bearing and uses forearm in cast within limitations of cast and healing time. Soft tissue edema and inflammation are resolving normally.
There are no neurovascular complications.	Color, temperature, and capillary refill are normal in injured tissues. Edema and pain or tenderness are minimal; no tingling or numbness is present. Motion is possible within limitations of cast or internal fixation device. All peripheral pulses are present.

PATIENT OUTCOME	DATA INDICATING THAT OUTCOME IS REACHED
Pain is largely resolved; rehabilitation exercises can be performed comfortably.	Patient has no moderate pain, only minimal and occasional pain. Patient needs only non-narcotic analgesics on prn basis and sleeps well all night. Patient performs rehabilitation exercises comfortably and as required to regain full function.
Circulatory, pulmonary, and peripheral tissue perfusion have been regained.	Patient's vital signs are within normal limits; pulse is full and regular. Weight and fluid balances are approaching preinjury levels. Hematologic data are within normal limits. Breath sounds are heard in all lobes and are clear; patient has no cough or sputum production. Skin is pink in color and not dry or wrinkled. All peripheral pulses are present. Capillary refill occurs in 2-4 sec.
No fat or pulmonary emboli developed.	Patient had no embolic episodes and no thrombophlebitis.
The patient had only mild anxiety.	Able to listen to and understand explanations, became calmer and relaxed over several days post injury; participated in self-care willingly.

PATIENT TEACHING

1. Teach the patient about inflammatory processes, bone healing and callus formation, and neurovascular checks.
2. Teach the patient about cast application and maintenance care or use of skin or skeletal traction, if appropriate. Prepare the patient for surgical implantation of internal fixation device or for placement in external fixator, when appropriate.
3. Teach the patient about stress responses; discuss the patient's usual responses to stress.
4. Teach the patient about nutritional needs to achieve bone healing; include information about necessary calcium and vitamins A, B, C, and D.
5. Teach the patient about the need to have a fluid intake of 3,000 ml minimum per 24 hours.
6. Teach the patient about the use of an ambulatory aid, splint, or sling as necessary.
7. Teach the patient about his rehabilitation pattern or planned program to regain full function. (Recovering function takes twice the amount of time spent immobilized; e.g., if the patient was in a cast for 6 weeks, it will take 12 weeks to regain full use of the affected joints.) Be sure the patient understands the exercise program and performs them as taught.
8. Teach the patient about gradual resumption of usual roles and responsibilities to prevent overtiring or added stress.

CHAPTER 5

Inflammatory Musculoskeletal Conditions

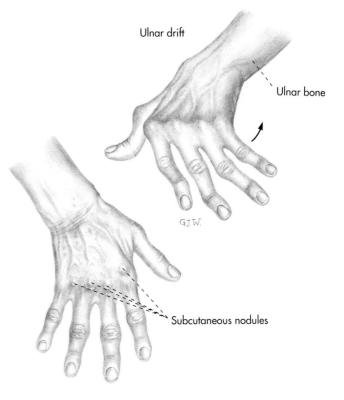

Ulnar drift

Ulnar bone

G.J.W.

Subcutaneous nodules

Rheumatoid Arthritis

Rheumatoid arthritis (RA) is a chronic, systemic, autoimmune inflammatory disease of the connective tissues of the body. It is one of the major rheumatic diseases.

RA is a very common condition. It has been estimated that up to 1.5% of the people in the United States have the disease, and as many as 200,000 new cases are diagnosed each year. Women are affected more often than men, at a 3:1 ratio between 30 and 50 years of age. A juvenile form of RA, called **Still's disease,** affects children from 8 to 15 years of age. People over 65 years of age can also develop RA, with a male peak over age 65. The disease is more prevalent in all age groups during the winter months, although climate alone has not been shown to have any specific effect on RA. The disease is predominently present in Caucasians, having a very low incidence in Oriental and Hispanic populations. The incidence among blacks in the United States is similar to that of Caucasians. There are no known consistent risk factors for RA, and the economic costs of the disease are marked because of the numerous treatments and systems involved.

PATHOPHYSIOLOGY

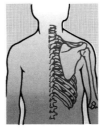

RA varies in onset from acute to insidious, being noted initially in the fingers, hands, and feet in more than 70% of patients. Joint pain and stiffness may be the initial symptoms, because even though RA is a systemic disease affecting many organs, the synovial lining of joints is one of the major tissues initially inflamed. The inflammation is noted by marked edema, tenderness, pain and limitation of motion. The involved joint becomes reddened and hot. As the inflammatory changes continue, the synovium thickens and proliferates (overgrows) inside and outside the joint, referred to as pannus formation of the synovium. Commonly, more than one joint becomes inflamed; those the most frequently affected are in the hands, wrists, feet, ankles, and knees. The joints are symmetrically inflamed bilaterally, a characteristic that aids in the diagnosis of RA. The disease also shows a familial trend.

As the joint inflammation progresses, other joint tissues become secondarily involved, especially the cartilage. Inflammatory changes lead to deterioration of the cartilage, and erosion of its surfaces leaves exposed bone surfaces; these in turn develop erosions, bone fissures, cysts, or bone spurs (osteophytes). Ligaments and tendons around or in the inflamed joints also become inflamed, leading to shortening and fibrosis (stiffening and scarring); consequently, contractures and subluxation (partial dislocation) of the joints are noted. Pain develops from the edema, inflammation, and grating of unprotected bone surfaces that rub against each other with movement and weight bearing.

Systemic manifestations of RA may be noted in the heart, lungs, kidneys, and skin. The changes in the functions of these organs are related to the degree or severity of the particular organ's involvement.

COMPLICATIONS

Cardiac degenerative conditions, including cardiomyopathy and congestive heart failure or pericarditis
Chronic renal failure
Chronic restrictive pulmonary diseases
Loss of range of motion (ROM) of several joints; multiple subluxations
Anemia
Repeated infections (pulmonary, renal, or other)
Ankylosis of joints
Deformation of several joints
Muscle wasting and atrophy
Amyloidosis (in up to 26% of patients)[88]
Septic arthritis
Avascular necrosis of hip joints

DIAGNOSTIC STUDIES AND FINDINGS

Diagnostic test	Findings
Laboratory tests	
Hematocrit (Hct) and hemoglobin (Hb)	Hct <35% and Hb <12g, indicating anemia (hypochromic is common)
Red blood cell (RBC) count	<3.5 million cells/ml, indicating anemia
White blood cell (WBC) count	Elevated in all differential cells, indicating inflammation (neutropenia, however, is associated with Felty's syndrome [renal involvement])
Erythrocyte sedimentation rate (ESR)	Elevated: moderate to severe elevation to 15 mm/h in males, 25 mm/h in females (normal: 0-9 mm/h in males, 0-20 mm/h in females)
Rheumatoid factor (RF) (an immunoglobulin)	Positive in 95% of patients with RA
Serum complement	Decreased, particularly during "flare" times
Immunologic assays	HLA-DR4 marker present in 55%-69% of persons with RA but is not a diagnostic marker because it is also present in 14%-31% of normal people[88]
C-reactive protein	Present during acute episode
Synovial tissue biopsy	Inflammatory changes; calcium hydroxyapatite crystals may be present
Synovial fluid analysis	Fluid clear or cloudy, has elevated WBC counts, and may have immune complexes
X-rays	Bone erosion, osteophytes, bone cysts, rarefaction of bones, subluxed bones
MRI	Help detect changes in femoral head before they appear on x-rays that indicate avascular necrosis; carpal tunnel inflammation (related to RA) also can be noted with MRI
CT	May show or help determine presence of synovial cysts

MEDICAL MANAGEMENT

GENERAL MANAGEMENT

Rest to specific joints.
Systemic rest: 1-h naps 1-2 times/day, plus 8-10 h nighttime sleep.
Alternating applications of heat and cold.
Physical therapy exercises adapted to individual.
Use of resting splints.
Occupational therapy to help the patient adapt to limitations of joints, muscles, or other tissues or organs.
Patient education.

DRUG THERAPY

Salicylate medications, usually aspirin, q 4 h.
Nonsteroidal antiinflammatory medications, 1-4 times/day.
Nonnarcotic analgesics, prn.
Administration of gold salts, PO or IM, daily or weekly.
Corticosteroids, in low dose, PO and occasionally intraarticularly; later higher doses of corticosteroids.
Antimalarial medications (type and dosage varies).
Immunosuppressive medications (type and dosage varies).
Chemotherapeutic medications (type and dosage varies).

OTHER THERAPIES

Lymphapheresis: 2-5 times/wk up to 20 treatments.
Thoracic duct drainage: 0.5-6 L of lymph drained per day and reinfused after removal of lymphocytes.
Lymphoid irradiation of subdiaphragmatic lymphoid tissues: 2,000-4,000 rads per treatment.
Plasmapheresis: 4 L of plasma drained and replaced with fresh-frozen plasma, dry reconstituted plasma, and albumin.

SURGERY

Arthroplasty of joint(s); Silastic implants to joints; Insertion of femoral shaft prosthesis; Total joint replacement; Arthrodesis of specific joint.

1 ASSESS

ASSESSMENT	OBSERVATIONS
Assess joints bilaterally	Symmetry; Signs of inflammation, angulation or deviation, and limpness
Assess ROM of joints	Stiffness or rigidity of joints and ligaments and for shortening or tightness of ligaments or tendons
Assess fingers and toes	Raynaud's phenomenon (color changes of fingers or toes)
Assess sensations	Numbness, tingling, pins and needles; painful joints (e.g., grimacing, withdrawal)

→ › › ›

ASSESSMENT	OBSERVATIONS
Assess systemic condition	Overall weakness or tiredness
Assess condition of oral tissues and conjunctivae	Moistness or dryness of oral mucous linings and conjunctivae; ulcerations or sores in mouth or eyes (if Sjögren's present)
Assess parotid gland	Observe for unilateral or bilateral enlargement (a sign correlated with Sjögren's syndrome)
Assess breath sounds and percuss all lobes	Breath sounds diminished in one or both lobes; percussion blunted if fluid is present
Assess bowel sounds (all four quadrants)	Low pitched and clearly heard; (RLQ), high-pitched bowel sounds or squeaks may be present
Assess abdomen	Abdominal girths may be same or increasing; abdomen may be tender when palpated; on percussion may have hollow or dull sounds
Assess for renal involvement	Correlate or compare intake with output; urine may be clear, cloudy, or blood-tinged; may have mild to moderate edema over body; weight may be increased or decreased from previous readings

2   DIAGNOSE

NURSING DIAGNOSIS	SUBJECTIVE FINDINGS	OBJECTIVE FINDINGS
Impaired physical mobility related to joint inflammation, deformity, or nodules	States joints are stiff and very tender	Joint(s) are edematous, red, hot, and tender on palpation; joints are enlarged and deformed with subluxed bones and angled and deformed bones (swan neck, boutonnière, or ulnar deviation); subcutaneous nodules are near joints; muscles, ligaments, and tendons are shortened and tight, with some muscle wasting
Self-care deficit related to joint deformities, inflammation, or systemic RA	States can't open jars, hold knives or other kitchen instruments firmly or comfortably; also states can't close buttons, comb hair easily, or go up and down stairs	Deformity of fingers with ulnar drift; wrist has limited ROM and fingers are stiff
Activity intolerance related to anemia and fatigue	States "wakes up tired" and becomes more tired during the day; becomes short of breath quickly; has to rest and nap several times a day	Sits with stooped shoulders; face looks "tired"; skin and conjunctivae are pale, nail beds are pale pink; breathes deeply with slight dyspnea; shortness of breath becomes more pronounced when going up stairs or walking short distances

NURSING DIAGNOSIS	SUBJECTIVE FINDINGS	OBJECTIVE FINDINGS
Pain (acute) related to inflammation and deformity of joints	States has dull, almost constant aching pain in joints, only somewhat relieved with analgesics; states pain increases when using hands (e.g., for activities of daily living [ADL]); states takes analgesics q 4 hr	Winces and withdraws hands when palpated; pain chart indicates amount of pain as 6-8 (on scale of 10); analgesic chart marked q 4 h
Impaired home maintenance management related to weakness and pain	Reports difficulty with activities such as preparing meals, cleaning, doing laundry because of weakness, tiredness, and pain	Moves slowly and sits "gingerly" to ease soreness (see above for other observations)
Sleep pattern disturbance related to pain, muscle or joint stiffness	States wakes frequently at night and has difficulty returning to sleep; states wakes up tired daily; states pain wakes her up	Has taken nighttime sedative for past several years since disease worsened; pain chart shows many nighttime entries
Body image disturbance and Altered role performance related to deformity	Complains of ugly hands and feet and difficulty buying shoes and gloves; may have had to quit a job because of finger and wrist conditions; other person may have had to take over cooking and household chores	Wears long-sleeved clothes covering subcutaneous nodules at elbows; keeps hands in lap, where they are less visible; in history, stated loss of employment and inability to do tasks at home
Impaired gas exchange related to pneumonitis and anemia	Reports becomes short of breath easily with minimum exertion; chest feels "tight," and has difficulty taking full, deep breaths; cough is present in morning	Respiratory rate 24-26 when ambulating; uses accessory muscles to breathe; opens mouth widely when taking deep breaths; cough produces thick, clear mucus; breath sounds diminished in both lower lobes; decreased fremitus; Hct ($<$35%) and Hb ($<$12 g) indicate anemia; skin pale, nail beds pale pink
Impaired renal function related to rheumatoid arthritis and secondary amyloidosis	States, "My urine is often cloudy when I pass it; my feet, legs, and hands are nearly always swollen; I don't pass as much urine lately; my weight has increased, and my appetite is way down"	Urinalysis shows 4$^+$ protein; cloudy specimen; 24-h specimen is only 960 ml (normal: 1,500-2,300 ml); edema around eyes, puffy cheeks, edematous fingers and hands; feet and ankles have 2$^+$ pitting edema; ate only about one third of foods served
Potential for injury related to gastrointestinal bleeding	States sometimes "coughs up blood, and water in toilet is pink at times"	Stool guaiac positive; Hct and Hb levels indicate possible blood loss

3 PLAN

Patient goals

1. The patient will regain satisfactory range of motion of joints after treatments.
2. The patient will do own activities of daily living with modified equipment.
3. The patient will regain a normal hemoglobin level and be relieved of anemia, tiredness, and malaise.
4. The patient will experience only minimum pain after treatments and medications.
5. The patient will learn alternatives to home management activities.
6. The patient will experience increased tolerance of daily activities.
7. The patient will develop a positive body image.
8. The patient will achieve satisfactory gas exchange.
9. The patient will retain satisfactory renal functions.
10. The patient will not experience major complications of RA for a prolonged period of time.
11. The patient will recover from surgical corrective procedures without complications.
12. The patient will attain a sound understanding of RA, compliance with its various treatments and their purposes, and the purposes and side effects of medications.

4 IMPLEMENT

NURSING DIAGNOSIS	NURSING INTERVENTIONS	RATIONALE
Impaired physical mobility related to joint inflammation, deformity, or nodules	Assess ROM of joints, overall mobility, joint deformities, and signs of inflammation (edema, heat, color changes, pain, and altered functions).	Provides the basis for subsequent care.
	Explain treatment regimen related to joints and ROM, such as use of heat or cold applications and paraffin packs.	Understanding of treatments may increase compliance with mobility aids; alternating applications of heat and cold help relieve inflammation; paraffin packs bring more heat, blood, and nutrients, and aid in removing wastes.
	Arrange consultation with physical and occupational therapists for individualized programs of exercise and home management.	Professional health team members provide vital services to aid care.
	Provide ROM exercises in conjunction with physical therapy.	Assures continuity of care.
	Apply splints or provide ambulatory aids such as cane or crutches.	Splint allows rest to an inflamed joint, as do a cane and crutches when weightbearing.
	Turn or reposition patient q 4 hr; provide back support when on side.	Repositioning prevents muscle tiredness and lessens joint stiffness; support to back lessens muscle strain.
Self-care deficit related to joint deformities, inflammation, or systemic RA	Assess patient's ability to do own ADL; assess effects of efforts at self-care on blood pressure (BP), pulse and respirations, strength, or complaints of being very tired.	Provides information to develop individualized care.

NURSING DIAGNOSIS	NURSING INTERVENTIONS	RATIONALE
	Assist with self-care and ADL as needed.	Providing assistance conserves patient's energy for additional activities.
	Provide modified utensils or equipment (e.g., grabbers, rubber-handled utensils, long cords to attach to zippers).	Modified utensils help joints and small muscles conserve their functions.
	Encourage ambulation q 4-6 h; help patient increase time and distance covered.	Ambulation helps maintain full body functions.
	If individual is an outpatient, discuss care with community health nurse at planned intervals.	May identify need for additional activities for continuity of care.
Activity intolerance related to anemia and fatigue	Assess conjunctivae and nail beds for color; check Hct and Hb data; assess complaints of fatigue and when they occur.	Anemia may be noted by pale nail beds and pale conjunctivae; Hct <40% and Hb <12g indicate anemia; fatigue accompanies anemia as a result of decreased oxygen to cells.
	Encourage rest periods of 30 min or longer in AM and PM.	Rest helps maintain or restore strength, lessens demands on body.
	Encourage patient to have 8-10 hr nighttime sleep; provide for uninterrupted sleep.	Continuous sleep over long periods helps body tissues regenerate strength and preserves available energy.
	Alternate rest periods with activities during day.	Activity helps maintain strength of tissues.
	Encourage intake of iron-rich foods daily; consult with dietitian to provide for patient's likes and dislikes.	Iron-rich foods help raise iron stores in body to overcome anemia; foods high in iron include dried fruits, green vegetables, raisins (see Table 5-1).
	Discuss need for iron replacement medications with physician; if ordered, teach patient when to take medication and its side effects, such as dark green stools, constipation, and gastric irritation.	Ferrous gluconate medications given after meals help restore iron levels more rapidly than foods alone; patient must be taught medication's side effects and how to deal with them.
	If iron replacement medications are given, encourage patient to increase fluid and fiber intake to prevent constipation and to note color of stools.	Cooperation helps lessen discomfort and increases tolerance of medication.
Pain (acute) related to inflammation and deformity of joints	Assess complaint of pain: severity, character, duration, what makes it worse or less, and effects on activities; discuss patient's recording of pain experiences.	Pain is usually related to the amount of inflammation, the joints involved, the patient's pain tolerance, and involvement with pain behaviors; objective data help health team members assist patient to a more comfortable daily existence.

NURSING DIAGNOSIS	NURSING INTERVENTIONS	RATIONALE
	Administer analgesics or nonsteroidal anti-inflammatory medications as ordered (see pages 280-283).	Analgesics and nonsteroidal antiinflammatory medications relieve pain by interrupting inflammatory products and pressure on nerve endings.
	Discuss effects of prescribed medications on patient's pain experiences; correlate with pain recordings.	May provide data regarding need to continue or change medications.
	Monitor patient's responses or reactions to medications, including monitoring for side effects (see pages 281-283).	All medications have specific responses and side effects; nonsteroidal antiinflammatory medications have numerous side effects that must be noted.
	Encourage patient activities when pain free; encourage use of diversionary activities such as music, art, and games when pain is less.	Activity helps patient maintain a positive outlook and customary roles; diversion takes patient's mind off pain experiences and may lead to longer pain-free periods.
	Provide back massage; apply moist compresses or ice to tender joints or muscles.	Massage eases tight muscles and aids removal of wastes, as do moist compresses; ice causes vasoconstriction, which lessens edema and pressure on nerve endings.
	Encourage patient to express feelings about disease or pain experiences and other concerns related to roles or responsibilities.	Ventilation helps patient clarify reactions and share concerns, lending assurance that concerns will be dealt with.
Impaired home maintenance management related to weakness and pain	Assess efforts for home maintenance: opening jars, preparing meals, handling dishes, vacuuming, etc.	Yields baseline data for necessary care or changes that might be required.
	Encourage participation in occupational therapy activities for home management; have modified utensils for use.	Using modified utensils saves tender, weak muscles and joints.
	Encourage compliance with therapy regimen and use of modified utensils.	Compliance preserves functions over time.
	Encourage exercises to facilitate movements in home environment (e.g., going up and down stairs).	Exercises help patient maintain or regain strength of muscles and joints.
Sleep pattern disturbance related to pain, muscle or joint stiffness	Assess sleep pattern over several days or weeks.	May indicate need to continue or change regimen.
	Encourage patient to take a warm bath before bedtime.	Warm water increases circulation to inflamed joints and relaxes muscles.
	Provide back massage at bedtime.	Relaxes tired muscles.

NURSING DIAGNOSIS	NURSING INTERVENTIONS	RATIONALE
	Position patient in bed with pillows to back and between legs; place bed in down position with head of bed flat.	Pillows support back to lessen muscle strain; bed should be flat and low for patient's comfort and safety.
	Straighten bed linens and change damp linens; place side rails up as needed.	Dry linens prevent skin maceration, and straight linens prevent pressure on tender skin areas; side rails may prevent a fall or injury.
	Administer medications to relieve pain or promote rest at bedtime.	Relief of pain and sedatives promote pain-free rest for long periods.
	Provide a snack or warm milk at bedtime.	Milk contains L-tryptophan, which produces sedation; hunger pangs may interfere with rest and prevent sleep.
	Provide a quiet environment.	Quiet atmosphere aids in sleep over long periods.
Body image disturbance and Altered role performance related to deformity	Assess concerns about body image, deformities, and usual roles.	Body image is related to an individual's physical boundaries; assessment yields understanding of patient's concerns.
	Encourage patient to ventilate feelings about deformed joints, limitations in role performance, or other concerns. Offer encouragement and understanding of concerns.	Ventilation clarifies feelings and concerns. Understanding helps patient regain or maintain a positive body image or a positive attitude about self and RA.
	Encourage family members to maintain open communication with patient.	Open communication helps reduce stress, maintains patient's roles, and enhances patient's positive outlook.
	Encourage patient to participate actively in usual roles and responsibilities.	Helps patient maintain a positive outlook.
	Discuss patient's concerns with health team members if appropriate.	Health team members can offer specialized guidance related to their expertise.
Impaired gas exchange related to pneumonitis and anemia	Assess respirations, respiratory rates, breath sounds and laboratory data.	Provides current data for care planning and interventions.
	Encourage deep breathing q 2 h. **Caution:** Coughing may not be ordered.	Deep breathing helps maintain respiratory functions and increases oxygen supply to cells; coughing may cause increased bleeding tendency.
	Administer antibiotics q 6 h as ordered.	Antibiotics help rid patient of pathogens to clear lungs if needed.
	Encourage use of respiratory aid, such as Respirex, q 2-4 h.	Use of a respiratory aid helps increase respiratory capacity by forcing air into as many alveoli as possible.

→ › ›

NURSING DIAGNOSIS	NURSING INTERVENTIONS	RATIONALE
	Monitor breath sounds q 4 h; note improvement or status quo of diminished breath sounds, if present; record and report findings to physician.	Breath sounds in all lobes indicate free passage of air; diminished or absent breath sounds indicate blockage of air to area, which can lead to infection and increase dyspnea; prompt attention from physician may prevent additional problems.
Impaired renal function related to rheumatoid arthritis or secondary amyloidosis	Assess intake and output q 8 h; assess color and other characteristics of urine.	In amyloidosis, insoluble protein substances are deposited in the extracellular matrix of specific organs (the kidneys are commonly affected, as are the liver and gastrointestinal [GI] tract); renal functions are diminished, and protein is excreted in the urine in increasing amounts; nephrosis could result in patient's death.
	Obtain 24 h urine for total protein, cellular content, and amount.	Proteinuria is a major indicator of renal function; urinary output in people with amyloidosis or nephrosis is lower than normal.
	Monitor daily weight, vital signs, and edema.	Body weight and edema are increased in renal failure; BP, pulse, and respirations rise as a result of increased fluid load.
	Assist with synovial biopsy if performed; biopsy will be done aseptically under local anesthesia using an arthroscope (may be done in outpatient or ambulatory surgery unit).	Biopsy of synovium may show proteinaceous deposits in synovium, along with hydroxyapatite crystals (calcium crystals) if amyloidosis is present.
Potential for injury related to GI bleeding	Assess vomitus and stools for blood.	Medications may cause GI bleeding.
	Monitor abdominal girth and bowel sounds q 4-6 h; monitor for abdominal tightness or complaints of tenderness or pain. Document findings.	Increasing abdominal girth or decreased bowel sounds indicate altered GI functions; tightness or tenderness may indicate peritoneal irritation.
	Monitor patient's appetite and intake at meal times.	Decreased appetite may be a sign of nausea or gastric distress.
	Note patient's complaints of sharp or dull abdominal pain (epigastric area) between meals or pain that wakes patient at night.	Pain associated with gastric ulcerations or bleeding may be sharp or dull, occurs about 2 h after meals, and wakes patient from sleep.
	Administer antacids q 2 h if ordered; monitor for side effects of antacids (diarrhea, constipation, or metabolic alkalosis).	Antacids neutralize acids secreted in the stomach and aid in coating irritated tissues. Antacids containing magnesium hydroxide may cause diarrhea; those containing aluminum hydroxide may cause constipation; increased intake of antacid (alkalis) may lead to metabolic alkalosis.
Knowledge deficit	See Patient Teaching.	

5   EVALUATE

PATIENT OUTCOME	DATA INDICATING THAT OUTCOME IS REACHED
Patient has regained satisfactory ROM of joints after treatments.	Following synovectomies of fingers (pages 232-233), total hip replacement (pages 220-222), and physical therapies, ROM of affected joints is in normal ranges.
Patient performs own ADL using modified equipment.	Patient dresses self using grabbers and strings attached to zippers; uses rubber cuff over handle of toothbrush and comb.
Patient has overcome anemia, tiredness, and malaise.	Hct raised to 40% and Hb >12 g consistently; patient states feels refreshed, stronger, and less tired.
Patient has only minimum pain with treatments and medications.	Charts show pain relief patterns with ordered medications; patient states that pain is markedly less after physical therapies.
Patient has learned alternative home management activities.	Patient participated in all home management classes and did all activities well; has modified home cabinets and furniture as needed.
Patient has increased tolerance of daily activities.	Following treatments, patient walks 2-3 miles every other day; walks with cane only following partial recovery from hip surgery; uses hands for personal and home activities since repairs and healing.
Patient has developed a positive body image.	Patient walks straighter with head up, usually with a smile; says feels much better about self.
Patient has achieved satisfactory gas exchange.	Patient's breath sounds are clear in all lobes; has minimum dyspnea on exertion.
Patient has retained satisfactory renal functions.	Patient's intake and output are approximately equal. Urinalysis shows few WBCs and RBCs; protein is within normal limits.
Patient has not experienced major complications at present.	Chest x-ray is clear; breath sounds are heard satisfactorily in all lobes; avascular necrosis is removed with total hip replacment; renal function is satisfactory with 1$^+$ protein excreted in urine and 24-h output steady at 1,200 ml/24 h.
Patient has recovered from surgical procedures without complications.	Patient uses hands and fingers for personal and home activities following surgery; walks with cane until healing period following hip or knee surgery will be completed.
Patient has achieved sound understanding of RA.	Patient can discuss manifestations of RA, correctly compare own patterns with patterns common to RA; is present and prompt for physical therapies, paraffin packs, and home management classes and activities; takes medications as ordered. Patients understands treatments and their purposes and the purposes and side effects of medications, and complies with treatment regimens.

→ › ›

PATIENT TEACHING

1. Reiterate the explanation of RA as a chronic disease that can be controlled through treatments and compliance with care goals.
2. Explain the purposes, actions, and common side effects of each medication; clarify which side effects should be reported to physician.
3. Teach the patient the specifics of hot and cold applications and cautions with each regimen.
4. Teach the patient and family members modifications in self-care or home maintenance specific for the patient's condition (initial teaching may be done by physical or occupational therapists; only reiteration may be required).
5. Discuss stress-reduction techniques, and teach relaxation exercises.
6. Teach the patient about the foods needed for a balanced diet and which foods are high in iron (see Table 5-1).
7. Teach the patient about pain and symptom recording and management.
8. Explain the specific surgical procedures for the patient's condition and the rehabilitation regimen.

Table 5-1

FOODS HIGH IN IRON*

Food	Serving size	Iron (mg)
Beef, ground chuck	3½ oz	3.3
Chicken	3½ oz	1.7
Lamb, loin chop	1	1.4
Liver, calf	3½ oz	14.2
Pork, loin chop	1	3.5
Egg, medium	1	1.2
Perch	3½ oz	1.3
Corn flakes	1 cup	1.4
Rolled oats	1 cup	1.7
Cream of Wheat	1 cup	1.4
Potato, white	1 medium	1
Spinach	½ cup	2
Raisins	¼ cup	1.6
Banana	1 medium	1
Tuna, in oil	3 oz	1.6

*Recommended daily allowance (RDA): men, 10 mg; women, 18 mg.
From Poleman CM and Capra CL: Shackelton's nutrition essentials and diet therapy, ed 5, Philadelphia, WB Saunders Co.

Ankylosing Spondylitis

Ankylosing spondylitis (AS) is an inflammatory disease of the spinal column, sacroiliac joints and, later, of the larger joints such as the shoulders, hips and knees; it leads to deformity and ankylosis of the affected bones.

Ankylosing spondylitis develops in late adolescence or early adulthood. It has a marked predominance in males with an 8:1 ratio over females. The peak age for AS is 20 to 40 years of age; it rarely occurs over age 50. Approximately 90% of people with AS have an association with the antigen HLA-B27, which is normally present in only 8% of the population. AS has a lower incidence in blacks than in other racial groups.

AS is also referred to as **Marie-Strümpell arthritis** and **Bechterew disease,** but the preferred term is ankylosing spondylitis, which describes its major pathologic lesions.

PATHOPHYSIOLOGY

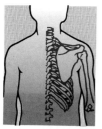

The exact initiating inflammatory process in AS is still unknown; however, the pattern of fibrosis and ankylosis is noted as the disease progresses. AS begins insidiously in an adolescent or young adult, primarily with morning backache in the lumbar area and both sacroiliac joints, with stiffness and aching in these areas. Activity eases the pain and stiffness, but they return with sitting in one position for long periods. The pain and stiffness worsen over several months and spread to other spinal components, ligaments, and muscles. Severe muscle spasms occur, which pull the vertebral column into forward flexion, obliterating the lordotic curves in the cervical and lumbar areas and leading to increases in thoracic rounding; this results in marked rounding or kyphotic curvature of the entire vertebral column and back. As these changes occur, the intervertebral disks also become inflamed and become infiltrated with vascular connective tissue that ossifies. These inflammatory changes slowly move up to involve all the spinal column. The pathologic changes in the vertebral column give rise to the term "bamboo spine," because the spine looks look like a bamboo cane on x-rays. The joints of the hips, knees, and shoulders also become involved and ossify, with progressive disease manifestations. Eventually patients with severe disease cannot extend their heads and necks upward, and the neck is ankylosed, with the head facing nearly horizontally.

Ossification of discs, joints, and ligaments of spinal column

Bilateral sacroiliitis

Ankylosing Spondylitis

COMPLICATIONS

Respiratory compromise
Fusion of vertebral bodies
Loss of ROM of joints

DIAGNOSTIC STUDIES AND FINDINGS

Diagnostic test	Findings
Laboratory tests	
Complete blood count (CBC)	RBCs decreased; Hct and Hb levels indicate anemia; differential WBCs elevated, indicating inflammation
Erythrocyte sedimentation rate	Elevated throughout disease, to 10-15 mm/h in males and 20-25 mm/hr in females (normal: 0-9 mm/h in males, 0-20 mm/h in females)
HLA-B27 antigen	Present in more than 90% of patients
Rheumatoid factor	Negative in most patients
Vital capacity determination	Below normal (normal: above 4 L for females; 4-5 L for males)

Continued.

DIAGNOSTIC STUDIES AND FINDINGS

Diagnostic test	Findings
Urine tests	
17-Ketosteroid levels	Increased in 24-h specimens
X-rays	
Vertebral column	Squaring of anterior portion of vertebral bodies with loss of anterior concavity of each body; loss of lordotic curve; development of vertebral ossification in annular areas and in paravertebral ligaments; as vertebral ossification proceeds vertically, "bamboo" spinal configuration is seen; increased thoracic kyphosis
Sacroiliac joints	Joint margins blurred with widening of joints; "rosary" effect develops, caused by subchondral erosions; subchondral sclerosis develops; osteoporosis of distal third of both sacroiliac joints is seen
Hips	Bony ankylosis of both joints is seen, as is osteoporosis of joints

MEDICAL MANAGEMENT

GENERAL MANAGEMENT

Physical therapy for exercises to entire back, hips, and other affected joints.
Deep-breathing exercises to preserve vital capacity.
Swimming and walking exercises to maintain joint mobility (rest is not beneficial in AS).
Use of a firm bed mattress, a small pillow, and flat position in bed to maintain straightness of spine.
Application of warm, moist packs to reduce muscle spasms.
Occupational therapy to identify possible modifications of home or job environments necessary because of rigidity and abnormal curvatures of spine.
Consultations with social service and community nursing personnel for long-term or follow-up care.
Application of skin traction (cervical head halter or Buck's extension [to legs]) to lessen muscle spasms and ankylosis.
Use of soft cervical collar to help neck muscles maintain neck positions.
Use of lumbar back brace to lessen muscle strain.

SURGERY

Total hip replacement bilaterally to correct fixed flexion; cervical spinal fusion to help patient maintain upright position of neck.
Osteotomy of thoracic or lumbar vertebrae to help prevent or correct severe kyphosis, which prevents patient from looking forward.

DRUG THERAPY

Analgesics: Antipyretic agents such as aspirin, 600 mg q 4 h.

Nonsteroidal antiinflammatory drugs (NSAIDs): Phenylbutazone (Butazolidin), 100-200 mg/day or up to 400 mg/day—patient must be monitored for toxic effects; indomethacin (Indocin), 100 mg up to 200 mg/day.

Antacids: 30 ml PO to counter side effects (gastric irritation of NSAID).

Cortisone: 10-40 mg/day, adjusted to patient's specific needs.

1 ASSESS

ASSESSMENT	OBSERVATIONS
Back and vertebral column	Pain, tenderness around entire spine, paraspinal ligaments, and muscles; pain around shoulders and hip joints with radicular pain in deltoid and shoulder areas or in groin
Physical appearance	Evidence of weight loss with loose skin folds; chest expansion is restricted; hips are firmly ankylosed (with advanced disease) in flexion and adduction positions
Posture and gait	Loss of normal spinal curves; head and neck are flexed forward; marked kyphosis is present; ankylosis of vertebrae; steps carefully with some sideways swaying when walking
ROM of joints	Limited flexion, extension, abduction and adduction, and circumduction of hips, knees, shoulders, and back
Pain, muscle spasms, or tender areas	Pain over and around paraspinal muscles and ligaments over entire spinal column, radiating into shoulders and hips
Skin color and characteristics of folds or turgor	Pink color of skin and nail beds; no tenting or dryness
Chest expansion and vital capacity	Chest expansion restricted; 2 L vital capacity; breath sounds diminished in all lobes
Eyes and eyesight	Eye tissues, especially iris, choroid areas, and pupil, have usual characteristics and tears; eyesight is within normal limits
Vital signs	Temperature, pulse, respirations elevated; and BP varies
Oral cavity and mucous membranes	Pink color; moist; no lesions, edema or tenderness in mucous membranes
Urinary system (with male patient)	Straw color and satisfactory amount of urinary output; some tenderness of glans penis, which is dry and slightly edematous
Risk factors	Age is 15-40 yr; history of weight loss; male

2 DIAGNOSE

NURSING DIAGNOSIS	SUBJECTIVE FINDINGS	OBJECTIVE FINDINGS
Impaired physical mobility related to inflammation of spine and major joints	States back and hip tenderness or pain frequently limits movements; can no longer play sports (e.g., softball or tennis); cannot do things such as gardening; can walk only short distances	Walks very slowly and hesitantly when asked with less arm swinging than usual (or normal); steps forward gingerly to go up steps, holding both rails for support; gait has "hitches" when walking on flat surfaces; appears to hold neck firmly when moving; has marked difficulty removing clothing and redressing

→ > >

NURSING DIAGNOSIS	SUBJECTIVE FINDINGS	OBJECTIVE FINDINGS
Pain (acute) related to inflammation of spine and major joints	States wakes up every morning with pain in lower back, hips, upper back, and shoulder joints; pain is dull and aching, and at times is sharper and prevents activities	On palpation, spinal column, shoulders, and hips are edematous and hotter than surrounding tissues; winces on palpation of areas; has decreased ROM of flexion, extension, adduction, and abduction of shoulders and hips; can slowly bend forward but holds lower back when straightening up; needs analgesic q 4 h to tolerate pain
Potential for injury related to associated Reiter's syndrome (conjunctivitis, urethritis, and arthritis)	**Arthritis:** See above assessment findings	See above findings
	Conjunctivitis: States has occasional periods when eyes feel dry and "scratchy"; states does not routinely wear glasses except for reading; states sometimes has lots of fluid in eyes and other times has very little fluid	Can do eye movements with normal results for oculomotor, trochlear, and abducens nerves; right pupil is slightly more dilated than left (right pupil 2.5 mm and left is 2 mm); conjunctivae are moist and slightly reddened, no edema is noted, and tears are present, and conjunctivae are moist
	Urethritis: States has occasional problems voiding, with some burning, frequency, and/or urgency; some tenderness or soreness of glans penis	Urinalysis: Clear, straw-colored urine; 1-3 RBCs, 4-6 WBCs; 4 mg protein; no crystals, sugar, or acetone; glans penis dry and slightly edematous; no open lesions noted
Body image disturbance related to inflammatory changes or development of abnormal curvatures	Complains of need to limit social activities because of inability to sit or stand for long periods; has to lie down frequently to ease back and joint pain and muscle spasms	No longer participates in sports and stays home on weekends instead of going out (e.g., dancing or playing bridge); (see above physical examination findings for additional objective data)
Altered role performance related to limitations in mobility and pain	Reports change in jobs to ease back strain; may report need to give up hobbies or household chores (e.g., gardening, mowing lawn)	See above physical findings for objective data

3   PLAN

Patient goals

1. The patient will maintain satisfactory physical mobility with minimum limitations or little marked ankylosis of vertebrae.
2. The patient will have long periods of pain-free activities.
3. The patient will not develop Reiter's syndrome of conjunctivitis, urethritis, and arthritis.
4. The patient will maintain a positive body image and self-concept.
5. The patient will experience minimum role disturbance.
6. The patient will understand the effects of AS.

4 IMPLEMENT

NURSING DIAGNOSIS	NURSING INTERVENTIONS	RATIONALE
Impaired physical mobility related to inflammation of spine and major joints	Assess posture, gait, and ROM of joints (see previous assessments for findings).	Individualized data are vital for care.
	Teach patient proper bedding (firm mattress, small pillow, light covers) and bed position (flat and recumbent positions); teach to turn side to side but to avoid lying prone.	Lying on firm mattress with small pillow helps prevent flexion contractures of inflamed joints. Lying recumbent and flat helps maintain joints in extension; turning helps maintain joint mobility; lying prone can hasten development of abnormal curves.
	Offer back massage several times daily.	Massage eases sore muscles and lessens muscle spasms.
	Encourage participation in prescribed exercise regimen (swimming and walking); assess results of exercises.	Exercises maintain joint mobility, vital for persons with AS; rest is contraindicated, because it increases development of ankylosis.
	Assist patient to apply body cast (bivalved), if used, to be worn as tolerated.	Use of body cast helps maintain posture and curvatures and eases muscle and ligament strain.
	Apply cervical traction to head or traction to legs, if used; remove traction at bedtime; check traction functioning q 4 h when in use.	Skin traction maintains extension of muscles and joints and lessens muscle spasms; traction should be removed at bedtime, since the patient could inadvertently increase muscle contractions instead of relaxations; frequent inspection of traction helps assure that it will function as required.
	Assist with ADL as needed.	Assistance conserves energy for daily activities and prevents strain or overtiredness.
	Assist with immersion in Hubbard tank 1-2 times/day.	Warm water increases circulation to inflamed tissues to ease inflammation; immersion removes effects of gravity, so joints can be moved easier and longer.
	Assist with ROM exercises 3-4 times/day.	ROM exercises maintain joint mobility over long periods.
	Teach deep-breathing exercises; have patient do them q 4 h.	Deep breathing maintains respiratory functions and increases oxygenation.
Pain (acute) related to inflammation of spine and major joints	Assess for presence of pain, its amount, character, and duration, and relief efforts.	Data determine extent of problem.
	Use moist applications to ease painful areas (see above interventions).	Warm, moist applications relieve pain by easing muscle spasms and increasing circulation.

→ › ›

NURSING DIAGNOSIS	NURSING INTERVENTIONS	RATIONALE
	Reposition patient or help him reposition himself q 4 h.	Changing positions eases tired or painful muscles and joints.
	Administer analgesics q 4 h; observe effects of medications for pain relief.	Analgesics interfere with pain pathways and lessen perception of pain sensations; noting effects of medications allows them to be continued or changed.
	Observe for side effects of medications (see pages 281-283 for side effects of analgesics or antiinflammatory medications).	Reactions to and severity of side effects may be harmful; medications may need to be changed.
	Instruct patient to record pain patterns and results of medications or other therapies such as exercises and hydrotherapy. Monitor activities to note changes.	Data indicate adequacy of pain relief or need for change.
Potential for injury related to associated Reiter's syndrome	Assess eye condition and functions (see assessment data above and on page 77).	Assessment determines care or need for additional treatments; conjunctivitis is associated with Reiter's syndrome.
	Assess oral cavity and condition of mucous membranes.	Oral ulcerations are associated with Reiter's syndrome.
	Assess intake and output, characteristics of urine, complaints of dryness or tenderness of glans penis.	Dryness of glans penis is associated with Reiter's syndrome.
	Discuss use of artificial tears if feasible.	Artificial tears provide moisture to dry conjunctivae.
	Discuss application of warm, moist compresses to closed eyes several times daily.	Warm, moist compresses increase circulation and lessen inflammation.
Body image disturbance related to inflammatory changes or development of abnormal curvatures	Assess statements of effects of condition on body image and self-concept (see assessment data above).	Data indicate lack or presence of a problem.
	Encourage participation in desired activities when pain or condition permits.	Participation helps enhance self-esteem.
	Apply soft collar to neck, if ordered.	Collar helps hold neck in more vertical position, allowing more direct vision and upright posture.
	Consult or secure guidance from mental health consultants if feasible.	Professional guidance offers specific suggestions for care.
	Discuss surgical options (after physician has done so) (see page 76 for options).	Surgical reconstruction may be needed for long-standing AS.
Altered role performance related to limitations in mobility and pain	Seek guidance of physical and occupational therapists for exercises and home management.	Optimum care may require help of all health team members.

NURSING DIAGNOSIS	NURSING INTERVENTIONS	RATIONALE
	Encourage family members to consult with patient frequently about daily activities.	Consultation enhances self-esteem and fosters maintenance of usual roles.
Knowledge deficit	See Patient Teaching.	

5 EVALUATE

PATIENT OUTCOME	DATA INDICATING THAT OUTCOME IS REACHED
Patient maintains satisfactory physical mobility with minimum limitations and without marked ankylosis of vertebrae.	Patient can maintain employment; spinal and hip ankylosis is minimal to moderate; abnormal curvature of cervical and lumbar areas of back have not progressed to require fusion or osteotomy.
Patient has long pain-free periods.	Patient tolerates corticosteroid and analgesic medications, with marked easing of pain; minimum residual pain is tolerable.
Patient does not have Reiter's syndrome (conjunctivitis, urethritis, and arthritis).	Patient has clear mucous membranes of eyes, oral cavity, and glans penis; has satisfactory supply of tears and saliva; has clear urine; has no difficulties during sexual intercourse.
Patient maintains a positive body image and self-concept.	Patient continues employment daily; supervises family members in garden and yard activities; participates actively in all family discussions.
Patient has undergone minimum role disturbance.	Patient delegates to family members when unable to do own care or other activities, as stated above.
Patient understands effects of AS.	See Patient Teaching.

PATIENT TEACHING ■

1. Discuss the processes of inflammation and the rationale for specific treatments; may need to repeat explanations several times; use pictures to clarify explanations.
2. Explain the purposes of specific exercises to maintain mobility (rest is contraindicated in AS, since rest may foster development of ankylosis of joints).
3. Explain the side effects of corticosteroids, analgesics, and antiinflammatory medications; encourage the patient to report untoward side effects, since medications can be changed.
4. Discuss techniques for conserving energy.
5. Discuss which foods are high in iron, to overcome anemia (see page 74 for foods).
6. Teach care to family members, as feasible, for continuity and home care.
7. Reiterate the options for surgical procedures, if the patient requires corrective repair (see page 76 for such procedures).

Epicondylitis and Tendinitis (Tenosynovitis)

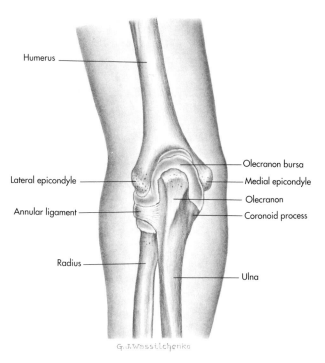

Humerus

Lateral epicondyle

Annular ligament

Radius

Olecranon bursa

Medial epicondyle

Olecranon

Coronoid process

Ulna

G.J.Wassilchenko

Epicondylitis is inflammation of the origins of tendons where they insert into condyles of bones, such as the epicondyles of the humerus, radius, ulna, patella, and other bones.

Gastrocnemius muscle

(Lateral head)

(Medial head)

Soleus muscle

Achilles tendon

Calcaneus

G.J.Wassilchenko

Tendinitis is inflammation of the tendon-covering sheath around one or a group of tendons. The terms *tendinitis* and *tenosynovitis* are synonymous, since the sheath is lined with a synovial layer.

Epicondylitis and tendinitis often occur together because of the proximity of these structures to one another. Each condition has been diagnosed more frequently in recent years, often related to sports injuries or overuse syndromes. Cases of epicondylitis commonly can be divided half and half between younger people with sports-related or other activity-type injury and older people with overuse problems, often work-related from repetitive motions, as in office workers, clerks, writers, and meat cutters. Epicondylitis is called **tennis elbow** when the lateral epicondylar area is involved and **golfer's elbow** when the medial epicondylar area is inflamed.

Tendinitis also occurs in the groups described above but in addition affects people with rheumatoid arthritis and diabetes. The condition occurs across age groups, from adolescents to the elderly.

PATHOPHYSIOLOGY

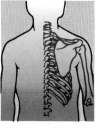

To date, the exact pathophysiologic entities in epicondylitis and tendinitis have not been clearly established, possibly because various changes have been noted in cases of epicondylitis. What is known is that repetitive motions and overuse contribute to microtraumatic changes in the affected tendons, causing microscopic tears, bleeding, edema, and pain. Pain in or around the epicondylar area (often point tenderness in which the patient can point to the tenderest area) is the presenting symptom. Epicondylitis usually occurs in the dominant arm; however, bilateral epicondylitis can also occur when supination and pronation motions of the forearm are done repetitively. Along with the microscopic tendon tears, pathologic signs include avascularity of the tendon and calcification at the tendon origin. Scar tissue is formed from the avascularity and microtrauma. In some cases the tendon ruptures as a result of the degenerative changes. Ischemia from the avascularity may account for the pain.

Pathophysiologically, tendinitis involves inflammation of the synovial-lined sheath around one or more tendons. Thickening of the sheath or sheaths, caused by inflammatory changes, limits movement and causes pain as the trapped tendon tries to glide within a thickened, tight sheath.

Epicondylitis and tendinitis can accompany bursitis and rotator cuff tears. Common sites of tendinitis include bicipital tendinitis of the shoulder, patellar tendinitis of the knee, Achilles tendinitis of the heel, and de Quervain's tenosynovitis of the radial area of the wrist.

COMPLICATIONS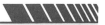

Chronic inflammation
Degenerative arthritis
Avulsion tears

MEDICAL MANAGEMENT

GENERAL MANAGEMENT

Judicious rest to affected part or parts for each condition.
Use of forearm band for lateral epicondylitis.
Application of splint to forearm for lateral or medial epicondylitis.
Applications of ice to inflamed area for 24-48 h.
Application of moist heat to area q 4 h after discontinuing ice applications.
Teaching patient different methods for use of arm and forearm.
ROM exercises after initial inflammation is resolved (may be isometric, isotonic, isoflexion, and isokinetic exercises).

For tendinitis: Achilles tendinitis: Use of heel pads or orthotics (shoe inserts).
Gluteus maximus tendinitis: Rest to hip and leg; Injections of corticosteroids into greater trochanter area.
Trigger finger (stenosing tenosynovitis): Injection of corticosteroids into site helps approximately 50% of those affected.
Surgical release of tightened tendon may be needed.
Bicipital tendinitis: Avoidance of activities requiring overhead reaching; application of heat to area; muscle exercises to aid rehabilitation of area; injection of corticosteroid in individualized dosage (care must be taken to ensure that injection is not intratendinous, or tendon could eventually rupture).

DRUG THERAPY

Nonsteroidal antiinflammatory medications: Ibuprofen (Motrin, Advil), 200-400 mg q 4 h.

Injection of corticosteroid into area in lateral or medial epicondylitis: 1-3 injections are given a month apart in individualized doses. (Injections of steroids are controversial, since they may cause complete tendon rupture or degenerative changes.)

Analgesic-antipyretic medications: Buffered aspirin, 600-1,000 mg q 4 h.

SURGERY (USUALLY RESERVED FOR LATER, IF CONSERVATIVE TREATMENTS HAVE FAILED)

Removal of calcified deposits; removal of exostosis (bone projection similar to a bunion) around lateral epicondyle; removal of granulation tissue from subtendinous area; resection of the origin of the extensor carpi radialis brevis and reinsertion in lateral epicondyle.

DIAGNOSTIC STUDIES AND FINDINGS

Diagnostic test	Findings
X-rays	May show calcified areas; tears may be noted in specific tendon, and degenerative changes in area

1 ASSESS

ASSESSMENT	OBSERVATIONS
Physical examination	
Lateral epicondylitis Lateral side of elbow	Patient can do motions that produce symptoms Tenderness and pain over and around lateral epicondyle of humerus; point tenderness; exostosis may be present
Medial epicondylitis Medial side of elbow	Tenderness and pain over and around medial epicondyle of humerus; point tenderness
Tendinitis Pain is usual symptom	Pain is poorly localized; patient can repeat motions that aggravate condition; resisted active motion of specific musculotendinous group can reproduce symptoms
History	
Presenting symptom: pain	Person states that doing the same movements repetitively produce the pain and tenderness, such as when reaching overhead (bicipital tendinitis)
Finkelstein's test for de Quervain's tendinitis	Positive if pain is reproduced when patient grasps thumb with the fingers into a fist, and wrist is ulnar deviated
Medial or lateral epicondylar areas	Patient does motions that produce pain in area; has point tenderness in epicondylar areas; small exostosis is present
Tendinitis (assess specific site)	
Bicipital area of humerus	Pain and discomfort in anterior shoulder; symptoms increase when reaching overhead; positive Yergason's test (see page 297)
Trigger finger	Digit is held in flexed or extended position; active and passive ROM of digit slightly limited
Gluteus maximus	Tenderness or pain in hip and upper thigh; tenderness in area of greater trochanter
Patella (jumper's knee)	ROM of knee is limited on flexion; upper portion of patella is tender; quadriceps muscle mass is slightly atrophied
Achilles tendon area	Heel area is tender and edematous with foot/heel pronation; soleus and gastrocnemius muscles have slightly decreased flexibility; shoes show abnormal wear at heels

2   DIAGNOSE

NURSING DIAGNOSIS	SUBJECTIVE FINDINGS	OBJECTIVE FINDINGS
Impaired physical mobility and pain related to trauma to specific muscle/ tendon area (medial or lateral epi- condyles)	Medial epicondyle (golfer's elbow): States has sharp pain in inner elbow area when swinging golf clubs; states has "nagging" tenderness in same area at rest	Has marked tenderness over medial epi- condylar area; can reproduce pain by go- ing through golf swing; area has slight edema
	Lateral epicondyle (tennis elbow): States has sharp pain in lateral elbow area when swinging tennis racket, or when ice fishing and scaling the fish, or when playing rac- quetball or squash.	Has acute pain when lateral epicondyle is palpated (point tenderness); pain is less when not using extremity; relieved by rest (NOTE: observe both elbow areas, medial and lateral—condition can be bilateral)
Impaired physical mobility and pain related to tendinitis	States has tenderness and pain (dull and at times sharp) in specific area:	
	Bicipital: Reports increasing pain in front of shoulder when reaching overhead	Pain is increased with Yergason's test
	Trigger finger: Reports cannot straighten out finger and has pain when attempts to do so	Palpate flexor tendon sheath—can have pain and tenderness; ROM will be limited by tightness of tendon
	Gluteus maximus: States has pain in hip and outside of thigh	Palpation elicits complaints of tenderness in hip area and upper thigh distal to the greater trochanter (at insertion of gluteus maximus tendon)
	Patella: Reports pain around top of knee when running, jumping, or climbing steps	Palpation elicits complaints of tenderness localized to upper or lower part of patella; may have hypermobility of patella; quadri- ceps muscle has signs of atrophy or wast- ing
	Achilles tendon area: Reports nagging pain in heel(s) when jogging; swollen foot/ heel	Palpation elicits localized tenderness at insertion of Achilles tendon at heel; slight edema is present; pain is increased when patient hops repeatedly on foot; one foot or both overpronate when standing or stepping; exercise shoes are worn in heel areas

3   PLAN

Patient goals

1. The patient will regain full function and mobility after treatment for epicondylitis.

2. The patient will have relief of pain in inflamed area.

➔ ❭ ❭

4 IMPLEMENT

NURSING DIAGNOSIS	NURSING INTERVENTIONS	RATIONALE
Impaired physical mobility and pain related to epicondylitis or tendinitis	Assess specific site(s) as indicated.	Data on specific condition are needed for planning care.
	Clarify the rationale for rest to affected part plus avoiding activity that precipitates symptoms.	Rest allows inflamed tissues to begin healing and inflammation to resolve.
	Teach patient how to do heat or cold applications as ordered; teach patient to cover heat or cold container with dry, cotton cover.	Temperature changes increase circulation (heat) or slow circulation and decrease edema (cold), to lessen pressure on inflamed nerve endings and thus lessen pain; covering container prevents excess heat or cold to skin, which could cause a burn; cold causes excess vasoconstriction, leading to marked ischemia and blister formation.
	Teach patient how to apply splint, immobilize, or use orthotic device as ordered.	Orthotic devices ease strain on inflamed tissues, aiding healing and relieving pain.
	Administer analgesic or nonsteroidal medication q 4 h as ordered.	Analgesics reduce perception of pain; NSAIDs aid resolution of inflammation.
	Assist with injection of corticosteroids as needed (usual dosage is 0.5-1 ml); explain that there may be some increase in pain in injected area for 12-24 h, after which time pain should decrease dramatically.	Corticosteroids hasten resolution of inflammation when injected into site; however, their use is controversial, because repeated use may predispose to rupture of the affected tendon. Increased pain is common because of increased volume in an enclosed area, causing pressure on nerve endings.
	Arrange consultation with physical therapist for teaching prescribed exercises.	Exercising properly and repetitively helps retain or regain functional muscles and joints; exercises performed over time strengthen the weakened tissues.
Knowledge deficit	See Patient Teaching.	

5 EVALUATE

PATIENT OUTCOME	DATA INDICATING THAT OUTCOME IS REACHED
Patient has regained full function after treatment for epicondylitis.	Patient returns to recreational or professional sports activities after resolution of inflammation and rehabilitation period. Patient can do full ROM of elbow and upper extremity when working or using arm. All pain and tenderness are gone.
Patient has not experienced a recurrence.	Over time patient has used both upper extremities without signs of inflammation or pain. Patient has adjusted wrist strokes for tennis, golf, baseball, or other sport. Patient has returned to full employment with no problems in extremities.

PATIENT OUTCOME	DATA INDICATING THAT OUTCOME IS REACHED
Patient has regained full ROM after treatment for tendinitis.	Patient could repeatedly raise arms overhead without pain or tenderness. Tendon release surgery has relieved trigger finger and fixed flexion, and affected joint can do normal ROM. Patient has no hip, knee, or heel pain or tenderness with weight bearing, hiking, or running. Patient has substituted fitness walking for jogging and has returned to full employment. Patient wears orthotic device in shoe to correct overpronation.

PATIENT TEACHING

1. Teach the patient about inflammatory processes and signs of resolution of inflammation.
2. With the assistance of the physical therapist, teach proper exercises to regain muscle/joint strength.
3. Teach the patient the side effects of medications and ways to prevent secondary effects such as gastric irritation and diarrhea; instruct the patient on which symptoms to report to the physician.
4. With the assistance of the occupational therapist, teach the patient alternate methods for using the extremities without increasing inflammation.
5. Instruct the patient about the effects of heat and cold and the cautions with use of each modality.
6. Teach the patient about orthotic devices, or repeat explanation if already given.

Bursitis

Bursitis is inflammation of a bursa.

A *bursa* is an enclosed sac found between muscles and tendons and bony prominences. A bursa can suffer trauma, infection, or inflammation, which is the most common condition. Since a bursa is enclosed within other tissues, those tissues also can become inflamed. Also, two or more bursae can become inflamed simultaneously. Bursae that are commonly inflamed are the subdeltoid and subacromial bursae of the shoulder; the olecranon (elbow) bursa; the greater trochanteric bursa, lateral to the hip; and the anserine bursa, located between the tendons of the sartorius, gracilis, and semitendinosus muscles and the tibia. Chronically inflamed bursae may develop calcifications.

PATHOPHYSIOLOGY

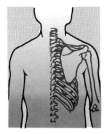

Bursitis can develop as a result of constant friction between the bursa and the musculoskeletal tissues surrounding it. Friction causes irritation, edema, and eventually inflammation. The bursal sac becomes engorged, and the area around the sac becomes exquisitely tender and

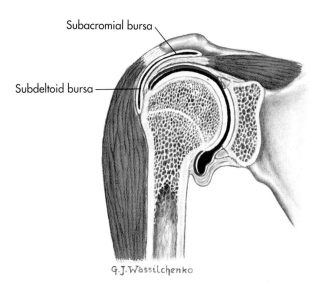

Subacromial bursa

Subdeltoid bursa

G.J.Wassilchenko

painful. Movement of the tissues around the bursa causes pressure and more pain. Flexion and extension of the joint near the inflamed bursa are affected and are limited by the pain. The area may be red, hot, and edematous, with pain radiating to contiguous tissues. Point tenderness may be present, in which the patient can point to the spot or area of greatest tenderness.

Bursitis can also develop from repeated microtrauma, which leads to effusion and thickening of the bursal sac. With continued irritation and inflammation, calcification of the bursa can occur, and adhesions may develop around the bursa that limit movement of the tendons.

COMPLICATIONS

Calcifications in joint(s)
Loss of ROM of joint(s)
Muscle weakness

DIAGNOSTIC STUDIES AND FINDINGS

Diagnostic test	Findings
X-rays	May show enlarged bursa with or without calcified deposits

MEDICAL MANAGEMENT

GENERAL MANAGEMENT Avoidance of activities, such as kneeling or repeatedly raising arms above head, that can lead to constant irritation.
Use of sponge rubber knee pads to lessen pressure when kneeling.
Avoidance of constant friction movements, such as throwing or hitting a ball, that cause the inflammatory reaction.
Application of moist heat to affected area(s) q 4 h.
Wrapping of area, if accessible, to reduce edema and provide support.
Performing ROM exercises to help maintain or regain motion.

DRUG THERAPY

Analgesic-antipyretic medications: Aspirin, 600-1,000 mg q 4 h; acetaminophen, 250-500 mg q 4 h for patients under 18 yr of age (aspirin has been associated with the development of Reye's syndrome).

Nonsteroidal antiinflammatory agents: Ibuprofen (Motrin, Advil), 200-400 mg q 4-6 h; indomethacin (Indocin), 25 mg tid or qid; injection of corticosteroids into bursal area in individualized dosage; antibiotics specific to offending organism after culture, if infection is present.

SURGERY Excision of the bursal wall and calcified deposits; aspiration of bursal fluid.

1 ASSESS

ASSESSMENT	OBSERVATIONS
Area of involvement (may be shoulder, knee, hip, elbow, or thigh area)	Edema, heat, redness, tenderness, limitation of motion, point tenderness

ASSESSMENT	OBSERVATIONS
Vital signs	Temperature, pulse, and respirations within normal limits
ROM of joints around area	ROM limited by pain; holds joint area with hand to lessen pain

2 DIAGNOSE

NURSING DIAGNOSIS	SUBJECTIVE FINDINGS	OBJECTIVE FINDINGS
Impaired physical mobility (ROM) related to inflamed bursa and surrounding tissues	Reports sharp pain when flexes (bends) elbow, knee, or shoulder	Area is red, feels hot, has edema and tenderness over bursa and in associated tendons; moves joint slowly and hesitantly through ROM; avoids full circumduction of shoulder or hip by stopping when pain occurs
Pain (acute) related to inflamed bursa	Reports sharp pain when doing extension or circumduction movements; pain is relieved when stops using involved joints; pain noticed when kneeling or reaching up	Has tenderness on palpation of area; holds affected arm at elbow to ease pain; winces when circumducting arm; points to sore area around affected joint

3 PLAN

Patient goals

1. The patient will regain full range of motion of affected musculoskeletal tissues.
2. Inflammation of bursa is relieved.
3. Inflammation does not recur.

4 IMPLEMENT

NURSING DIAGNOSIS	NURSING INTERVENTIONS	RATIONALE
Pain (acute) related to inflamed bursa	Assess pain, its amount, duration, characteristics, and relief or exacerbation.	Provides data for planning care.
	Apply moist compresses to inflamed areas.	Moist compresses increase circulation to help relieve inflammation.
	Help patient into as comfortable a position as possible.	Comfortable position can relieve strain on weakened tissues.
	Administer analgesics as ordered q 4 h.	Analgesics relieve pain perception and responses to pain.

NURSING DIAGNOSIS	NURSING INTERVENTIONS	RATIONALE
	Assist with injection of corticosteroids into site, if done; explain temporary increase of pain after injection.	Corticosteroids are antiinflammatory medications that relieve pain and inflammation; Pain at the site is increased temporarily (8-12 h or longer) because of increased pressure of fluid in an enclosed space.
	Monitor effects of medications and injection of corticosteroids.	Determining effects of treatments may indicate need for change.
	Support inflamed tissues, and handle gently. Support joints above and below area, if feasible.	Careful, gentle handling lessens stress and helps prevent additional trauma.
Impaired physical mobility (ROM) related to inflamed bursa and surrounding tissues	Assess bursa and surrounding area for ROM or limitation of movements.	Provides data for planning care.
	Monitor resolution of inflammation with treatments.	Determining current condition indicates need to continue treatments or to add new ones.
	Apply moist, warm compresses to area q 4 h.	Warm, moist compresses increase circulation to help resolve inflammation.
	Encourage ROM exercises q 4 h.	ROM exercises help maintain or regain functions of inflamed tissues.
	Apply sling or elastic bandages to inflamed area.	Support to affected joints lessens strain and gives external support.
	Caution patient to avoid activities that could prevent healing of present inflammation or cause a recurrence.	Recurrence can lead to development of a chronic inflammatory process, which can restrict or permanently damage affected tissues.
	Suggest use of aids to lessen pressure on inflamed joints (e.g., use knee pads when kneeling; use a step stool when reaching for high shelves).	Use of an aid lessens strain on inflamed tissues, can prevent development of bursitis or a recurrence.
Knowledge deficit	See Patient Teaching.	

5 EVALUATE

PATIENT OUTCOME	DATA INDICATING THAT OUTCOME IS REACHED
Patient has regained full ROM of affected tissues.	Patient uses affected joints and tissues normally through all ROM without hesitation; has had no recurrence.
Patient's bursal inflammation has resolved.	Area is no longer reddened, hot, or edematous. All pain is gone without use of medications.

PATIENT TEACHING

1. Clarify the site and purposes of bursae; use pictures to locate bursal sites.
2. Teach the patient range-of-motion exercises to maintain function.
3. Alert the patient to the possibility of increased pain for 8 to 24 hours after injection of corticosteroids into the bursal sac, followed by dramatic relief of pain and inflammation.
4. Teach the patient how to use aids such as pads or stools to ease pressure on vulnerable tissues.
5. Caution the patient to curtail activities that could cause reinflammation of incompletely healed tissues (full healing may take 4 to 6 weeks.)

Lyme Disease

Lyme disease is caused by a spirochete bacterium carried by a tick, rodent, or animal such as a deer. It causes flu-like symptoms and can masquerade as arthritis, gastritis, or encephalitis.

Lyme disease was first diagnosed in 1975 and was named after the Connecticut city in which it was first noted. It is one of the fastest growing infectious diseases in the United States, along with acquired immune deficiency syndrome (AIDS). No one is immune to infection, which occurs in all age groups.

Lyme disease is more prevalent in the northeastern sections of the United States, particlarly in New York, New Jersey, and Connecticut, although the disease has been found in 43 states and on five continents.[57] Precautions against contracting the disease include wearing sturdy boots, long pants, and bug repellants when in woods, fields, or areas where the disease is known to be more prevalent. The use of lawn sprays is being studied to determine their effectiveness in eradicating the ticks. People who have been in areas where ticks are common should check their bodies thoroughly. If a tick is found, it should be removed and the person should consult a doctor.

PATHOPHYSIOLOGY

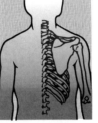

The pathogenic organism is carried by a tick in its insect, rodent, or animal vector. It is transmitted to humans through a bite and can infect any organ in the body, which often causes a delay in diagnosis. It can also be carried through the placenta to the fetus.

Approximately half the people with Lyme disease develop a reddish rash with a characteristic red circle, called a target lesion because of its resemblance to a bull's eye target. This lesion aids in making a positive diagnosis. Other people develop flulike symptoms such as a headache, aches, pains, and polyarthritis; some may develop encephalitis, gastritis, or carditis. Low-grade fevers accompany the flulike condition.

COMPLICATIONS (if disease is long-standing or undiagnosed)

Muscle weakness
Paralysis
Patient-specific neurologic deficits such as learning difficulties, coordination problems, and excessive drowsiness

DIAGNOSTIC STUDIES AND FINDINGS

Diagnostic test	Findings
Laboratory tests	
Blood serum	Positive for antibodies for Lyme disease (test may not become positive for 4-6 wk after exposure)
Urinalysis	Under development

MEDICAL MANAGEMENT

GENERAL MANAGEMENT

Bed rest if neurologic symptoms are present; Physical therapy for muscle weakness, paralysis, or arthritis; Removal of tick if found on clothing or skin.

DRUG THERAPY

Benzathine penicillin, 7.2 million U IM 3 times/wk; **or** penicillin G, 20 million U IV qid; **or** tetracycline, 250 mg qid; Ceftriaxone (Rocephin) (for long-standing, previously undiagnosed disease, or if in brain tissues, since ceftriaxone crosses the blood-brain barrier; given for 2 wk or longer in age-related doses); Acetaminophen, 300-1,000 mg (age-related doses) for headache and fever.

PREVENTION

Wear boots and long pants if going into wooded areas; apply bug repellants before going into wooded areas; check clothing and body after being in wooded areas; vaccinate dogs (currently only vaccine available, but others are being developed).

1   ASSESS

ASSESSMENT	OBSERVATIONS
Signs or symptoms of infection (e.g., vital signs, temperature elevation, systemic signs, or localized symptoms)	Variations in blood pressure; fever; flulike symptoms such as aches and pains, headache, joint tenderness, and edema; confusion and disorientation; muscle weakness; heart irregularities; changes in renal functions; respiratory complaints with cough or cold symptoms; nausea and vomiting; constipation or diarrhea
History of being in woods, fields, or areas ticks may inhabit	Ask patient to describe sites in woods or fields; ask about visits to northeastern United States, especially New York, New Jersey, or Connecticut
Entire body (for ticks, rash, or target lesion)	Tick(s) on body or clothes; reports mice and other rodents, deer, or birds were in immediate area; hairline, groin, and areas behind knees have bite marks of ticks; reddish rash with targetlike circular area

2   DIAGNOSE

NURSING DIAGNOSIS	SUBJECTIVE FINDINGS	OBJECTIVE FINDINGS
Hyperthermia related to inflammatory process	States feels warm or hot	Temperature above 37° C (98.6° F)

NURSING DIAGNOSIS	SUBJECTIVE FINDINGS	OBJECTIVE FINDINGS
Activity intolerance related to muscle weakness and arthritis	States feels weak, tired and achy	Weakness, aches and pains, joint soreness, muscle weakness, or paralysis with movement by examiner
Impaired physical mobility related to arthritis and neurologic problems	States joints are very sore and painful; complains of difficulty moving	Arthritis of more than one joint, with edema and tenderness on palpation; movement painful
Impaired skin integrity related to rash and pruritus	States skin itches	Rash on skin surfaces; target lesion
Impaired gas exchange related to dyspnea and pneumonitis	States is short of breath at times	Dyspnea, cough and production of sputum, tachypnea; nail beds are pink
Sensory-perceptual alteration related to encephalitis-like symptoms	States has headache, is sleepy	Disorientation, confusion, headache; falls asleep easily
Pain related to headache, joint pain, and muscle soreness	States muscles and joints ache; headache	Aches and pains, headache, joint pain, and disorientation; joints and muscles tender on palpation; holds involved tissues immobile

3 PLAN

Patient goals

1. The patient will regain normal vital signs and temperature.
2. The patient will return to usual activities after treatments.
3. The patient will regain usual physical mobility with no permanent arthritis.
4. The patient will have normal skin integrity.
5. The patient will have normal gas exchange.
6. The patient will regain normal sensory and neurologic functions.
7. The patient will have no lingering discomfort or pain.

4 IMPLEMENT

NURSING DIAGNOSIS	NURSING INTERVENTIONS	RATIONALE
Hyperthermia related to fever	Assess for temperature elevations q 2-4 h; notify physician of elevations of temperature.	Temperature readings can fluctuate (up to 38.3-38.9° C [101-102° F])

→ › ›

NURSING DIAGNOSIS	NURSING INTERVENTIONS	RATIONALE
	Administer ordered antipyretics q 4 h if needed; use acetaminophen, not aspirin, for children and teenagers.	Antipyretics aid in thermoregulation by reducing fevers through their effect on the heat-regulating center in the hypothalamus; do not give aspirin to children and teenagers because of the drug's association with Reye's syndrome.
	Change gowns and bed linens as needed if patient has diaphoresis.	Diaphoresis is one method the body uses to cool itself as temperatures return to normal or when fevers "break"; moisture allowed to remain on the skin may cause maceration.
	Increase fluid intake as tolerated, to 3,000 ml or more per 24 h.	Increased intake decreases the possibility of dehydration from fluid loss through perspiration and diaphoresis.
Activity intolerance related to arthritis and muscle soreness	Assess patient's ability to participate in ADL and self-care activities; provide assistance with ADL or self-care as needed.	Assistance conserves patient's energy and strength for fighting infection and helps maintain patient's physical strengths.
	Offer rest periods during day.	Rest helps patient regain homeostasis and fight infection.
	Assist patient to be out of bed and to ambulate as permitted.	Activity and ambulation help patient retain musculoskeletal functions and other body functions.
Impaired physical mobility related to arthritis and neurologic problems	Consult with physical and occupational therapists if patient has muscle weakness, arthritis, or neurologic problems (eye muscle weakness, paralysis of muscles).	Special therapies may be needed to help restore full functions or to prevent additional losses.
Impaired skin integrity related to rash and pruritus	Assess for characteristic rash with bull's eye target configuration (some individuals do not develop a rash).	Presence of the target lesion helps confirm a diagnosis of Lyme disease.
	Caution patient not to scratch areas with rash.	Scratching may cause skin breaks, which could lead to infection if not already present.
	Help patient bathe or shower if assistance is needed.	Bathing and cleansing skin help maintain its health.
	Obtain physician's order for antipruritic if itching is severe.	Antipruritics lessen itching through action on nerve endings.
	Note spreading or disappearance of rash.	State of rash gives evidence of disease activity.
Impaired gas exchange related to dyspnea and pneumonitis	Assess for signs of dyspnea, cough and production of sputum, and soreness in thoracic tissues.	Dyspnea, cough and production of sputum, and thoracic soreness are some signs of extent of Lyme disease.

NURSING DIAGNOSIS	NURSING INTERVENTIONS	RATIONALE
	Encourage deep-breathing exercises q 2-3 h.	Deep breathing aids oxygenation and helps pulmonary tissues retain their strength and functions.
	Check sputum color; note color change, if present.	"Normal" sputum is clear; if pulmonary infection is present, sputum may be yellow or green.
	Check vital signs q 2-4 h.	Respiratory changes are reflected in increasing dyspnea or tachypnea.
	Check nail beds and skin color periodically.	Hypoxia may be noted in dusky nail beds or skin color.
Sensory-perceptual alteration related to encephalitis-like symptoms	Assess level of consciousness q 4 h (or q 1-2 h if changes are noted); note restlessness.	Level of consciousness is a major indicator of cerebral oxygenation and functioning.
	Monitor vital signs q 2-4 h.	Changes in vital signs, such as elevation in systolic blood pressure, tachycardia, and tachypnea, are signs of increased intracranial pressure.
	If patient becomes confused, provide a safe environment: observe patient more frequently; raise side rails; check for orientation to time, place, and person; remove sharp objects or unsafe furniture from area.	Confused or disoriented patients may injure themselves through falls, unsteadiness, unsafe handling of utensils, and tripping over furniture or falling out of bed. Efforts must be made to provide for safety while patient is unable to protect self.
	Attempt to orient patient and lessen confusion by explaining where he is, time of day, date, or other information to lessen confusion.	A confused patient may need cues to lessen confusion or disorientation; cues help restore reality and aid orientation.
Pain related to headache, joint pains, and muscle soreness	Assess for aches and pains, headache, joint soreness or stiffness, and nausea or vomiting.	Lyme disease causes flulike symptoms and can affect any organ system; symptoms vary depending on the organ or tissues involved. Inflammation causes soreness, tenderness, and pain because of edema and increased metabolism.
	Help patient into comfortable position, which may be lying flat, propped up at 45-degree angle, or sitting upright.	Muscle and joint soreness and aches and pains make patient uncomfortable; frequent changes in position aid comfort.
	Administer prescribed analgesics q 4 h if needed.	Analgesics help relieve pain; regular administration maintains therapeutic blood levels.
	Note effects of physical therapies to ease muscle or joint soreness.	Increased muscle activity increases circulation to remove wastes and bring nutrients to tissues, thus aiding healing.
Knowledge deficit	See Patient Teaching.	

➜ ❯ ❯ ❯

5 EVALUATE

PATIENT OUTCOME	DATA INDICATING THAT OUTCOME IS REACHED
Patient has regained normal vital signs.	Vital signs are within normal ranges for size, age, and sex (body temperature, 36.7°-37° C [98°-98.6° F]; pulse, 68-80 beats/min; respirations 12-16/min; BP: systolic, 100-140 mm Hg, diastolic, 68-80 mm Hg).
Patient has returned to usual activities after treatments.	Patient goes about usual activities such as school, employment, exercise programs, and hobbies.
Patient has regained usual mobility with no permanent arthritis.	Patient has no residual pain.
Patient has regained normal skin integrity.	Patient has no rash or pruritus.
Patient has normal gas exchange.	Patient has no cough, dyspnea, or chest soreness; respiratory rates are normal.
Patient has regained normal sensory and neurologic functions.	Patient has no numbness or tingling, no headache, and no disorientation or altered consciousness.
Patient has no lingering discomforts or pain.	Patient needs no analgesics for pain nor additional treatments for soreness or joint weakness.

PATIENT TEACHING

1. Instruct the patient and family about the characteristics of Lyme disease, its cause and course.
2. Instruct the patient and family about the side effects of medications.
3. Clarify possible sequelae the patient should watch for, such as muscle weakness, joint pain, excessive drowsiness, or altered mental functioning (these should have been discussed previously by the physician).
4. Teach the patient and family ways to prevent future infection; i.e., wearing long pants and boots when in fields or wooded areas; checking clothing and body thoroughly for ticks or bites after being in tick-infected areas; removing ticks from the body with tweezers, as close to the skin as possible, then saving the tick and notifying the physician immediately.

CHAPTER 6

Degenerative Musculoskeletal Conditions

Degenerative conditions are associated with life and living; with aging, and "wear and tear" resulting from use; with abuse, trauma, and developmental or other influences on tissues in and around joints. Degenerative conditions tend to become progressively worse over time and can become incapacitating, even after treatment.

The primary musculoskeletal tissues involved in degenerative conditions are the multiple layers of cartilage covering the ends of bones. As cartilage deteriorates other joint tissues are secondarily affected, leading to the condition referred to as degenerative joint disease. Although the degenerative changes are really *processes* of change, they are called *diseases* when they produce symptoms.

Osteoarthritis

Osteoarthritis (OA) is a condition noted by degenerative changes in articular cartilage mainly in the major weight-bearing joints although other joints are also affected.

OA is referred to as primary (idiopathic) if there is an absence of any known underlying predisposing factors, and secondary if there is a clearly defined, underlying condition contributing to its etiology. The incidence of primary OA is higher in whites, whereas secondary OA is found among southern Chinese.[46]

OA is a condition of older adults. It is the most common form of arthritis, with estimates of up to 50 million Americans affected. It is more prevalent in men under the age of 45 but is more common in women over age 55. OA occurs worldwide in all climates. The incidence

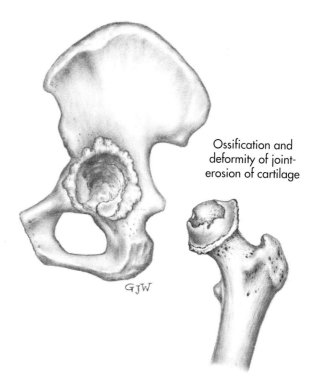

Ossification and deformity of joint-erosion of cartilage

GJW

of OA increases as people age and is almost universal in persons 75 or older. Obesity is thought to play a part in the development of OA, although controversy as to its role persists. The degenerative changes may not be due to the weight itself but rather to mechanical alterations in the mode of walking, e.g., change in heel strike or valgus deformity caused by heavy thighs or foot deformities.[1]

Overuse of joints has been indicated as contributing to the presence of OA, particularly those joints involved with repetitive movements such as throwing, repeated depression of pedals while standing, and others.

PATHOPHYSIOLOGY

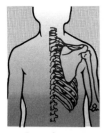

OA is a progressive deterioration of the cartilage within the joint, characterized by microfissures, uneven eroded surfaces, fraying and fibrillation, and loss of some cells. Fragments of cartilage may become unattached into the joint, setting up a low-grade, chronic inflammation within the joint or synovial lining. As the articular cartilage continues to degenerate, the underlying bone produces spurs of new bone, called osteophytes, which may affect joint mobility as they increase in size. Pain or aching discomfort in the affected joint may also be noticed as osteophytes develop. Cysts may develop in the subchondral bone due to infiltration of synovial fluid through the fissured joint cartilage. The joint (articular) cartilage attempts to repair itself in the early stages of OA, but the repair processes slow and eventually fail in the later stages of the condition.

The progression of the changes in articular cartilage vary, and OA may persist for long periods without becoming severe. Pain is not present early but may become noticeable when the chronic inflammatory changes develop, and pain may be present with joint movement or activity. The range of motion of the affected joint may be affected as the osteophytes increase in size or as pain becomes a more prominent symptom.

The major weight-bearing joints such as the hip and knee are the two most commonly affected joints, but the joints of the fingers, especially the distal interphalangeal (DIP), proximal interphalangeal (PIP), and metacarpophalangeal (MCP) (Figure 6-1), the glenohumeral, and the elbow, wrist and ankle all are affected to lesser degrees. Degenerative changes in the vertebrae and facet joints and sacroiliac joints can also occur in OA. OA may develop secondary to trauma in some patients.

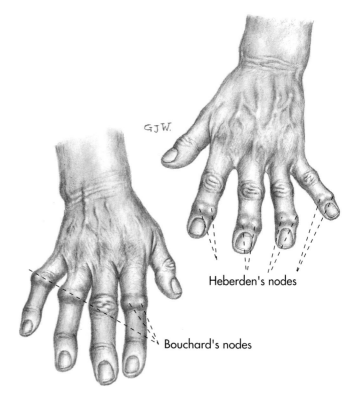

FIGURE 6-1
Osteoarthritis. Heberden's nodes and Bouchard's nodes.

Symptoms of OA vary with the severity of the condition. Joint soreness, stiffness, and aching, dull pain are some common complaints. Joint swelling and deformity may be noted later, as well as reduced range of motion (ROM) and bony enlargements within the affected joints. Tenderness, joint instability, and increasing pain on use or weight bearing are also commonly noted.

Although the exact cause of OA has not been positively determined, it may be due to a defective gene in the joint cartilage, causing it to repair itself less effectively or to become degraded (worn) more easily. Such a gene was discovered and reported in 1990.

COMPLICATIONS

Ankylosis of joints
Deformity of one or more joints
Loss of sensation and decreased mobility

MEDICAL MANAGEMENT

GENERAL MANAGEMENT

Supportive care

Use of a cane or walker and, at times, crutches to lessen pressure and strain on the joints; Weight reduction to ease joint strain; Rest to inflamed or tender joint to increase comfort; Use of orthotic devices to alter pressure and/or maintain joint strength

Nutritional management

Weight reduction diet: lower in fat and calories; Diet high in vitamins A and C.

Physical therapy

Moist heat applications to relieve soreness and aching—may alternate with cold applications; ROM exercises to help maintain joint functions within limits to avoid excess pressure on joint surfaces; Massage around joint to lessen stiffness and relax tight muscles or ligaments; Application of supportive splint to rest a tender joint or prevent progressive deformity; Use of elastic bandages, or supportive elastic cuffs to ease edema or soreness; Use of a girdle, corset, canvas belt or brace to relieve back strain or soreness; Sturdy, well-fitting shoes to help maintain posture and ambulation.

DRUG THERAPY

Antiinflammatory analgesics to relieve pain and soreness and reduce inflammatory changes, if present; medications are given four times daily with antacids to lessen gastric irritation.
Muscle relaxants to relieve muscle spasms.
Nonsteroidal antiinflammatory drugs (such as phenylbutasone or indomethacin) may be used briefly to lessen pain or inflammation; newer NSAIDS are also used.
Intra-articular steroid injections may be used to relieve soreness in enlarged, inflamed joints (systemic steroids are not used in OA).

SURGERY

Total joint replacement is commonly done for OA, such as total hip, knee, shoulder elbow, wrist and ankle replacement to relieve pain, restore motion, or maintain motion (page 97).
Arthrodesis (joint fusion) may be done in adjacent cervical or lumbar segments to relieve pain and increase joint stability. Fusion of other joints is less commonly done (see pages 97-98).
Osteotomy to change weight bearing surfaces in involved or distant joints, such as hallux valgus.

DIAGNOSTIC STUDIES AND FINDINGS

Diagnostic Test	Findings
Radiologic studies	Confirm diagnosis by presence of osteophytes, narrowing (or obliteration) of joint spaces; also may show sclerosis of subchondral bone surfaces, subchondral cyst formation, "lipping" of osteophytes into joint, and calcification of ligaments, especially along vertebrae
CT	Same as x-rays; also may show impingement of spinal canal (stenosis) or narrowing of neural foramina

Continued.

Diagnostic Test	Findings
MRI	Confirms findings of CT and x-rays
Gait analysis	May show leg length discrepancy, positive Trendelenburg sign (see inside back cover); varus malalignments
Muscle testing	May show weakness of muscles supporting joints
Laboratory analysis	
Synoval fluid analysis	Fluid usually clear and colorless (or may be yellow tinged); no crystals present; an occasional white blood cell may be noted (mainly mononuclear cells); glucose levels of blood and synovial fluid are usually equal
Bone scan	May show increased nuclide uptake in area of OA
Arthroscopy (not usually needed for diagnosis of OA, but may be done if additional diagnosis is suspected)	OA cartilage appears frayed, yellow, irregular, and ulcerated (normal cartilage is smooth, white, and glistening)

1 ASSESS

ASSESSMENT	OBSERVATIONS
Posture and gait	"Hunched" shoulders with excessive dorsal kyphosis; feet placed wider apart than normal; lists to one side; abdomen protruberant; walks slowly with limp, steps in shorter steps, and foot "plants" in varus position to offset changed angle in hip joints; guards amount of weight applied to particular joints; positive Trendelenberg sign (see inside back cover); may use a cane and walker
ROM of all joints	Moderate degree of limitation of motion; active ROM less than passive related to patient's concern for pain
Joints	DIP joints have deformity and Heberden's nodes; PIP joints show Bouchard's nodes; knee joints deformed, enlarged, and edematous with varus deformity; hip joints deformed, enlarged, and slightly edematous; affected joints warmer than unaffected joints; skin thinner and redder than normal; skin surfaces usually intact
Pain and/or muscle spasms	Pain may be dull, aching, sore, or sharp on weight bearing (may be relieved with rest or non-weight bearing); guarding when moving joints through ROM; muscle spasms of lower back and cervical posterior muscles occur periodically with use and position changes; pain of hip OA referred to inner thigh or knee; cervical OA pain referred to posterior shoulders with some numbness and tingling of shoulder area and radiation to fingertips (some fingertips numb due to pressure on specific cervical nerve areas); pain centered in lower back with radiation to buttocks and hip areas, down thighs to feet and toes associated with pressure on specific spinal nerves, or the sciatic nerve
Weight	May be overweight or obese with much weight carried on abdomen, buttocks, and thighs
Vital signs	Normal temperature, pulse rate, and respirations; BP slightly elevated due to stress or pain
Usual roles and ability to do own ADL	Roles vary per individual; may be slow and deliberate when doing own ADL; sits in shower on stool; needs assistance to close or button shirts, belts, etc

2 DIAGNOSE

NURSING DIAGNOSIS	SUBJECTIVE FINDINGS	OBJECTIVE FINDINGS
Impaired physical mobility related to OA and limited ROM	Reports limited ability to walk distances; pain when bearing weight; aching in affected joints when non-weight bearing; stiff fingers	Noticeable limp and altered gait; knee joints deformed and edematous; feet closer together or farther apart than normal when standing; hunched shoulders, loss of lumbar lordosis, protruberant abdomen; deformed finger joints with nodes in DIP and PIP joints; moves fingers slowly and stiffly; slight edema of joints; wrists have some deformity and some limited ROM
Pain (acute) related to muscle spasms	Reports aching pain, which increases to sharp pain with full weight on affected joints or when using fingers; reports muscle spasms of shoulders, neck, lower back to buttocks, which are sharp, irritating, and tiring; pain in hip radiates down thigh to knee; some numbness and tingling of fingers and fingertips; sometimes wakes up from muscle spasms	Has facial grimaces, frown, and "look of pain" when moving joints; draws in breath when walking; clasps lips tightly or bites lips and limps; cautiously closes fingers when lifting objects; quickly drops items when reaches ROM
Fatigue related to disturbed sleep or rest	States feels tired nearly all the time; sleeps poorly at night and joints are painful when turning self; sleeps only 5-6 h in entire night; naps 30 min during day when able	Begins to breathe more quickly after walking short distances; rests after short distance; breathing slowly returns to resting rates
Self-care deficit related to osteoarthritis	Reports difficulty doing ADL	Is slower, more deliberate in doing ADL

3 PLAN

Patient goals

1. The patient will regain satisfactory mobility and joint ROM with treatments.
2. The patient will be relieved of joint and muscle pains with treatments.
3. The patient will regain energy for ADL and have undisturbed sleep.
4. The patient will be able to perform own self-care following treatments.

4 IMPLEMENT

NURSING DIAGNOSIS	NURSING INTERVENTIONS	RATIONALE
Impaired physical mobility related to OA and limited ROM	Assess mobility and ROM of all joints.	Assessment determines which joints are affected and to what extent.
	Observe patient's use of ambulatory aid.	Ambulatory aid relieves pressure on inflamed or painful joint by resting and reducing the amount of weight borne by the joints.

→ → →

NURSING DIAGNOSIS	NURSING INTERVENTIONS	RATIONALE
	Observe patient during postural changes; suggest changes, if needed, while rising, sitting, turning, or lying down.	Professional guidance provides ways to lessen stress or strain on affected joints.
	Discuss weight-reduction programs if feasible; consult with dietitian if appropriate.	Weight loss lessens load on all musculoskeletal tissues.
	Discuss medical plan of care with physician, patient and family or significant others.	OA is a progressive degenerative condition. Joint replacement increases mobility and arrests progression of OA.
Pain (acute) related to muscle spasms	Assess for expressions of pain, its amount, character, frequency; factors that increase or ease pain; presence of muscle spasms, numbness, tingling, radiation, or other pain experiences.	Knowledge of exact patient status helps professionals develop individualized plan of care.
	Assist patient to positions of comfort; adjust position with bed rest, pillows, or blankets.	Changes in positions ease sore, tired or aching muscles or joints by removing wastes and increasing oxygenation.
	Apply ice or warm, moist applications as ordered to affected joints.	Ice applications constrict blood vessels to lessen edema and relieve pain. Warm moist applications cause vasodilation, bring more blood and nutrients to the area, aid in removing wastes, lessen edema, and relieve pain.
	Discuss use of ambulatory aid with physician, if patient not using one.	Ambulatory aids relieve joints of weight bearing.
	Administer ordered medications q 4 h.	Analgesics of NSAIDs relieve pain through specific actions (pages 281-283). Regular administration maintains therapeutic blood levels.
	Consult with physical therapist; use suggestions for on-unit exercises.	Collaboration with health team members helps provide optimal care.
Fatigue related to disturbed sleep or rest	Assist patient to position of comfort for bedtime rest and sleep; place bed in low or flat position if tolerated; place pillows to back and between legs when on side; straighten bed linens and replace damp linens.	Placing body in comfortable positions aids sleep and rest. Skin tissues remain intact with clean, dry, wrinkle-free linens; propping with pillows lessens strain on musculoskeletal tissues.
	Avoid discussing stressful or upsetting topics with patient before bedtime; discuss with family members ways to lessen patient's concerns or stress; avoid stimulating activities and exercises immediately before bedtime.	Wakefulness may be precipitated by stressful situations, anxiety, or other emotional responses or muscular activities.
	Administer analgesic and/or sedative or muscle relaxant 30 minutes prior to desired hour of sleep.	Sleep can be enhanced and prolonged by pain-free musculoskeletal tissues. Sedatives lessen neurologic responses.

NURSING DIAGNOSIS	NURSING INTERVENTIONS	RATIONALE
	Encourage planned periods of rest during day.	Rest restores energy and maintains strength.
Self-care deficit related to degenerative condition	Assess effects of OA on roles and ADL.	Assessment determines needs.
	Encourage patient to do own ADL and other usual activities.	Doing own care helps maintain active ROM and enhances self-esteem.

5 EVALUATE

PATIENT OUTCOME	DATA INDICATING THAT OUTCOME IS REACHED
Patient has regained satisfactory mobility and joint ROM.	Patient walks easily without use of ambulatory aid after appropriate time period following treatment.
Patient is relieved of joint pains.	Patient uses only occasional nonnarcotic analgesic for occasional pain or soreness.
Patient is regaining energy for ADL and has undisturbed sleep.	Patient is increasing ADL and other activities daily; sleeps well for 6-7 h at night.
Patient has regained ability to perform own ADL.	Patient states is able to function well at home; can bathe and dress self; can do light housework.

PATIENT TEACHING

1. Explain progression of OA to patient, family or significant others.
2. Explain actions of medications to relieve symptoms; explain side effects of medications.
3. Explain purposes and actions of heat or cold applications; caution about decreased sensitivity to temperature extremes.
4. Clarify surgical care and postoperative recovery course if surgery is to be done (see pages 261-263 for operative care, rehabilitation, and nursing care).

Carpal Tunnel Syndrome

Carpal tunnel syndrome is compression of the median nerve at the wrist, although compression may occur at other levels along the pathway of the median nerve. The word *carpal* refers to wrist.

Carpal tunnel syndrome is one of the three most common industrial or work-related conditions, resulting from the increasing use of computer-related data processing, word processing, computer programming, and other computer uses. Repetitive motions involving twisting or turning of the wrist and fingers, such as during assembly-line activities, also may cause compressive symptoms of the median nerve. Construction sites, with percussive jack-hammer-type activities, account for other work-related injuries or compressive signs. Approximately one third of all traumatic injuries for which people seek medical attention involve the hand and upper extremity.

Carpal tunnel syndrome results from compression of the median nerve in the tendon sheath as it passes under the transverse ligament on the ventral surface of the wrist where the canal is snug and any swelling will usually bring on compressive symptoms (Figure 6-2).

Carpal tunnel syndrome is more common in women (more women are computer word processors) than men. It is also more common in persons with rheumatoid arthritis, menopausal women, and pregnant women in their last trimester.

PERIPHERAL NERVE ENTRAPMENT SYNDROMES

Nerve entrapment syndromes are conditions that produce symptoms indicative of pressure—pain, sensory changes, and motor functional loss—of one or more peripheral nerves. Peripheral nerve entrapment syndromes are becoming increasingly more common as causes of disability, loss of work time, and personal suffering. Entrapment may be of upper or lower extremity nerves, and may be of only one nerve or may involve two or more nerves. Many injuries may be sports-related or work- or industrial-related conditions or may stem from home, recreation, or other causes. Two common peripheral nerve entrapment syndromes are carpal tunnel syndrome in the upper extremity and sciatic nerve syndromes in the lower extremity.

Peripheral nerve entrapment syndromes

Nerve	Site	Characteristic patterns
Brachial plexus	Shoulder, arm, forearm, hand	Weak shoulder abduction and extension; weak hand grasp; weak supination; weak external rotation of arm. Erb's palsy noted by above patterns.
	Lower trunk of plexus	Thoracic outlet syndrome noted by weak grasp, arm, and shoulder pain. Klumpke's paralysis.
Ulnar	Across elbow	Cubital tunnel syndrome with weak intrinsic hand muscles from ulnar palsy. May be from direct trauma with edema and fibrosis; numbness of ring and little fingers.
Median	Across wrist	Carpal tunnel syndrome with numbness of thumb, index finger, and medial portion of middle finger; atrophy of hypothenar muscles with thumb-palm abduction deficits.
Median	Across pronator teres muscle	Anterior interosseous and pronator syndromes, causing deficits of flexor policis longus.
Radial	In the spiral groove at wrist	Weak wrist with ultimate wrist drop; deficit of brachoradialis and palsy.
Peroneal	Across head of fibula (lateral surface upper fibula).	Numbness and tingling lower leg and into foot; foot drop with continued compression.
Tibial	Across medial ankle and proximal foot areas	Tarsal tunnel syndrome of numbness, tingling, pain, and weakness of intrinsic foot muscles.
Sciatic	Lumbar or sacral areas of back.	Compression of spinal sensory nerves at exit foramina from lumbosacral areas with pressure on sciatic nerve dermatomes.

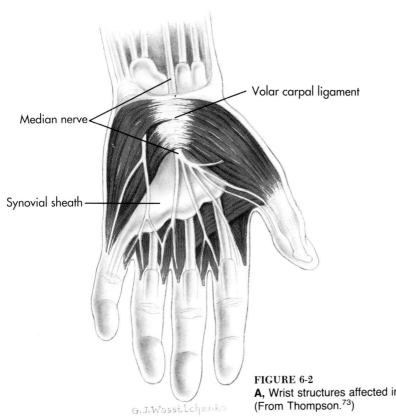

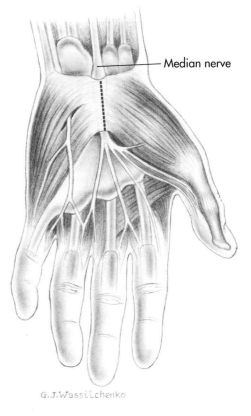

FIGURE 6-2
A, Wrist structures affected in carpal tunnel syndrome. **B,** Decompression of median nerve. (From Thompson.[73])

Labels: Median nerve, Volar carpal ligament, Synovial sheath, Median nerve

PATHOPHYSIOLOGY

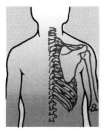

The carpal tunnel is a canal through which nine flexor tendons and the median nerve pass to the hand. The carpal (wrist) bones bind the tunnel on the dorsal and lateral sides and the transverse carpal ligament binds it on the ventral (volar) side. When the injury or inflammation of the median nerve is low (in wrist area) on the median nerve, the person experiences sensory changes with numbness or tingling in the thumb, index finger, and lateral-ventral surfaces of the middle fingers of the affected hand. Pain may be present also, mainly noticed at night when it wakes the person. Shaking the hand or massaging the fingers may ease the pain, numbness, or tingling. Itching in the numbed fingers may also be noticed. Motor weakness makes the hand feel weaker and clumsy, and the person is unable to hold utensils such as a cup or perform activities that require precision movements. Some person's symptoms may persist for months (or longer) before they become severe enough to demand medical care, but other persons have such rapid progression of symptoms that they seek medical attention early in the pathologic process.

COMPLICATIONS

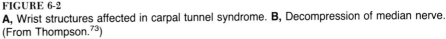

Prolonged muscle weakness and atrophy
Rupture of tendon sheath from inadvertent injection of corticosteroid
Keloid formation after surgery

DIAGNOSTIC STUDIES AND FINDINGS

Diagnostic Test	Findings
Electroconductive tests	
Electromyogram	May be within normal limits or it may show denervation of thenar muscles
Nerve conduction velocity test	May show delayed nerve response
X-ray	May show bony pressure on tunnel area

MEDICAL MANAGEMENT

GENERAL MANAGEMENT

Application of wrist splint to prevent flexion of wrist during repetitive activities and at night; wrist is splinted in 20 degrees to 25 degrees of dorsiflexion.
Ice applications to volar (ventral) wrist PRN.

DRUG THERAPY

Systemic administration of nonsteroidal antiinflammatory medication such as ibuprofen, naproxen, or piroxicam in dosage individualized for patient.
Injection of corticosteroid into carpal tunnel: may use 1.5-2 ml of 50/50 combination of triamcinolone or betamethasone and 1% xylocaine[33a]; reinjection may be done 3 to 4 months later if first injection provided marked relief.

SURGERY

Surgical decompression: Resection and surgical decompression of the carpal tunnel (resection [division] of the transverse carpal ligament).

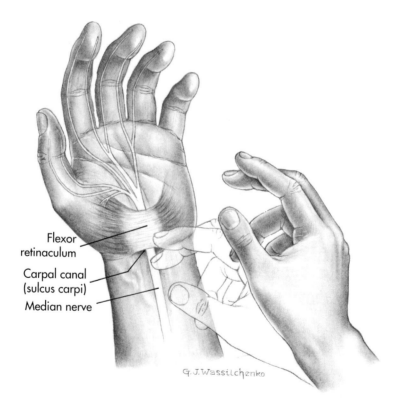

Flexor
retinaculum

Carpal canal
(sulcus carpi)
Median nerve

G.J.Wassilchenko

FIGURE 6-3
Elicitation of Tinel's sign. (From Seidel.[91])

1 ASSESS

ASSESSMENT	OBSERVATIONS
History	May use computer for extended periods daily; may use percussive equipment, hammers, screwdrivers or other requiring repeated turning or twisting of wrist; may be engaged in sports activities such as gymnastics, cycling, weight lifting, tennis, or golf; may do hobbies with repetitive wrist actions such as crocheting, knitting or painting; gives history of recent numbness, tingling and itching of fingers, swollen, painful fingers and wakening at night because of numbness or pain in hand and fingers; history of radial bone fracture, or rheumatoid arthritis
Physical examination	Sensory exam may be normal or may have abnormal two-point discrimination (normal is distance less than 6 mm); thenar eminence may be smaller than opposite hand indicating some atrophy of muscle; ability to abduct thumb against resistance is less in affected hand; Phalen's test (see inside back cover) may be and usually is positive (presence of numbness and tingling); Tinel's sign (Figure 6-3 and inside back cover) is positive (tingling and electric shock sensation); hand may be warmer or cooler than opposite hand; may have mild to moderate edema of affected hand

2 DIAGNOSE

NURSING DIAGNOSIS	SUBJECTIVE FINDINGS	OBJECTIVE FINDINGS
Altered peripheral tissue perfusion (musculoskeletal and neurologic) related to compression of carpal tunnel	Complains of pain that is "burning" that wakes him/her at night; hanging hand over mattress and shaking hand relieves pain; has numbness and tingling of thumb, index finger, and ventral and lateral sides of middle finger; may do word processing 8 h daily	Skin of affected hand is slightly swollen and cooler than opposite hand; has atrophy (mild) of thenar eminence of affected hand; sensory changes—area touched is numb; 2-point discrimination abnormal; pinprick felt but states feels "funny"; Phalen's and Tinel's signs positive
Impaired physical mobility (of hand and fingers) related to motor and sensory deficits	States hand feels big, swollen, and clumsy and can't hold or lift heavy items because of soreness, pain, and weakness	Muscle strength of push, pull, and grip weaker than other hand; thenar eminence has less mass and is atrophied compared to other hand
Pain related to compression of nerve and edema	Pain in hand and fingers wakes patient at night; has soreness at times when working during day	Palpation elicits statements regarding pain; soreness and pain when joints moved, turned, or twisted

3 PLAN

Patient goals

1. The patient will experience relief of altered peripheral tissue perfusion.
2. The patient will regain full mobility of muscles of hand and fingers.

3. The patient will have relief of pain after treatments.

4 IMPLEMENT

NURSING DIAGNOSIS	NURSING INTERVENTIONS	RATIONALE
Altered peripheral tissue perfusion (musculoskeletal and neurologic) related to compression of carpal tunnel	Perform neurovascular checks (see inside front cover) and compare with opposite hand and fingers. Document findings.	Data indicate severity of condition. Increase in numbness and tingling is untoward sign.
	Monitor complaints of increasing numbness and tingling.	Sensory changes are indicative of increasing compression of median nerve.
	Apply ice bags to ventral wrist if ordered.	Ice decreases inflammation and edema.
Impaired physical mobility (of hand and fingers) related to motor and sensory deficits	Assess ROM of wrist, thumb, and fingers.	Decreased ROM indicates decreased motor function.
	Explain inflammatory processes and need to limit flexion of wrist.	Carpal tunnel area has very little space; flexion increases compression and tension on inflamed nerve.
	Elevate hand if edematous.	Elevation increases venous return and lessens edema.
	Assist with and teach patient ROM exercises if ordered.	ROM helps maintain strength of musculoskeletal tissues.
Pain related to compression of nerve and edema	Assess site, amount, type, severity, and duration of pain.	Increase in pain indicates progression of condition.
	Assist with injections of corticosteroids into site of carpal tunnel.	Corticosteroids are antiinflammatory medications and relieve the compressive symptoms in the majority of patients. Caution is required in their use because injection into the tendon area may weaken the tendon and lead to rupture; if the injection is into the nerve itself, it may cause permanent damage to the nerve.
	Administer oral antiinflammatory medications as ordered.	Systemic antiinflammatory medications aid resolution of inflammation around nerve. Medications may already be in use for rheumatoid arthritis (carpal tunnel is common condition in these patients).
	Monitor patient's response to systemic and local medications.	Relief should be almost immediate after injection and pain relief should continue with systemic medications.
	Apply and teach patient application of splint to wrist.	Splint will limit wrist flexion, especially at night. Flexion during night and while doing activities contributes to pain.

NURSING DIAGNOSIS	NURSING INTERVENTIONS	RATIONALE
If pain and numbness continue over time, surgical reduction with release of the transverse ligament is the next logical step.	**Postoperatively:** Continue to monitor neurovascular status q 1-2 h initially, then q 4 h.	Findings should return toward normal limits soon after surgery. Numbness should be greatly lessened or be completely relieved.
	Elevate operative wrist and hand.	Elevation decreases edema formation and enhances venous return.
	Teach patient and significant others about self-administered analgesics and/or antiinflammatory medications prior to discharge.	Medications will be given in early postop period because of trauma and inflamed nerve. Healing is rapid after surgical release of carpal tunnel.

5 EVALUATE

PATIENT OUTCOME	DATA INDICATING THAT OUTCOME IS REACHED
Patient experiences relief of altered peripheral tissue perfusion.	Patient expresses complete return of sensitivity of thumb, fingers, and hand following injection or surgical release of transverse ligament; pain does not wake patient at night and requires only prn analgesic intake.
Patient regains full mobility in muscles of hand and fingers.	States hand feels stronger and less clumsy since injection or section of transverse ligament. (Full strength will only return over time with exercises and resolution of inflammation).
Patient has relief from pain.	Patient states does not need analgesic medications.

PATIENT TEACHING

1. Explain resolution of inflammatory processes to relieve symptoms.
2. Teach use of splint, ice and elevation to relieve symptoms.
3. Discuss trying to maintain neutral wrist positions to prevent recurrence or progression of symptoms.
4. Discuss rest and conditioning exercises to strengthen wrist and fingers.
5. Teach ways to manage use of wrist and grip while doing work, hobbies, and other activities.
6. If areas injected with steroids, discuss symptoms to report to physician (increased pain, loss of motor strength, or increased numbness).
7. If surgical release done, instruct about wound-healing processes and recovery phases, plus exercises to regain strength and full use of affected hand.

Sciatic Nerve Injury

Sciatic nerve injury is a pathologic condition caused by trauma, degenerative conditions, or pressure external to the nerve.

Sciatic nerve trauma or pressure may be primary, from a fall, gunshot wound, stabbing, or other cause, or it may result from pressure on it or closely positioned other peripheral nerves caused by rupture of an intervertebral disc. The degenerating or ruptured nucleus pulposus of the intervertebral disc exerts pressure on the spinal nerves as they exit the spinal canal, and impulses travel down the sciatic nerve (see Figure 6-4 for nerve pathways). Ruptured or rupturing nucleus pulposus and pressure on the sciatic nerve cause low back pain, an entity that causes as much morbidity as any other single cause of musculoskeletal morbidity. Low back pain is the most expensive health difficulty for people 30 to 50 years old—people at their peak of earning potential. It produces, or can produce, severe disability. Major factors associated with costs of low back pain include temporary disability, permanent disability, and direct medical costs related to diagnosis and treatment of the back pain and injured nerves. Men are more often affected than women and older persons are more often affected than younger persons.

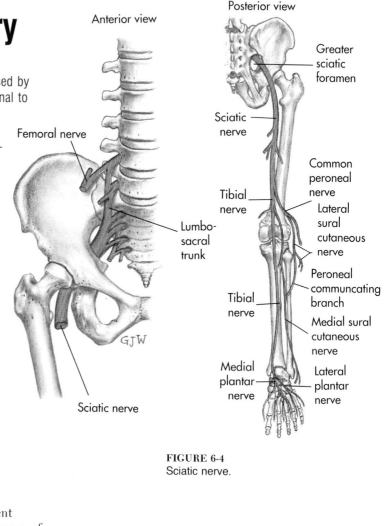

FIGURE 6-4
Sciatic nerve.

PATHOPHYSIOLOGY

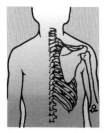

During early decades of life the intervertebral disc maintains its full height with a thickened, laminated (layered) annulus and a tense (preloaded) nucleus.[105] Protection to the disc and nucleus pulposus come from the vertebral bodies above and below each disc and nucleus, the long vertical ligamentum flavum, and the openings (foramina) between the facets that permit exit of the spinal nerves from the cord area.

With aging, the intervertebral disc experiences degeneration of the annulus that could lead to herniation of disc nuclear material through posterior tears; or the annulus can remain intact and the nucleus pulposus can degenerate; or lastly there can be simultaneous degeneration of both the annulus and the nucleus. As the disc's insufficiency progresses, more load (stress) is placed on the facets, and there may be more articular cartilage fibrillation and bone spurs may develop. The ligamentum flavum will need to carry more loads, but will become redundant (longer) as the disc(s) degeneration progresses and the total spine length decreases.

As the disc degenerates and pressure builds on the nucleus pulposus, the nucleus may rupture inward toward the canal. If the canal area is small, the herniation will compress the spinal nerves and the patient will experience pain. Lateral or posterior ruptures may or may not produce symptoms, depending upon the severity of the rupture, the proximity of the nerve to the ruptured nucleus, and the strength of the ligaments and muscles.

Intervertebral discs are prone to rupture after the age of 30 due to many reasons. First, by the age of 30, the major blood supply to the disc comes through peripheral annular vessels, resulting in a relatively avascular structure by early middle age. Nourishment to the disc subsequently comes from passage of nutrients and elimination of wastes through the central portion of the cartilaginous end-plate and peripherally through the annulus. Additionally, the fluid content inside the nucleus decreases to approximately 65% of that of a full-term baby. The collagen fibers of the disc age over time. With an increased load on the aging collagen fibers, and on the relatively avascular, water-deficient

disc, its ability to dissipate energy is markedly decreased and disc herniation is possible and even probable. Rupture of one or more discs can produce severe, sharp pain with radiation to the sciatic nerve and down the leg to the foot. Pain may be continuous, and numbness of the dermatome areas ennervated by the affected nerve(s) may become troublesome and aggravating. Persons with ruptured discs may be unable to sit or stand comfortably, but will want to lie on one side or in a back-lying position to achieve a measure of relief.

Lastly, recent studies have determined that the relatively avascular disc may trigger an autoimmune response as the avascular tissues act as antigens leading to an inflammatory autoimmune response that promotes a more rapid degenerative process within the disc itself.[105] It is little wonder that discs rupture with aging, loading (stressing), and with inflammatory changes. Signs of sciatic nerve pressure follow the rupture.

COMPLICATIONS

Paresis	Sensory changes
Motor weakness	Foot drop

MEDICAL MANAGEMENT

GENERAL MANAGEMENT

Bed rest in position of comfort (may be side-lying or recumbent with pillow under knees); mattress should be firm.
Application of skin traction with pelvic belt; Ice massage to lumbosacral area; Ultrasound diathermy several times daily with back massage; Application of back support or back brace; Exercise regimen (after acute pain and inflammation have abated) to strengthen back and abdominal muscles; Teach body mechanics and principles of lifting, moving, and carrying; Referral to "back school" for consultation and care.

DRUG THERAPY

Analgesic-antipyretic agents: Aspirin, 600-1000 mg q r h; Acetaminophen (Tylenol, Panadol, Datril, and others), 600-1000 mg q 4 h

Muscle relaxant medications: Diazepam (Valium), 2-10 mg PO q 4-6 h; Methocarbamol (Robaxin), 1 g qid; Cyclobenzaprine (Flexeril), 10 mg tid

Anti-inflammatory (nonsteroidal) medications: Piroxicam (Feldene), 20 mg PO daily; Ibuprofen (Motrin); Advil or Nuprin are non-prescription strengths; of ibuprofen), 400-800 mg q 4-6 h; Naproxen (Naprosyn), 250 mg bid

Narcotic analgesics (used only for severe pain uncontrolled by above medications): Oxycodone (Percodan), 30-60 mg q 4 h; Meperidene (Demerol), 100-150 mg IM q 3 h

SURGERY

Percutaneous discectomy; Hemilaminectomy; Spinal fusion (see pages 228-230 for discussion); Chemonucleolysis (see pages 243-248 for discussion); Microdiscectomy.

DIAGNOSTIC STUDIES AND FINDINGS

Diagnostic Test	Findings
Roentgenogram	Decreased disc space, L_3-L_4 and L_5-S_1 (not necessarily diagnostic)
CT scan	Will show anterior, lateral, or posterior rupture of disc
MRI	Shows soft tissue structures clearly and site(s) of pressure on spinal nerves
Myelogram	Shows site(s) of rupture by impaired flow of contrast agent
Discogram	Should show disc degeneration/rupture (for differential diagnosis)
Blood serum studies	Rheumatoid factor negative; HLA-B27 negative

1 ASSESS

ASSESSMENT	OBSERVATIONS
History	Reports sudden pain following an unexpected cough, sneeze while bent over, shift in load while carrying, or other sudden change in routine lifting, moving, or carrying activities; a common finding is that persons rising from bed in the morning experience sudden, severe low back pain and numbness when turning or rising to a standing position from a lying one; reports that sitting or lying on side or with knees propped up with pillows are more comfortable than standing; may also give history of urinary retention
Physical examination	May have prominent abdomen with increased lordotic curve or lordotic curve may be decreased; may stand listing to one side; May walk using shoulders and arms to help when stepping forward; when standing appears to tense back muscles to hold pelvis immobile; Appears tense and not able to relax when standing or sitting. Back exam: shoulders even at same height; vertebral column straight and in midline; iliac crests even and level; lumbar lordotic curve diminished; has positive Trendelenburg sign (see inside front cover); the thighs, knees, legs, and feet appear straight and "planted" evenly; ROM of hips and flexion of back slowly done with gasping and holding of lower back with moderate limitation of flexion, complaint of pain, soreness and numbness radiating down left leg to side of foot and toes; forward flexion 35 degrees; extension 20 degrees; right side flexion 20 degrees; left side flexion 10 degrees; rotation 10 degrees (see Chapter 2, pages 21-34 for normal ROM of various joints); palpation of sacroiliac joints shows fixation of sacroiliac joint (normal: posterior superior iliac spine will drop; elevation means fixation); hip extension causes pain in lumbosacral area on left as does knee extension; reflexes: straight leg raise limited on left leg; knee jerk 2+ on left, 3+ on right; Achilles reflex absent on left; has paresthesia on lateral two toes and lateral foot, lateral leg and plantar aspect of foot; has muscle spasm in lumbar area of back (examine tender areas last)

2 DIAGNOSE

NURSING DIAGNOSIS	SUBJECTIVE FINDINGS	OBJECTIVE FINDINGS
Pain related to possible ruptured disc and compression of sciatic nerve	Reports severe pain when trying to change positions; pain is in lower back and spreads to left hip, "tailbone" and down left leg to foot and toes	Has marked guarding and muscle spasms of lumbosacral area; areas of tendernes in left hip, gluteus muscles and coccyx area; SLR (straight leg raising) increases pain and SLR decreased; lists to left side when standing; positive Trendelenburg sign; has decreased sensations over lateral leg, lateral, and plantar areas of foot

NURSING DIAGNOSIS	SUBJECTIVE FINDINGS	OBJECTIVE FINDINGS
Impaired physical mobility related to compression of sciatic nerve and possible ruptured disc	Reports severe pain when changing from lying to sitting to standing positions; can hardly bear weight on left leg, and foot and leg feel numb and have tingling; can only walk a short distance, then has to rest because of pain and numbness; is unable to work because of pain on standing	Requires assistance to adjust positions without severe discomfort; walks with list to left side; only takes a few steps before stopping to rest; steps forward slowly, deliberately, gingerly to avoid pain; steps are small; covers short distance before resting
Self-care deficit related to pain and possible ruptured disc	States significant other has to help with self-care and ADL since acute pain has started; is unable to work	Uses assistance to move to new position; leans on someone's arms to move at times; has been on bed rest since acute pain began

3 PLAN

Patient goals

1. The patient will experience relief of back pain and sciatic neuritis following treatments.
2. The patient will regain satisfactory physical mobility and ROM of back, hips, and legs.

3. The patient will resume responsibility for self care.

4 IMPLEMENT

NURSING DIAGNOSIS	NURSING INTERVENTIONS	RATIONALE
Pain related to compression of sciatic nerve and possible ruptured disc	Assess types, amount, severity, duration, and characteristics of pain.	Provides basis for care; pain is common symptom.
	Maintain on bed rest, if ordered, with position of greatest comfort. Position may be side-lying on right side or recumbent with 45° flexion of hips and knees (Williams position) and pillow under knees.	Bed rest decreases inflammatory responses and eases pain and pressure. Williams position relaxes lumbosacral muscles, thereby decreasing muscle spasms and pain.
	Apply ice bags to lower back if desired.	Ice causes vasoconstriction and lessens edema; ice may not help some patients, therefore is individual choice.
	Offer back massage prn.	Massage increases circulation and aids removal of waste products; however, masage may increase muscle spasms for some patients.
	Administer muscle relaxants as ordered.	Muscle relaxants ease muscle spasms by decreasing response times to stimuli.
	Administer nonnarcotic analgesics as ordered (order should be for q 4 h to maintain therapeutic blood levels).	Analgesics relieve pain, soreness, and help decrease inflammation.
	Do "laminectomy checks": assess color, temperature, edema, movement, sensation, and capillary refill times.	Laminectomy neurovascular checks provide data related to progression or regression of pressure on nerves.

→ › ›

NURSING DIAGNOSIS	NURSING INTERVENTIONS	RATIONALE
	Apply pelvic belt traction if ordered; remove if pain or spasms increase.	Traction usually helps ease muscle spasms (see pages 192-203).
Impaired physical mobility related to compression of sciatic nerve and possible ruptured disc	Assess ROM, limitations of movement.	Indicates severity of condition and presence of muscle spasms.
	Encourage use of bed rest.	Bed rest decreases inflammation.
	Secure physician's order for use of diathermy (ultrasound), massage, exercise programs.	Ultrasound treatments and massage reach deeper muscles and joints to ease muscle tension and remove waste products. Exercise programs strengthen back, thigh, and abdominal muscles.
	Assist patient to apply back brace or canvas support when allowed up; teach self-application.	Brace or support may be used to provide external support for weak or injured muscles and joints. Self-application increases independence and activity.
	Remove and reapply pelvic belt traction as ordered (order may read in 2 h, out 2 h, out at night).	Pelvic belt traction helps ease muscle spasms to help person regain mobility.
Self-care deficit related to pain and possible ruptured disc	Assess effects of condition on ability to perform self-care.	Back spasms and pain limit patient's ability and/or willingness to perform self-care.
	Encourage discussions with family members or significant others about needed changes in roles or responsibilities.	Clarifying needed changes eases patient's concerns or lessens stress.
	Seek guidance from health team members to meet specific needs (social worker, occupational or physical therapists, vocational or educational counselors).	Specialists can provide vital information and guidance that others may not have.

5 EVALUATE

PATIENT OUTCOME	DATA INDICATING THAT OUTCOME IS REACHED
Patient experiences relief of back pain and sciatic neuritis following treatments.	Can move easily through various positions without pain or discomfort. Can do own ADL and is looking forward to return to employment.
The patient regains satisfactory physical mobility and ROM of hips, back, and legs.	Moves freely, goes up and down stairs; normal lordotic curve has returned; has no limitations of ROM of hips, lumbosacral joints, or knees.
Patient performs own self-care.	Patient is able to perform own hygienic care, dressing, and grooming; participates in household activities as needed.

PATIENT TEACHING

1. Teach patient/family members processes of and resolution of inflammation.
2. Teach patient/family members about purposes of bed rest, positions to relieve pain and inflammation, pelvic belt traction, and massage.
3. Teach patient/family members about purposes, effects, and side effects of medications.
4. Teach patient about proper exercises to strengthen back and abdominal muscles.
5. Teach principles of body mechanics to lessen chance of recurrence of disc problems.
6. Teach lifting, moving, and carrying techniques (or have them taught by proper therapists).

Hallux Valgus

Hallux valgus is a deformity in which the great toe (hallux) angulates away from the midline (valgus angulation) toward the second and other toes. At times the great toe may deviate over or under one or more of the toes.

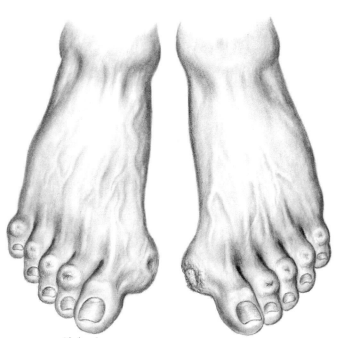

G.J.Wassilchenko

Hallux valgus is an osteoarthritic degenerative condition of the great toe. It becomes progressively worse and more painful, being aggravated by wearing shoes that are improperly fitting, are high heeled, or do not properly support the foot. Hallux valgus is more common in women, and there is a familial tendency for the condition. Adolescent girls also develop hallux valgus. The condition can also be associated with rheumatoid arthritis and osteoarthritis. Additionally, in nearly all cases of hallux valgus, a bunion develops at the first metatarsophalangeal (MTP) joint, which can become inflamed and then is very painful.

PATHOPHYSIOLOGY

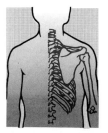

Hallux valgus develops secondary to OA of the first metatarsophalangeal (MTP) joint or to medial angulation of the first metatarsal bone. A "flat" foot also contributes to HV because a fallen or dropped longitudinal arch causes dorsiflexion of the first cuneiform-metatarsal joint, with the distal end of the first metatarsal bone becoming displaced dorsally and medially, causing the adductor hallucis tendon to draw the big toe laterally or in a valgus direction. The great toe may ride over or under the second toe, and the other toes are crowded, leading at times to the development of hammer toe, claw toe, or mallet toe. The angulation and degeneration of the first MTP joint may lead to development of a bunion on the medial side of the first MTP. A bunion is an inflamed bursa, which forms adventitiously at the first MTP because of pressure and inflammation. There may also be valgus deviation of the heel.

Hallux valgus can progress to become hallux rigidus, which is narrowing and rigidity of the MTP joint, making joint flexion extremely painful and subsequently lost from bone spurs in the MTP joint. Hallux rigidus is more common in men.

COMPLICATIONS

Development of bunion
Stress fracture
Degenerative joint disease

DIAGNOSTIC STUDIES AND FINDINGS

Diagnostic Test	Findings
X-rays	Lateral (valgus) displacement of great toe; degenerative arthritic joint changes; varus displacement of first metatarsal bone; splaying of metatarsal bones; bone spurs may be noted; first metatarsal deviated away from second metatarsal.

MEDICAL MANAGEMENT

SURGERY*

Osteotomy to realign bones; Wedge resection or arthrodesis of affected joints
Transfer of insertion of abductor hallucis tendon to a more medial and distal position; Removal of medial bony prominence, if present; Arthroplasty of first metatarsal joint; Bunionectomy.

DRUG THERAPY

Analgesic-antipyretic agents: Aspirin, 600-1000 mg qid, Acetaminophen, 600-1000 mg qid

Intra-articular injection of corticosteroids, doses individualized.

GENERAL MANAGEMENT

Wearing shoes with enlarged toe portions or lower heels; Placing felt ring or covering cap around bunion area may relieve pressure; Taping pads under metatarsal heads to change weight bearing pressure; Application of moist compresses to bursitis area; Foot exercises to lessen splay foot; Application of ice to site of bunion to lessen pain and inflammation; Rest to affected joints; Application of felt pads over corns.

*Over 100 different or variations of techniques are available for correction or treatment of hallux valgus.

1   ASSESS

ASSESSMENT	OBSERVATIONS
Posture and gait	Stance is slouched; walks favoring one side or foot; steps somewhat hesitantly at a normal pace

ASSESSMENT	OBSERVATIONS
Feet (bilaterally)	Deformities: valgus deviations of forefoot bones and heels; has hammer, claw, or mallet toes; corns and callouses; bunion—has redness, heat, and edema; fallen longitudinal arch and splay foot
Age and sex	Women have more hallux valgus; men have more hallux rigidus
OA in other joints	OA may be present in weight-bearing joints of hip, knee and in fingers (DIP and PIP joints) and spinal column
Complaints of pain	Pain in great toe, hip, and down to knee, worse with use

2 DIAGNOSE

NURSING DIAGNOSIS	SUBJECTIVE FINDINGS	OBJECTIVE FINDINGS
Impaired physical mobility related to pain and deformity	Reports pain and soreness when standing or walking; tires with minimal mobility; shoes increase pain and tenderness around metatarsal joints.	Walks with limited flexion of metatarsal joints; forefoot splays when walking; valgus deviation of great toe with varus deformity of first metatarsal bone; flatfooted; corns on toes and metatarsal joints.
Pain related to bunion and bursitis	Reports exquisite, throbbing pain when standing, walking, and at times at rest; pressure of shoes increases pain and tenderness.	Redness, edema, and bulging of first MTP joint; area hot to touch; shoe bulged outward at first MTP joint.
Body image disturbance related to deformities	States is ashamed of "ugly" feet; is reluctant to go barefoot; also states it's difficult to find comfortable, stylish shoes.	Covers feet quickly and frequently during examination.

3 PLAN

Patient goals

1. The patient will have painless ambulation after treatment of hallux valgus.
2. The patient will be relieved of pain from bunions and bursitis.

3. The patient will have an improved body image.

4 IMPLEMENT

NURSING DIAGNOSIS	NURSING INTERVENTIONS	RATIONALE
Impaired physical mobility related to pain and deformity	Assess effects of condition on mobility.	Assessment aids in developing care.
	Assist with application of felt rings, felt pads, or other orthoses to affected areas.	Pliability of feet lessens pressure over tender areas and changes weight-bearing surfaces.

→ > >

NURSING DIAGNOSIS	NURSING INTERVENTIONS	RATIONALE
	Encourage ambulation and standing when soreness is lessened.	Increased mobility improves patient's outlook and ability to perform ADLs.
	Encourage consultation with physician for possible surgical corrective procedures.	Surgical correction may be needed to prevent further degenerative changes, to lessen pain, and to correct deformities to increase mobility.
	Encourage use of analgesic medications (aspirin is commonly prescribed).	Analgesics relieve pain and are antiinflammatory to lessen bursitis.
	Encourage wearing of proper footwear (e.g., low heels, soft shoe materials).	Lower heels lessen pressure on balls of feet and joints to lessen aggravation of condition.
Pain related to bunion and bursitis	Assess for redness, edema, heat, and amount and duration of pain.	Assessment aids in care. Bursitis is secondary to increased pressure, leading to development of protective bursa around MTP joint of great toe. Pain results from pressure on nerve endings and is usually intermittent in hallux valgus when person is not actively putting pressure over inflamed area.
	Encourage rest or cessation of weight bearing during acute pain episodes.	Rest and removing pressure by temporarily ceasing weight bearing lessens inflammation and pain.
	Administer analgesic medications qid.	Analgesics relieve pain, and if antiinflammatory, lessen inflammation of bursa.
	Apply ice bag to MTP joint; elevate foot if edema present.	Ice relieves edema and lessens pain by relieving pressure on nerve endings.
Body image disturbance related to deformities	Assess effects of deformities on body image. Encourage patient to verbalize concerns about deformities of feet.	Visible deformities can adversely affect patient's body image. Verbalization helps clarify patient's understandings and feelings.
	Encourage consulting with physician about management of deformities; encourage patient to perform exercises or other measures suggested by physician.	Seeking professional advice and guidance is a positive step toward patient's acceptance of condition.
	Clarify proposed surgical procedure if needed; provide preoperative and postoperative care and explanations.	Understanding of benefits and risks aids patient's participation in and positive outlook on recovery and rehabilitation.

5 EVALUATE

PATIENT OUTCOME	DATA INDICATING THAT OUTCOME IS REACHED
Patient has painless ambulation.	Patient ambulates easily and comfortably (after healing or treatment) and needs no analgesic medications.
Patient has relief from pain.	Padding and orthoses heal corns and callouses; bunion removed surgically.
Patient has positive body image.	Patient states feels more positive about "better-looking" feet; is more outgoing and active and returns to usual activities; wears well-fitting shoe with heel height according to physician's guidelines; goes barefoot at appropriate times.

PATIENT TEACHING

1. Explain deformities, presence of bunion and bursitis.
2. Teach application of felt rings or pads or other orthoses to prevent progression of deformities.
3. Instruct about use of proper footwear and exercises.
4. Clarify surgical options previously discussed with physician if needed. Explain that surgical wounds should heal fully with minimal scarring after maturation. Condition should not recur if proper footwear is worn (some adolescents may have recurrence in later years).

CHAPTER 7

Infectious Musculoskeletal Conditions

Osteomyelitis

Osteomyelitis is an infection of the bone and its marrow.

The development of osteomyelitis is of great concern in any patient with an open wound, sore throat, or other systemic infection that can be transmitted to bones. The infection can remain undetected for months, during which time it establishes a firm hold in the affected bone and surrounding tissues. With diagnosis, osteomyelitis usually requires long-term, extensive treatment and follow-up to prevent recurrent flares.

Osteomyelitis may develop from blood-borne pathogens deposited at a site, usually in the metaphyseal area of a bone. Hematogenous spread secondary to a sore (strep) throat is most common in infants and children who develop osteomyelitis. Young or older adults who develop the infection usually have experienced open trauma or have a debilitating, systemic disease such as diabetes or peripheral vascular disease. People with sickle cell disease and those with malignancies also are at increased risk for osteomyelitis.

The organism that causes most cases of osteomyelitis is *Staphylococcus aureus*, which accounts for 90% of osteomyelitic infections. Streptococci cause the second largest number; other agents are *Pseudomonas aeruginosa, Haemophilus influenzae, Escherichia coli, Clostridium perfringens, Salmonella typhi,* and *Neisseria gonorrhoeae.*

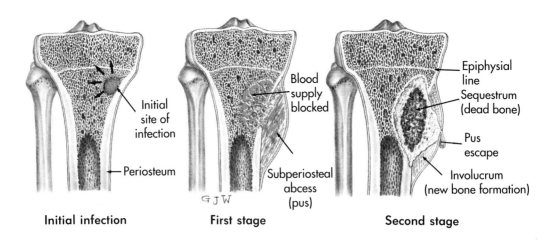

Initial site of infection

Periosteum

Initial infection

GJW

Blood supply blocked

Subperiosteal abcess (pus)

First stage

Epiphysial line

Sequestrum (dead bone)

Pus escape

Involucrum (new bone formation)

Second stage

ANATOMIC TYPES OF ADULT OSTEOMYELITIS

Type I   Medullary osteomyelitis: Primary lesion is endosteal.

Type II   Superficial osteomyelitis: Surface of bone is infected.

Type III Localized osteomyelitis: Bone cortex and osteum are infected; there may be cortical sequestration and cavity formation; possible extension to medullary portion of bone.

Type IV   Diffuse osteomyelitis: Disease spreads through bone and soft tissue; it is circumferential and permeative through bone.

PATHOPHYSIOLOGY

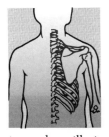

The infection develops in the metaphyseal area in direct proportion to the rate of growth and the size of the bone; i.e., the longer and larger the bone, the more susceptible it is to osteomyelitis. The infection develops as the pathogenic organisms become trapped in small end arteries and capillaries in the metaphyseal area. As the organisms proliferate, they block blood flow, causing an area of the bone to become necrotic. An inflammatory reaction occurs with hyperemia, an influx of polymorphonuclear leukocytes into the area to combat the pathogens. Because of these reactions, pain may be noted, as the exudate and purulent material enlarge and cause pressure in the rigid walls of the infected bone. More blood vessels are compressed, and more bone cells become necrotic. There is flow of exudate and purulent material by "least resistance" into subperiosteal spaces. The periosteum of the involved bone attempts to keep the infection localized and walled off by forming new bone trabeculae. Deprived of its periosteal blood supply, the cortex of the bone becomes necrotic, the purulent material breaks through to the soft tissue around the bone, and the infection spreads along fascial planes into the surrounding area. As the quantity of purulent material and exudate grows, it eventually forms a track through the soft tissues to the skin surface, or it may spread inside the bone to the bone marrow through the medullary canal. Dead pieces or parts of bone may become surrounded by purulent material. The dead bone is called sequestrum. Small pieces of sequestrum can be absorbed by osteoclastic activity and by granulation tissue. If the sequestra are large, they must be removed or they become sources of continual infection. New bone, called involucrum, may surround the sequestra in an attempt to heal the area; however, sequestra prevent full healing in most instances. Occasionally, the invading pathogens are insufficient in number or of lesser virulence and may form only a small abscess, which can be walled off and surrounded by fibrous tissue and a ring of dense bone. Such an area is called Brodie's abscess. The organisms within the abscess may remain alive and virulent, causing a flare-up reinfection at any time, or they may die, with the resultant cavity being filled with serum and blood.

The bones most commonly involved in osteomyelitic infections are the lower end of the femur, the upper ends of the tibia and humerus and, less often, the vertebrae. The knee is the joint most often involved, but the hip joint can also develop osteomyelitis secondary to total joint replacement.

Osteomyelitis most frequently develops from hematogenous spread, but it may also develop from lowered oxygen tension associated with sickle cell anemia, from open wounds, or from soft tissue infections that spread to bones.

Acute infections may become chronic with insufficient or inadequate treatment, and when sequestra separate and become extruded through draining sinuses to the exterior of the infected area. Chronic infections can drain repeatedly or may become active many years after previous infections.

COMPLICATIONS

Chronic osteomyelitis, which may require amputation

Brodie's abscess

DIAGNOSTIC STUDIES AND FINDINGS

Diagnostic test	Findings
Laboratory Tests	
White blood cell count	Markedly elevated (up to 30,000 total WBCs; normal: 5000-9,000); polymorphonuclear neutrophils are increased to 80% of total WBCs (normal: 50%-70%)
Culture of drainage or purulent material	Usually determines infecting pathogens
Blood culture	Bacteremia or septicemia
Teichoic acid antibody test	Antibodies appear two weeks after infection (Teichoic acid is a cell-wall component of *S. aureus*); test may remain positive even with antibiotic use
Erythrocyte sedimentation rate	Elevated above normal range
Tuberculin skin test	Positive if osteomyelitis is caused by tubercle bacillus
X-rays	May be negative in first 7-10 days; thereafter may show localized destruction with surrounding zone of decalcified bone; Eventually reveal raised periosteum, destruction of trabeculae, and moth-eaten appearance of bone with multiple erosions; sequestrum, if present, appears denser than surrounding bone
CT scan	Findings same as with x-rays; CT may detect bone changes when standard x-rays appear normal or unremarkable; CT also can show spread to contiguous soft tissues[107]
MRI	Aids in determining extent of acute or chronic osteomyelitis
Bone scintigraphy	Technetium-99m (^{99m}Tc) scan shows increased uptake if done in three-phase scan

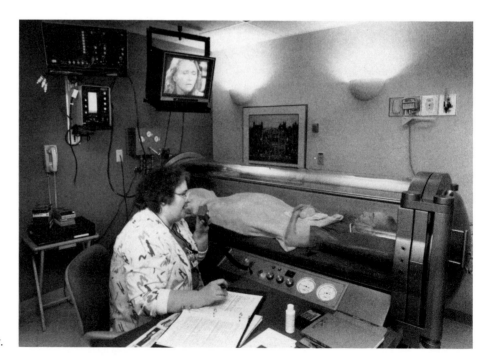

FIGURE 7-1
Hyperbaric oxygen chamber.

MEDICAL MANAGEMENT

GENERAL MANAGEMENT

No smoking (causes vasoconstriction and decreases blood flow to area).

Splint or sling to support joints and extremity to prevent fracture of weakened bones.

Nutritional supplementation: Increased intake of proteins, and vitamins A, B, and C to enhance cell regeneration.

Control of chronic conditions: Regulation of blood glucose level for diabetes; corrective arterial procedures for arteriosclerosis obliterans; elimination or treatment of drug abuse and alcohol intake, if possible; use of gamma-globulin to increase immune competence, if feasible.

Bed rest as needed to conserve energy or decrease venous stasis.

SURGERY

Holes are drilled into affected bone to localize sites of exudate; overlying infected bone is removed; cavity is loosely packed for drainage purposes and to keep the wound open.

Catheter(s) are inserted into site of osteomyelitis for instillation or irrigation with antibiotics.

External fixation devices such as Hoffman apparatus (see page 204) may be used to stabilize bones to prevent fracture.

Scraping (saucerization) of necrotic bone cells and scar tissue to provide a healthy surface for regeneration of bone or a site for bone grafts, which will be done after bone is "sterilized" of pathogens.

Hyperbaric oxygen treatments of 100% oxygen, 2 atmospheres (atm) pressure, 2 h duration, 1 dive/day, 6 dives/wk—30 used for chronic refractory osteomyelitis (Figure 7-1).

or oxygen therapy to 2.4 atm with humidified 100% oxygen for 90 min divided into three 30-min sessions daily.[30]

Microsurgical free-muscle transfer to cover wound and obliterate dead space.[109]

Amputation of limb for life-threatening, refractory, persistent infections (fortunately, less often needed in recent years because of more vigorous initial treatment).

DRUG THERAPY

Antibiotics (Type and dosage individualized according to patient's age, pathogenic organism, and patient's sensitivity or allergy): Aqueous penicillin, 500,000-1 million U, IV q 6 h continuously for 10-30 days or longer; cephalosporin (cephalothin or Keflin), 1 g IV q 6 h; erythromycin (Erythrocin), 1-2 g IV q 6 h (for penicillin-sensitive patients) or tetracycline, 500,000 U to 1-2 g, IV q 6 h; ampicillin (Omnipen), 1 g IV q 6 h.

If patient is severely ill or compromised: Ticarcillin (Ticar), 3 g IV q 4 h; cefazolin (Ancef), 2 g IV q 6 h or garamycin (Gentamicin), 5 mg/kg/day IV.

Tetanus toxoid, hyperimmune serum, or tetanus antitoxin, given at time of initial open wound to prevent tetanus infection.

Aspirin, 600 mg q 4 h, for pyrexia, (adult); if child, acetaminophen, 300-600 mg for pyrexia > 39° C (102° F).

1 ASSESS

ASSESSMENT	OBSERVATIONS
Area over involved bone (for signs of inflammation)	Tender, reddened, warm, edematous area over involved bone; mass felt at site; purulent drainage
Position of part	Part involved held in flexion; hesitant to move part
Possible systemic signs of infection	Fever ranging from 39-40° C (103-104° F), chills, diaphoresis, fatigue or malaise, headache, and nausea

ASSESSMENT	OBSERVATIONS
Presence of chronic disease	Blood sugar in normal values, weak peripheral pulses, skin over area shiny and atrophic with purulent drainage present
Spread to distant sites	Complains of backache, tender knee joint, and weak leg muscles

2 DIAGNOSE

NURSING DIAGNOSIS	SUBJECTIVE FINDINGS	OBJECTIVE FINDINGS
Impaired physical mobility related to presence of infection (osteomyelitis)	States area is very tender and painful; hurts to use the extremity	Holds affected extermity in flexion; very hesitant to straighten limb or put weight on it; limps when using leg
Pain related to pressure of expanding mass and purulent material	States area is very sore and painful to touch; can feel a bulge in area	Fluctuant mass can be palpated; winces when area is palpated and when joint distal to site is extended
Altered peripheral tissue perfusion related to infection and mass	States area is redder and hotter than normal and area around bulge is swollen	Skin around area is red and hot on palpation; moderate edema around area; peripheral pulses are all weakly palpated in affected limb; capillary refill in 2 sec (normal)
Impaired skin integrity related to infection, drainage, or surgical intervention (insertion of catheter at site)	States dressings and catheters make limb feel heavy and hard to move	Has extensive dressing over site with two catheters visible outside dressing; skin distal to dressing is cool and pale but intact
Hyperthermia related to local and systemic infection	States feels hot all over body and has chills at times; has headache and feels very tired and weak at times	Temperatures 38.8-39.5° C (102-103° F); pulse rates 88-96; respiratory rates 24-28/min; skin flushed; appears very tired and weak
Body image disturbance related to extent of pathology	Expresses concern about how long infection was present; how long treatment will last; whether infection will go away or if there will be lingering infection; possible loss of job because of length of time off work	Keeps limb covered when in halls; has been on continuous IV antibiotic therapy for 10 days; catheters visible when up in wheel chair; frequently noticed looking out windows of nursing unit with distant look in eyes; asks questions of health team members on each contact

3 PLAN

Patient goals

1. The patient's osteomyelitis will be eradicated, and physical mobility will be regained.
2. The patient's pain and discomfort will be relieved.
3. The patient will regain normal tissue perfusion.
4. The patient will regain intact skin tissues.
5. The patient's body temperature will return to normal.
6. The patient will regain a healthy body image.

4   IMPLEMENT

NURSING DIAGNOSIS	NURSING INTERVENTIONS	RATIONALE
Impaired physical mobility related to presence of infection	Assess ROM of joints and ability to bear weight.	Activity maintains musculoskeletal strength. Rest to affected part decreases spread of purulent material.
	Help patient move affected tissues.	Assistance maintains comfort and use of part.
	Encourage ROM for unaffected parts.	ROM movements maintain strength of muscles and joints and prevent atrophy of tissues.
	Encourage self-care as able; assist as needed.	Self-care maintains independence and strength.
	Assist with use of ambulatory aid if allowed out of bed.	Ambulation maintains body functions, prevents loss of strength, and helps patient maintain interactions and socialization.
	Encourage hobbies and diversionary activities.	Helps maintain interactions, interest, hopefulness, and positive outlook.
Pain related to pressure of expanding mass and purulent material	Assess type of pain, amount, duration, character, constancy, and site.	Helps determine degree or type of pain.
	Maintain rest/activity patterns as required.	Rest and activity moderate stress on involved tissues to permit healing.
	Handle affected tissues gently; use splint or sling as needed.	Careful handling of tissues, plus supporting the joints above and below, help the patient deal with pain by showing care and concern.
	Help the patient modify position in bed or chair; help him to move q 2 h.	Altering positions relieves tired muscles and joints and maintains circulation.
	Administer analgesics as ordered and needed; monitor responses to medications.	Analgesics relieve pain; they must be given in sufficient doses and in continuous patterns (q 3-4 h) to maintain therapeutic blood levels.
	Administer antibiotics as ordered; monitor responses to antibiotics per laboratory tests, vital signs.	Antibiotics rid the body of pathogens; they must be given IV to maintain constant, high therapeutic blood levels for 6 wk or longer; when infection is relieved, pain is relieved (WBC count, temperature, pulse rates, and respirations should return to normal).
	Carefully initiate IV therapy for administration of antibiotics; use aseptic technique; monitor therapy over time.	Careful insertion of IV needle or catheter lessens pain, helps patient accept therapy, and maintains venous integrity; aseptic technique prevents nosocomial infections (patient is more susceptible because of presence of infection).

→ ➤ ➤

NURSING DIAGNOSIS	NURSING INTERVENTIONS	RATIONALE
	Encourage activities to divert attention, (e.g., go to playroom, if patient is a child; take patient to lounge, lobby, or outside; use puzzles or games).	Diversion and change of scenery can take patient's mind off present situation and lessen pain responses.
Altered peripheral tissue perfusion related to infection and mass	Perform neurovascular checks (see inside front cover).	(See Appendix for rationale of checks).
	Encourage deep-breathing and coughing exercises q 4 h; monitor pain and pain relief.	Deep breathing and coughing increase oxygen intake to enhance tissue perfusion; pain is frequently caused by ischemia or anoxia, signs of altered tissue perfusion.
Impaired skin integrity related to infection, drainage, or surgical interventions	Assess skin tissues over body.	Helps determine present condition and need for corrective measures.
	Perform wound care or catheter irrigations as ordered with strict aseptic technique.	Wound care cleanses tissues of drainage to help skin regain tissue integrity; irrigations remove exudate to clear infection and remove drainage from site; aseptic technique prevents nosocomial infections.
	Turn or reposition patient q 2 h.	Turning increases circulation to tissues and relieves pressure.
	Remove splint or sling q 2-4 h; adjust as needed.	Equipment must be removed to check skin tissues for signs of pressure.
Hyperthermia related to local and systemic infection	Assess vital signs q 1-2 h as needed; note presence of chills and diaphoresis; recheck vital signs during and after chill or diaphoresis.	Fever is a sign of presence of pathogens; it may rise and fall quickly, necessitating frequent checks; chills may accompany bacteremic or septicemic situations before rises in temperature; diaphoresis indicates a drop in temperature to help body rid itself of higher temperature.
	Administer antibiotics as ordered.	Antibiotics rid body of pathogens to permit return to normal vital signs.
	Administer antipyretic medications if ordered (may be ordered for temperatures over 39-40° C (102-103° F).	Antipyretic medications lower body temperatures; lower temperatures lessen possibility of convulsions, especially with children.
	Change patient's clothing or bed linens after diaphoresis.	Diaphoresis causes mild to severe perspiring, which dampens clothing and linens and can cause skin maceration.
Body image disturbance related to extent of pathology	Assess concerns related to condition, treatments, or possible outcomes.	Treatment must be aggressive and continue for long periods for complete cure; recurrences are common with repeated antibiotic therapy, surgical removal of infected bone and soft tissues; at times (although less commonly now) amputation may be required; patient may suffer long-term disability.

NURSING DIAGNOSIS	NURSING INTERVENTIONS	RATIONALE
	Listen to patient express feelings about new or additional treatments; explain need for and purposes of treatments over time. Repeat as necessary.	Recurrence of infection may require additional therapy; anxiety may prevent patient from hearing or totally understanding explanations at times.
	Monitor patient's reactions to treatments.	Helps determine or need for change in treatment
Knowledge deficit	See Patient Teaching.	

5 EVALUATE

PATIENT OUTCOME	DATA INDICATING THAT OUTCOME IS REACHED
Patient's osteomyelitis has been eradicated, and patient has regained physical mobility.	Blood and local wound cultures are negative for pathogens; x-rays show no remaining foci of infection; no sequestra remain in site; patient walks easily without ambulatory aid; vital signs are within normal ranges.
Patient's pain and discomfort have been relieved.	Patient uses no analgesics.
Patient has regained normal tissue perfusion.	Skin is pink, firm, and without edema or ischemic changes; peripheral pulses and capillary refill are normal.
Patient has regained intact skin tissues.	Skin wounds are well approximated; there is no drainage.
Patient's fever has disappeared.	Body temperature is approximately 37° C (98.6° F).
Patient has regained a healthy body image.	Patient expresses positive feelings about past infection; is forward looking.

PATIENT TEACHING

1. Explain the disorder osteomyelitis, using appropriate pictures as needed.
2. Describe and explain the purposes for each treatment.
3. Explain long-term antibiotic therapy and the side effects of antibiotics.
4. Explain aseptic technique and its purpose (i.e., preventing nosocomial infections in a compromised patient).
5. Explain what symptoms require medical attention after the patient has been sent home.
6. Explain the technique for and purposes of range of motion (i.e., exercises to maintain strength of musculoskeletal tissues).

Wound Infections

Superficial or deep wound infections are severe complications of the patient's injuries or diseases or are secondary to the treatments of the patient's conditions. Wound infections can lead to osteomyelitis of involved skin and bones or can lead to deep joint infections.

SUPERFICIAL WOUND INFECTIONS

Superficial infections include wound infections, abscesses, carbuncles, and cellulitis. A *wound infection* is one that is localized at the site of an open wound caused by traumatic penetration or a surgical incision. An *abscess* is a localized collection of purulent material that may be in or near skin surfaces, such as in a surgical wound; an abscess also may develop in visceral tissues, as in the case of a subdiaphragmatic or pelvic abscess. A *carbuncle* is a localized abscess around a hair follicle or sweat gland. *Cellulitis* is inflammation of the interstitial cells around an open area, usually as a result of direct inoculation through the skin opening. Cellulitis may be only an inflammatory condition, or the inflamed tissues may become infected, as in gas gangrene.

The infecting organism is most commonly is *Staphylococcus aureus* (see also box below). Treatments include the following:

Warm compresses or warm soaks
Incision and drainage of purulent material
Irrigation and packing of wound q 4-6 h prn
Administration of oral antibiotics (may or may not be given, depending on extent of wound infection)

DEEP WOUND INFECTIONS

Deep infections may be the result of surgical exposure itself or secondary to an undiagnosed, occult infection such as a sore throat, infected sinuses or tooth, pneumonia, or urinary tract infection. Predisposition to the development of a deep wound infection includes diabetes or arteriosclerosis because of compromised immune competence and circulation.

Signs of deep wound infection include red, edematous wound in and around operative area; drainage from wound that may be serous or purulent; elevated temperature at site and systemically; pain at rest, aggravated by ambulation; elevated WBC counts; wound culture may or may not reveal offending organisms. The diagnostic studies include sinogram and injection of radiopaque dye, should show presence of purulent material around and in joint.

Treatments are similar to those discussed for osteomyelitis and superficial wound infections with some differences: A cephalosporin antibiotic will be used instead of a penicillin-type medication; it is initially given intravenously and then orally for 6-9 mo. Joint or wound internal fixation or implant devices are removed, since they are foreign bodies that resist antibiotic therapy; after infection has cleared up (wound cultures must test negative or be sterile), replacement surgery may be performed.

NURSING CARE

See pages 123 to 127

PATHOGENS ASSOCIATED WITH WOUND INFECTIONS AND OSTEOMYELITIS

Staphylococcus aureus
Streptococcus pyogenes
Pseudomonas aeruginosa
Escherichia coli
Clostridium perfringens
Salmonella typhi

Neisseria gonorrhoeae
Mycobacterium tuberculosis
Staphylococcus epidermidis
Treponema pallidum
Coccidioides immitis

CHAPTER 8

Metabolic Musculoskeletal Conditions

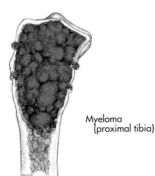

Myeloma
(proximal tibia)

Proximal
humerus

Proximal
femur

Fractures

Multiple myeloma
spine

Metabolic bone diseases are those that result in loss of or inadequate bone mineralization, bone mass, bone structure or shape, or an increased rate of demineralization. These diseases are of endocrine, dietary, or disuse origins primarily, although trauma may also be involved.

Osteoporosis

Osteoporosis is a systemic condition of overall reduction in bone mass or density when bone resorption is more extensive than bone deposition, upsetting the normal balance.

Osteoporosis is the most common human metabolic bone disease. It occurs in approximately 30% of all women over 45 years of age and is present in 70% of women over age 45 who experience bone fractures. Os-

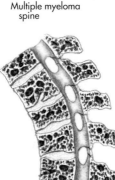

Bone marrow
tumor (femur)

GJW.

teoporosis is most common in postmenopausal women; however, younger people can also develop osteoporosis secondary to immobility following severe injuries and paralysis. Men develop osteoporosis in a ratio of 1:4 (men:women).

The annual cost of osteoporosis is more than $6 billion for acute and convalescent care.[59] More than a million fractures occur each year; about 40% are vertebral fractures, 20% are femoral (hip) fractures, 15% are distal forearm fractures, and the remainder occur in other skeletal sites.[59] Femoral fractures about the hip are fatal in approximately 10% to 20% of patients.

PATHOPHYSIOLOGY

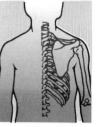

People with osteoporosis have normal bones but have less overall bone quantity and less bone density. This relative loss of bone density leads to frequent bone fractures, even with minor trauma or routine activities (Figure 8-1). In bones with osteoporosis, trabecular (cancellous) bone is more porous, and cortical bone is thinner. Recent estimations indicate that, over a lifetime, a woman loses about 35% of cortical bone mass

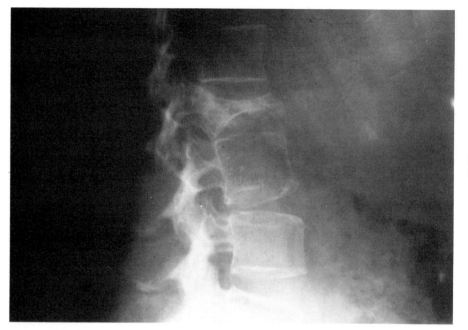

FIGURE 8-1
Compression fracture.

DIAGNOSTIC STUDIES AND FINDINGS

Diagnostic test	Findings
X-rays	May not show changes until more than 30% of skeletal calcium has been lost[46a]
Single-photon absorptiometry (SPA) or dual-photon absorptiometry (DPA)	Can measure skeletal "density" in two dimensions to show loss of trabecular bone (DPA), cortical bone in distal forearm (SPA); DPA can detect early loss of trabecular bone even with normal SPA: may show wedging, compression
Quantitative computed tomographic (QCT) scanning	Measures density of vertebral bone to correlate trabecular bone strength with strength of whole vertebral bodies
CT	Possibly vertebral fracture, herniated intervertebral disk, biconcave vertebral bodies, and increased curvature of thoracic vertebrae (kyphosis) or lumbar vertebrae (excess lordosis)
Blood serum study	Low levels of alkaline phosphatase

and 50% of trabecular bone mass. Beginning in the third and fourth decades, there is a yearly loss of 0.3% to 0.5%, which is accelerated to 2% to 3% with menopause. Continued loss of 0.3% to 0.5% is associated with aging over the latter years of a person's life. The age-related bone loss is the result of impaired osteoblastic functions, with less bone formation for a given degree of resorption. Also, with aging, calcium absorption is impaired, and vitamin D formation decreases because of lack of estrogen.[86] Parathyroid hormone activity also is somewhat altered, possibly because of high phosphate intake. A decrease in dietary intake of calcium, leading to calcium deficiency in the body, is a major contributing cause to the development of osteoporosis. Lack of weight-bearing activities and exercise and physical inactivity are other contributing factors; however, excessive exercise (e.g., running more than 40 miles per week) in young women may cause low bone mineral (calcium) density because of altered menstrual function and estrogen levels. Other risk factors for osteoporosis include smoking (women who smoke an average of 12 cigarettes a day have lower serum estrogen, even when taking oral supplements); alcohol abuse, which may lead to osteoporosis in some alcoholic individuals; and use of corticosteroids, which induce osteoporosis because they depress activity of osteoblasts (the bone-building cells)—these drugs account for more loss of trabecular bone than cortical bone. Lastly, caffeine intake affects bone loss (2 cups of caffeinated coffee per day can cause a net daily loss of 6 mg of calcium).[59] Also, people who have red or blonde hair and freckles run a greater risk of developing osteoporosis.[46a]

COMPLICATIONS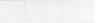

Fractures of vertebrae, hip, wrist
Respiratory compromise

Table 8-1

CALCIUM CONTENT OF SELECTED FOODS

Produce or food	Serving size	Calcium (mg)
Cheese, cottage	½ cup	90
Cheese, cheddar	1 oz	213
Cheese, Swiss	1 oz	262
Ice cream	½ cup	97
Ice milk	½ cup	102
Milk, 2%	1 cup	297
Milk, skim	1 cup	296
Milk, nonfat dry	1 Tbsp	52
Yogurt, low fat, plain	1 cup	400
Yogurt, low fat, with fruit	1 cup	350
Broccoli	1 stalk	158
Collard greens, cooked	1 cup	289
Salmon, canned, with bones	3 oz	167
Sardines, in oil, with bones	3 oz	372
Spinach, cooked	1 cup	167
Tofu, bean curd	3½ oz	128
Beans, navy, cooked	1 cup	95
Beans, red kidney	1 cup	74
Farina, cooked	1 cup	147
Muffin, bran	1 muffin	57
Shrimp, canned	3 oz	100
Molasses, blackstrap	1 tbsp	135
Milk chocolate bar	1 oz	65

MEDICAL MANAGEMENT

GENERAL MANAGEMENT

Nutritious diet with at least 1 g of elemental calcium per day.[59]

Individualized program of moderate exercise such as walking, swimming, stationary bike riding, or physical therapy exercises for those who are immobilized or paralyzed.

Application of back corset or neck support to prevent stress fractures.

DRUG THERAPY

Nutritional supplements: Calcium intake to 1,500 mg/day (see Table 8-1 for dietary sources of calcium); calcium carbonate (Os Cal) or with sodium fluoride, 40-60 mg/day (Os Cal-Fluor); vitamin D, 50,000 IU, 1-2 times/wk.

Estrogen/progestin combinations (estrogen, 0.625 mg/day for 25 days, with medroxyprogesterone, 10 mg for last 10 days of cycle [norethindrone, 2.5-5 mg may be used in place of medroxyprogesterone]). **NOTE:** There is an increased risk of endometrial and breast cancer with the use of estrogens, as well as cardiovascular complications.

Calcitonin, 100 U qid IM

Experimental therapies: Coherence therapy or ADFR (A, Activate osteoblasts; D, Depress activity of osteoclasts; F, Free osteoblasts to form bone; and R, Repeat the treatment). Medications used for ADFR include phosphates to activate osteoblasts and induce release of endogenous parathyroid hormone; calcitonin and sodium diphosphonate to depress the osteoclasts; and calcium or vitamin D or both to calcify newly formed bone.[2] Etidronate (Didronel), currently under study, has been shown to strengthen bones and help prevent fractures in menopausal women (used during the "D" phase of ADFR therapy).

1   ASSESS

ASSESSMENT	OBSERVATIONS
Risk factors	Menopausal woman; positive family history; red or blonde hair (although may be graying); freckles; prolonged immobility or decreased physical activity; decreased calcium intake; intake of alcohol or caffeine; smoking
Posture and gait	Increased thoracic kyphotic curve and lumbar lordotic curve; varus position of legs and feet; steps guardedly and slowly; hands used to aid walking and pressed to lower back as if to ease pain
Height, weight, and body build	Loss of height (e.g., ½-inch loss compared with 3 years ago); thin; low weight and bone mass
Complaints of pain	Moderate to severe pain in thoracic, vertebral, or lumbar areas (may radiate to neck, arms, hips, or legs); may have fractures of distal radius, vertebrae in lower back or hip; may have herniated intervertebral disk

2 DIAGNOSE

NURSING DIAGNOSIS	SUBJECTIVE FINDINGS	OBJECTIVE FINDINGS
Impaired physical mobility related to presence of osteoporosis	States has difficulty walking easily because of back and neck aches and pains; complains of difficulty rising from bed or chairs and getting in and out of cars	Has marked kyphosis and excessive lordosis; has increased varus angle of hips and legs (feet very close together when standing, and foot is placed directly in front of opposite foot when stepping); rises slowly from chair, supporting self with hands on chair or table
Pain related to vertebral body density loss	Reports burning pain in upper chest and neck, plus aching, constant pain in lumbar area of back; takes prescribed medications to ease pain	Winces when neck (nape), ribs, and spinal column are palpated
Anxiety related to fear of possible fracture	Reports participation in activities (e.g., lifting) and/or jobs that require strenuous physical activity	DPA shows marked loss of bone density in vertebral bodies, with concavity and loss of vertebral body mass and height.
Body image disturbance related to kyphosis and lordosis	States can't wear close-fitting clothes because of deformity of back; states clothes don't hang right; reports difficulty holding head upright without pain	Hemlines noticeably uneven; dress shorter in back; curvature easily noted even with loose gown; head flexed forward; unable to stand straight
Impaired gas exchange related to kyphosis	Reports difficulty taking deep breaths and coughing	Diminished breath sounds in all lobes; weak cough producing small amount of clear mucus; mild dyspnea; respiratory rate 24/min

3 PLAN

Patient goals

1. The patient will have satisfactory physical mobility.
2. The patient's pain will be relieved.
3. The patient will reduce risk of bone fractures.
4. The patient will accept altered body image.
5. The patient will maintain satisfactory gas exchange.

4 IMPLEMENT

NURSING DIAGNOSIS	NURSING INTERVENTIONS	RATIONALE
Impaired physical mobility related to presence of osteoporosis	Assess mobility, gait, ability to rise from bed or chair.	Assessment is the basis for care.
	Help patient change positions as needed.	Assistance is a safety measure since minor twists or turns can precipitate a fracture in osteoporotic bones.

→ › ›

NURSING DIAGNOSIS	NURSING INTERVENTIONS	RATIONALE
	Offer use of cane or crutches; teach patient safe use of each aid.	A cane or crutch eases muscle soreness or strain on ligaments and bones.
	If ordered, apply neck support, back belt, or corset.	Othotic devices aid mobility by easing strain on weakened bones and joints. (Use of supports is controversial, since they limit muscle movements and can lead to weakening of muscles.)
	Do ROM exercises actively with patient or do passive ROM exercises if needed; exercises may include quadriceps or gluteal setting, ankle/foot dorsiflexion, plantar flexion, and rotation and triceps setting.	Exercises help maintain muscle strength and ROM of joints, and help retain calcium in bones.
Pain related to vertebral body density loss	Assess type, amount, degree, duration, and constancy of pain in each site.	Determines extent of discomfort and provides data for care.
	Monitor effects of pain on mobility and ability to do self-care and to participate in daily activities and usual roles or responsibilities.	Pain often limits patient's activities, either through the pain itself or through fear of pain recurrence with activity.
	Administer ordered pain medication q 4 h as needed; monitor relief of pain.	Relief of pain requires maintenance of therapeutic blood levels.
	Encourage patient to participate in self-care, hobbies, or other active movements; encourage ambulation as able.	Diversion from concentration on pain lessens pain experiences; change of surroundings alters perceptions and self-attention to inner feelings.
Potential for injury related to fear of possible fracture	Assess concerns or fears about possible fracture.	Determines patient's concerns.
	Instruct patient about having safe home area (e.g., no loose rugs or long, uncovered cords), instruct on how to rise or sit.	Preventive measures provide security and mental peace.
	Discuss specific sites of patient's osteoporosis and use exercises to joints and muscles; discuss activities to aid calcium retention (e.g., walking, swimming, jogging if able, and repetitive exercise regimens).	Exercise helps maintain strong muscles and joints and aids retention of calcium in bones.
	Instruct on dietary intake of 1,500 mg of calcium per day; discuss likes and dislikes and alternative high-calcium foods; discuss dietary influences of intestinal absorption of calcium (see Table 8-1, page 131).	Recommended Daily Allowance (RDA) of calcium is 1,500 mg to prevent osteoporosis;[96] high intake of dietary fiber may inhibit intestinal absorption of calcium.
	Discuss patient's estrogen requirements related to menopause, age, or sex; refer patient to physician to discuss pros and cons of replacement estrogen or other medications (see page 132).	Lack of sufficient hormonal estrogen is a major cause of osteoporosis; replacement may be an option for many women.

NURSING DIAGNOSIS	NURSING INTERVENTIONS	RATIONALE
Body image disturbance related to kyphosis and lordosis	Assess effects of excessive curvatures on clothing types and fit; discuss patient's likes or dislikes of current fashions, fit, or specific types of clothes; refer patient to a fashion consultant if desired.	Particular styles and alterations in clothing can enhance fit and wearability of clothes, leading to a more positive self-concept.
	Discuss ways to lessen noticeability of curvatures with scarves, color schemes, etc.	Lessening obviousness of specific "deficit" enhances patient's self-concept and self-esteem.
Impaired gas exchange related to kyphosis	Assess respiratory functions.	Determines care needs.
	Listen to breath sounds; check chest expansion with respirations.	Breath sounds help evaluate respiratory competence and oxygenation.
	Monitor spirometry with vital capacity measurement.	Vital capacity results show whether or not patient has a deficit in intake.
	Monitor skin color, nail bed color, and capillary refill.	Skin should be pink and appear healthy-looking. nail beds should be pink with 2-4 second capillary refill.
	Monitor cough for sputum production and color; determine if cough produces pain, and if so, determine site, type, and severity of pain.	Cough should be nonproductive, but if productive, sputum should be clear and of small amount. Pain should not accompany cough; if pain is present with cough, it may signify rib or vertebral trauma.
Knowledge deficit	See Patient Teaching.	

5 EVALUATE

PATIENT OUTCOME	DATA INDICATING THAT OUTCOME IS REACHED
Patient has satisfactory physical mobility.	Patient can perform adequate self-care and exercises regularly (e.g., walks 1-2 miles daily, tends garden, maintains household); may walk with cane.
Patient has adequate pain relief.	Patient uses nonnarcotic analgesics once or twice daily; sleeps 7 hours nightly; no longer has burning pain.
Patient feels only mild anxiety about bone fractures.	Patient uses caution when going up or down stairs; is careful with unfamiliar surfaces such as waxed floors; practices safety measures at home.
Patient has accepted altered body image.	Patient has consulted experts for proper clothing to lessen evidence of kyphosis; has adjusted hemlines for evenness.
Patient has maintained satisfactory gas exchange.	Patient performs deep-breathing exercises several times daily; has no dyspnea or shortness of breath while going up stairs, walking, or swimming; has no cough.

➡ ❯ ❯

PATIENT TEACHING

1. Teach the patient and significant others about the nature of osteoporosis, possible causes, and ongoing care activities, including diagnostic examinations.
2. Teach the patient about the effects of estrogen on the body and the effect of its decrease on various organs and tissues.
3. Teach the patient the purpose of active exercise, which is to increase the uptake of calcium in the bones.
4. Teach the patient and significant others about dietary sources of calcium, its metabolism and/or absorption in the body, the effects of vitamin D, and the effect of other foods on calcium absorption.
5. Teach the patient about her medication regimen, expected side effects, and possible complications.
6. Teach the patient about safety factors for home maintenance to prevent falls, injuries, or pulmonary complications, or to cover patient-specific needs.

Gout

Gout is a hereditary disease involving overproduction or decreased excretion of uric acid and urate salts, leading to a high level of uric acid in the blood. The disease is thought to result from lack of an enzyme needed to completely metabolize purines for renal excretion. This incomplete metabolism causes the buildup of uric acid, which is a breakdown product of purines.

PATHOPHYSIOLOGY

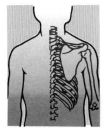 Urate salts of the excess uric acids are sluggishly excreted by the kidneys, causing them to build up in the body. They may be deposited in various tissues to lower the blood serum level of uric acid. Tissues with urate deposits include the joints, ear cartilages, and kidneys. Deposits of urate crystals form masses in the tissues called tophi. In the kidneys these crystals cause uric acid or urate-based calculi. Uratecrystals have very

pointed, sharp spicules that irritate and inflame the joints in which they are deposited. Characteristically, gout affects the first metatarsal joint of the great toe, causing severe and at times excruciating pain during an acute attack. The joints of the metacarpal bones and the wrist also frequently have large deposits of urate crystals, causing deformed, inflamed, edematous, hot, and painful joints.

Gout is uncommon in children, and men are affected more often than women. Gout may also develop secondary to increased cell breakdown from drug therapy, as with drugs used for leukemia and other malignant diseases.

COMPLICATIONS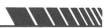

Renal calculi
Gouty arthritis

DIAGNOSTIC STUDIES AND FINDINGS

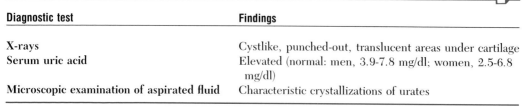

Diagnostic test	Findings
X-rays	Cystlike, punched-out, translucent areas under cartilage
Serum uric acid	Elevated (normal: men, 3.9-7.8 mg/dl; women, 2.5-6.8 mg/dl)
Microscopic examination of aspirated fluid	Characteristic crystallizations of urates

Table 8-2

FOODS HIGH IN PURINES

High (150-1,000 mg/100 g)	Moderate (50-150 mg/100 g)	Negligible
Liver	Lentils	Vegetables
Kidneys	Whole-grain cereals	Fruits
Sweetbreads	Meat	Cheese
Brains	Poultry	Eggs
Anchovies	Beans	Milk
Sardines	Peas	Refined cereals
Herring	Asparagus	Butter
Consommé	Cauliflower	Sugar
Heart	Mushrooms	Vegetable soups
Mussels	Spinach	

MEDICAL MANAGEMENT

GENERAL MANAGEMENT

During acute attacks: Bed rest to lessen pressure on inflamed joint(s); ice applications to joint (patient may not be able to tolerate pressure of ice bag over inflamed joint); bed cradle to keep covers off inflamed joint.

Dietary modifications: Low-purine diet.

Other: Weight loss if the patient is obese.

DRUG THERAPY

During acute attack: Colchicine (Colsalide), 1 mg po followed by 0.5-mg tablet every hour until pain is relieved or diarrhea occurs; then discontinue.

Maintenance therapy: Probenecid (Benemid) or allopurinol (Zyloprim) given daily, dose individualized.

Analgesic: Mild analgesics such as aspirin q 4 hr to ease pain.

1 ASSESS

ASSESSMENT	OBSERVATIONS
History	History of gout in family members
Joints	Presence of inflammation—reddened, hot, edematous joint; deformity of joints; tophi (rounded, pealike deposits in ear cartilage or large, irregularly shaped deposits in other joints); ROM limited by deformity and pain

⇥ ⟩ ⟩ ⟩

ASSESSMENT	OBSERVATIONS
Pain	Acute attacks cause sharp, excruciating pain (especially in joint of great toe or other joints)
Other symptoms: fever, nausea, headache	Temperature elevated to 37.5° C (99.6° F); pain causes temporary hypertension; headache and nausea present during acute episode

2 DIAGNOSE

NURSING DIAGNOSIS	SUBJECTIVE FINDINGS	OBJECTIVE FINDINGS
Pain (acute) related to urate deposits in joints	States pain is very severe in affected joints, joints feels very tender, can't put weight on joints	Writhes around in bed, trying to find comfortable position; calls out for pain relief
Impaired physical mobility related to inflammation of joints	States can't put weight on foot because of pain and swelling; states is using crutches to move about	Uses crutches to move about in room before bed-rest order; holds affected foot off floor; slight decreased ROM of some joints
Altered nutrition: greater than body requirements related to purine foods and total calories per 24 h	States has been eating "lots of chicken livers" and drinking one or two beers daily; also, eats sardines and mincemeat pie at least once a month	Serum uric acid level is above normal (normal: 2.8-7.8); weight is more than 20% above desired for body size, height, and sex; tophi noted in several joints and ear cartilages

3 PLAN

Patient goals

1. The patient's pain will be relieved with medication.
2. The patient's joint inflammation will be relieved.
3. The patient will change his eating habits to lower purine intake.
4. The patient will receive maintenance drug therapy to prevent acute exacerbations.

4 IMPLEMENT

NURSING DIAGNOSIS	NURSING INTERVENTIONS	RATIONALE
Pain (acute) related to urate deposits in joints	Assess type, degree, sites and duration of pain, locally in joints or systemically (e.g., headache).	Helps individualize care.
	Help patient to comfortable position in bed; elevate affected joint on pillow.	Bed rest lessens weight-bearing pressure and inflammation.

NURSING DIAGNOSIS	NURSING INTERVENTIONS	RATIONALE
	Maintain bed rest during acute exacerbations.	Bed rest eases pressure on tender, inflamed joints.
	Apply ice bag to inflamed joints; place bag so it does not put intolerable pressure on joint.	Ice causes vasoconstriction, decreasing edema and lessening pain.
	Administer ordered antigout medication: Colchicine (Colsalide), 0.5-1 mg/h, until patient has diarrhea or nausea—may give up to 8 mg.	Colchicine helps remove urates and eases pain in inflamed joints; diarrhea indicates that a therapeutic blood level has been reached, and drug is discontinued to avoid toxic levels.
	Administer nonnarcotic analgesic if ordered—may have order for aspirin, q 4 h prn.	Aspirin relieves pain in affected joints or other tissues.
Impaired physical mobility related to inflammation of joints	Assess ability to move about with ambulatory aid.	Helps individualize care.
	When patient is allowed up, help to ambulate with crutches, if needed; help with ROM exercises to uninflamed joints.	Prolonged bed rest causes musculoskeletal tissues to lose strength; ROM exercises help maintain muscle strength.
Altered nutrition: greater than body requirements related to purine foods and total calories per 24 h	Assess intake of purine foods (see Table 8-2) and calorie intake per 24 h; review dietary restrictions on purines and foods containing purines; discuss effects of excess urates on body tissues.	Purine-containing foods are common foods that should be restricted; understanding may increase compliance with restrictions.
	Discuss low-fat foods and techniques for reducing weight.	Decreasing weight lessens stress on inflamed or deformed joints.
Knowledge deficit	See Patient Teaching.	

5 EVALUATE

PATIENT OUTCOME	DATA INDICATING THAT OUTCOME IS REACHED
Patient's acute pain has been relieved.	Patient reports that pain is now gone. Can walk easily. Analgesics are not required.
Patient's joint inflammation has been relieved.	Affected joints are no longer edematous, reddened, or hot; weight bearing is not painful.
Patient has adopted a low-purine diet.	Patient and family choose allowed foods from menu; have list of foods high in purines and say they will not serve them.
Patient is taking medication daily for maintenance therapy.	Patient can explain need to take medication daily to prevent acute attacks and is taking medication as ordered.

➔ ❯ ❯

PATIENT TEACHING

1. Discuss gout and its effects on body tissues with the patient.
2. Teach the patient about foods high in purine, the effects of high levels of purine, and the need to restrict intake.
3. Discuss with the patient ways to prevent acute attacks and inflammation of affected joints.
4. Instruct the patient about his medication regimen, its purposes, and the side effects explain that gout cannot be cured but can be controlled with medication.
5. Discuss preventive measures with the patient (e.g., increasing fluid intake for renal health, ROM exercises for joint health, and weight loss for overall health).

Osteomalacia

Osteomalacia is a disease of adults characterized by loss of mineralization of bones, causing the bones to soften and become flexible, brittle, and deformed.

Osteomalacia is the adult form of rickets in children, which is caused by vitamin D deficiency and which leads to reduced absorption of calcium and phosphorus, so that these substances are not available for depositing in bone matrix. Vitamin D deficiency can result from poor absorption of the vitamin in the intestine, inadequate dietary intake of vitamin D, or insufficient exposure to sunlight; it can also be a consequence of chronic liver or kidney diseases, which impair vitamin D metabolism.

PATHOPHYSIOLOGY

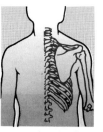

Without vitamin D, the amount of calcium and phosphorus available for bone calcification is inadequate to maintain bone strength. The balance of bone growth and resorption is disrupted. Defective growth and replacement of rigid bones are first noted in immature skeletal bones at sites of growth and in mature bones at points of stress, where turnover is most rapid. Defective replacement at these sites mentioned is noticed because of the increased demand for new bone formation. Failure of mineralization and the bones' resultant lack of rigidity lead to the symptoms of soft bones and deformities.

COMPLICATIONS

Degenerative joint disease
Bone deformities
Bone fractures

DIAGNOSTIC STUDIES AND FINDINGS

Diagnostic test	Findings
Laboratory tests	
Serum calcium level	Level is normal or below normal levels (normal: 4.5-5.5 mEq/L)
Serum alkaline phosphatase	Above 13 King-Armstrong units
Glucose	Elevated in urine
Serum amino acids	Elevated
Vitamin D level	Below normal
Parathyroid hormone level	May be elevated
Sedimentation rate	May be slightly elevated
X-rays	Areas of demineralization of bones, generally over body; pseudofractures (Looser's zones) strongly suggest osteomalacia; fractures may be in varying stages of healing
Bone biopsy	Absence of calcification with wide osteoid seams

MEDICAL MANAGEMENT

GENERAL MANAGEMENT

For patients with chronic renal failure: Diet low in phosphate-containing foods, along with administration of nonmagnesium phosphate—binding gel (such as Amphojel); calcium supplements and foods high in vitamin D are added when serum phosphate level is normal.

Incorporation of vitamin D—fortified milk into diet.

Exposure to sunlight, if feasible, to increase vitamin D metabolism and absorption, especially for older patients.

DRUG THERAPY

Administration of high doses of vitamin D, individualized to patient's age and severity of disease (doses may be 400-600 USP units/day).

If patient has chronic renal failure, calciferol may be used, because it accumulates faster due to decreased renal clearance; patient must be watched for signs of toxicity and renal calculi.

1 ASSESS

ASSESSMENT	OBSERVATIONS
History	Gastric or intestinal surgical resections; liver disease or alcoholic history; renal disease; decreased intake or absorption of vitamin D (low-fat or vegetarian diet)
Posture and bony structures	Abnormal bowing of bone, especially in rib area, pelvis, long bones, and vertebral column
Bones (for sore or tender areas or pain)	Areas of tenderness or pain (mild to severe, depending on site and severity of disease) in rib cage, vertebral column, pelvis, and limbs (pain in rib cage especially when turning or coughing)
Muscle strength and joint ROM	Muscle strength less than normal for age or physical status; joint ROM less than normal; fatigue common
Possible fractures	Stress fractures or pathologic fracture resulting from demineralized areas of bone

2 DIAGNOSE

NURSING DIAGNOSIS	SUBJECTIVE FINDINGS	OBJECTIVE FINDINGS
Impaired physical mobility related to weakened or deformed bones and pain	Complains of bones that bend more than normal and are deformed and unsightly; can't move around easily because of weak bones	Has malformed bones of limbs, kyphosis of thoracic vertebrae, and ribs are not in parallel curves; moves slowly and somewhat gingerly, as if expecting pain

→ > >

NURSING DIAGNOSIS	SUBJECTIVE FINDINGS	OBJECTIVE FINDINGS
Body image disturbance related to deformities	States feels "odd" because bones bend in unusual shapes; states people stare because of "bowlegs" and abnormal curve of upper back	Has pronounced genu varum (bowlegs) and marked kyphosis; rib cage not symmetrically shaped and ribs not curved similarly
Altered nutrition: less than body requirements related to inadequate intake or absorption of vitamin D	States is on vegetarian diet and rarely drinks milk or eats cheese; has had intolerance to gluten foods and milk intolerance (milk causes bloating) states has had intestinal resection for regional ileitis	Review of food likes/dislikes corroborates lack of milk and vitamin D intake

3 PLAN

Patient goals

1. The patient will regain satisfactory physical mobility and mineralization of bones.
2. The patient will regain a positive body image.
3. The patient will have normal intake of vitamin D to regain normal levels of serum calcium, alkaline phosphatase, glucose, and blood urea nitrogen.

4 IMPLEMENT

NURSING DIAGNOSIS	NURSING INTERVENTIONS	RATIONALE
Impaired physical mobility related to weakened or deformed bones and pain	Assess posture, gait, mobility, and musculoskeletal tissues.	Helps individualize care.
	Assist with repositioning, getting into or out of bed, and with ambulating, if needed; provide pillows for use to maintain positions.	Weakened or deformed bones or joints provide inadequate support for muscular activity; pillows provide support to lessen pain or tenderness.
	Assist with ROM and muscle-strengthening exercises q 4 h.	Exercises help maintain muscle and joint strength.
	Administer ordered analgesics q 4 h, if needed.	Maintaining therapeutic blood level of analgesics enables patient to be more active.
	Provide gentle massage to sore area; use caution to prevent injury as a result of weakened or deformed bones.	Massage increases circulation to painful or tender area, removes cellular debris, and provides comfort and a sense of well-being.
	Offer use of ambulatory aid, such as a cane or crutches; consult with physical therapist per physician's order.	An ambulatory aid lessens load and strain on weak bones and joints.

NURSING DIAGNOSIS	NURSING INTERVENTIONS	RATIONALE
	Discuss ways of using muscles, joints, and entire body to avoid injury.	Proper posture, gait, and exercises prevent injury to weakened bones and joints.
Body image disturbance related to deformities	Discuss patient's concerns about deformed and weakened bones and the effect on self, body image, and social and familial roles and responsibilities. If necessary, refer patient to image consultant or fashion coordinator.	Being different or unable to keep up with peers affects each person in varying degrees; understanding these effects is the basis for acceptance of change. Professional guidance assures patient of maximum benefits from resources.
	Encourage adherence to medical plans for strengthening or straightening musculoskeletal tissues.	Deficiencies must be corrected to aid recovery and healing.
Altered nutrition: less than body requirements related to inadequate intake or absorption of vitamin D	Assess intake of foods with vitamin D and calcium; administer vitamin D and calcium supplements if needed and ordered.	Additional vitamin D and calcium may be needed to restore levels to normal more quickly. Calcium is needed for every neuromuscular action; without vitamin D, inadequate calcium and phosphorus are available for bone calcification.
	Consult with dietitian about patient's likes and dislikes.	Intake should improve if likes are considered.
	Monitor intake for 24 h.	Totals help determine if intake is sufficient to overcome deficiencies.
	Discuss possible drug interactions or medications to avoid; consult with clinical pharmacist if necessary.	Medications high in magnesium, such as some magnesium-based antacids, limit absorption of calcium and phosphate; medications with little or no magnesium may be substituted.
Knowledge deficit	See Patient Teaching.	

5

PATIENT OUTCOME	DATA INDICATING THAT OUTCOME IS REACHED
Patient has regained satisfactory physical mobility and mineralization of bones.	X-rays show normal mineralization; bones gradually regain normal shapes.
Patient has a positive body image.	Patient reports that she no longer has bone pain, tenderness, and muscle and joint weakness and pain; feels positive about self and future.
Patient has normal intake of vitamin D.	Serum levels of calcium, vitamin D and its metabolites, and glucose and alkaline phosphatase are within normal limits.

→ > >

PATIENT TEACHING

1. Teach the patient about the causes of the condition related to deficiency or inadequate metabolism of vitamin D.
2. Teach the patient about dietary sources of vitamin D and calcium.
3. Explain the medication regimen for vitamin D and calcium and the side effects or drug interactions as needed.
4. Discuss an exercise regimen for retaining calcium in bones.
5. If pertinent, discuss hepatic or renal conditions and ways to improve health (e.g., stop smoking or drinking alcohol, use proper fluids or water for hydration, renal dialysis if appropriate).
6. Discuss follow-up care over lifetime. Osteomalacia may predispose to degenerative conditions in later life if not adequately treated or because of patient's specific condition.
7. Teach the patient dietary controls to prevent the disease in other family members, especially children and elderly people.

CHAPTER 9

Curvatures of the Spine

The spine develops its characteristic curves during fetal development and early postnatal growth. Spinal curves may develop abnormally because of defects in bone, muscle, nerve, or other growth factors or secondary to tumors or injuries. Abnormal curves are called kyphosis (excessive curvature of the thoracic spine), scoliosis (lateral and rotary curvature of the thoracic or thoracolumbar spine), or lordosis (excessive curvature of the lumbar spine).

Kyphosis

Kyphosis is excessive posterior curvature of the thoracic vertebrae.

Kyphosis can occur in various age groups. In young children, it is usually a congenital anomaly. In adolescents, it may be related to juvenile kyphosis (Scheuermann's disease), tuberculosis, or tumors, or it may be a compensatory mechanism for lumbar lordosis. Kyphosis is also a classic symptom of ankylosing spondylitis. Older, postmenopausal women also may develop kyphosis, which is called senile kyphosis.

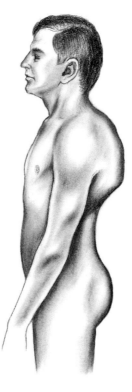

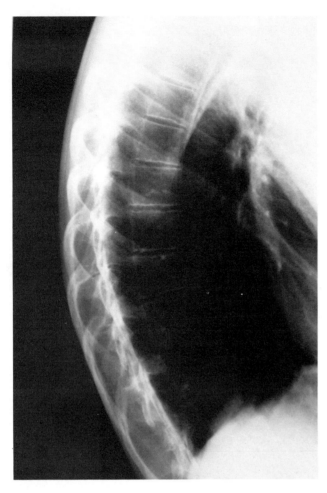

FIGURE 9-1
Kyphosis associated with Scheuermann's disease.

PATHOPHYSIOLOGY

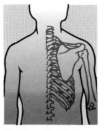

There are four types of kyphosis: (1) round back, characterized by a long, rounded curve with decreased pelvic inclination (less than 30 degrees) and thoracolumbar kyphosis[64]; (2) humpback (or gibbus), characterized by a localized, sharp posterior angulation in the thoracic spine; (3) flat back, characterized by pelvic inclination of less than 20 degrees and a mobile lumbar spine; and (4) dowager's hump, usually found in older, postmenopausal women and caused by osteoporosis (Figure 9-1).

Younger children with kyphosis may have no specific cause that can be determined and no noticeable pathologic condition except for the excessive kyphotic curve. As children become adolescents, they may develop an exaggerated curve related to Scheuermann's disease, which is inflammation of the bone and cartilage around the epiphysis of the vertebral body. The condition can lead to anterior wedging of the vertebrae, most commonly between the T6 and L2 vertebrae, thus producing an exaggerated curve. Approximately 10% of the population may have this growth disorder.[64] Tumors or tuberculosis that has spread to or begun in vertebral bodies and ankylosing spondylitis (see pages 74-75 for discussion) can lead to deterioration of vertebral bodies and kyphosis. In older people, osteoporosis can cause degeneration and anterior wedging, leading to excessive curvature.

COMPLICATIONS

Respiratory compromise
Degenerative joint disease

DIAGNOSTIC STUDIES AND FINDINGS

Diagnostic test	Findings
X-rays	Concave curvature of thoracic spine; wedging and narrowing of anterior portions of thoracic vertebral bodies (T6-T10); older people: possible osteoporosis, loss of bone density
Histocompatibility testing	Serum HLA-B27 antigen in young adults with ankylosing spondylitis
Erythrocyte sedimentation rate	Within normal limits
White blood cell count	Within normal limits

MEDICAL MANAGEMENT

GENERAL MANAGEMENT

Orthotic braces or various devices for adolescents; back corset for older adults; exercise programs to strengthen muscles and ligaments.

DRUG THERAPY

Older adults may be given hormonal treatment or mineral supplements for osteoporosis (see page 132). Patients with ankylosing spondylitis may receive several medications (see page 76). Antitubercular medications may be used to treat tuberculosis of the vertebrae.

SURGERY

Spinal fusion with or without metallic rods for severe kyphosis or removal of tumor.

1 ASSESS

ASSESSMENT	OBSERVATIONS
History	May be a history of trauma or injury, resulting in kyphosis after treatment or healing; may have tiredness or pain in shoulders or other areas of back, associated with Scheuermann's disease or ankylosing spondylitis; in older people, may be a history of gradually losing height with an increased thoracic curve developing, or a history of tuberculosis or tumors previously treated
Physical examination	Preteen, premenarchal, or postmenstrual (menopausal) individuals may have excessive thoracic curvature, or a gibbus; shoulders more prominent anteriorly when standing, with marked rounding of shoulders
Tiredness or back pain	Tires easily; upper (thoracic) or lower (lumbar) back pain; stiffness or soreness when rising or daytime pain

2 DIAGNOSE

NURSING DIAGNOSIS	SUBJECTIVE FINDINGS	OBJECTIVE FINDINGS
Body image disturbance related to excessive thoracic curvature	States people are always saying, "Stand up straight; put your shoulders back"; states it's hard to find clothes to cover hump; states it hurts to keep trying to hold shoulders back	Has rounding and forward-appearing shoulders; head slightly flexed forward; noticeable increased curvature of thoracic spine; may or may not have gibbus; pelvic inclination less than 30 degrees; legs appear (and measure) equal in length

→ > >

NURSING DIAGNOSIS	SUBJECTIVE FINDINGS	OBJECTIVE FINDINGS
Pain related to muscle strain and tiredness in back muscles	States has difficulty holding shoulders back because of tired, sore muscles; states has soreness in neck and upper back several times daily; states has occasional burning pain in upper back	Winces and twitches when paravertebral muscles and vertebrae are palpated; increased tightness and tension in all paravertebral muscles; sensory dermatomes in normal range
Potential for injury related to osteoporosis and kyphosis	States menses ceased about 10 years previously; has noticed gradual loss of height and hump in upper back	Measured height is about 1 cm less than stated height; thoracic curve more pronounced than normal; breath sounds normal in all lobes

3 PLAN

Patient goals

1. The patient will regain satisfactory thoracic curvature of the spine.
2. The patient will regain a pain-free existence relative to back condition.

3. The patient's kyphosis will not progress.

4 IMPLEMENT

NURSING DIAGNOSIS	NURSING INTERVENTIONS	RATIONALE
Body image disturbance related to excessive thoracic curvature	Assess posture and thoracic curvature.	Data are vital for planning nursing care.
	Discuss principles of proper posture.	Improving posture may lessen strain on muscles, ligaments, and bones.
	Ask physical therapist to help plan special exercises patient can do over time.	Exercises can strengthen back muscles to lessen strain.
	Assist with application of brace or other orthotic device, if used.	Brace or orthoses may be used to help muscles support vertebral column.
	Discuss effects of kyphosis on life's goals and future plans.	Condition may require some adjustment or alteration in goals or plans.
	Discuss clothing to make orthoses less noticeable.	Loose clothing is best.
Pain related to muscle strain and tiredness in back muscles	Assess degree, amount, severity, and duration of pain.	Provides basis for individualizing care.
	Palpate thoracic area of back to determine sites of tenderness.	Tender sites may be over vertebrae or along paravertebral muscles; pain may radiate to shoulders and may be burning or dull, depending on cause of kyphosis.

NURSING DIAGNOSIS	NURSING INTERVENTIONS	RATIONALE
	Administer ordered nonnarcotic analgesic or muscle relaxant if needed q 4 h.	Medications may be needed to ease muscle strain or frank pain, depending on cause of pain and kyphosis.
	Monitor prescribed exercise program.	Exercises ease strain and increase muscle strength.
Potential for injury related to osteoporosis and kyphosis	Assess serum calcium level and daily calcium intake.	May provide data related to development of osteoporosis.
	Encourage activities and exercises as condition permits.	Exercise helps keep calcium in bones.
	Assist with application of orthotic device if ordered.	Device may be used to ease muscle strain. (Use of orthotic devices is controversial, because it use may weaken muscles further.)
	Teach patient to use bannisters to ease muscle strain.	Bannisters provide support to aid weak muscles and joints.
Knowledge deficit	See Patient Teaching.	

5 EVALUATE

PATIENT OUTCOME	DATA INDICATING THAT OUTCOME IS REACHED
Patient has regained satisfactory thoracic curvature of spine.	Measurement of curvature is closer to normal as a result of exercises, postural adjustment, and surgical correction (if needed).
Patient has regained a pain-free existence relative to back condition.	Patient no longer needs analgesics or muscle-relaxant medications.
Patient's kyphosis has not progressed.	Kyphotic curve is closer to normal, as are back and shoulder alignments; respiratory functions have been maintained.

PATIENT TEACHING

1. Explain the development of kyphosis, spinal and muscle development, and the patient's particular condition.
2. Explain the purposes and techniques of the patient's exercise regimen.
3. Explain the possible side effects of the patient's medications.
4. Explain or clarify the patient's surgical procedure, if one is proposed or was done to correct kyphosis.
5. Explain the medication regimen for osteoporosis, if pertinent.
6. Explain safety factors to prevent injury if osteoporosis is present.
7. Teach the patient techniques for improving posture.

Scoliosis

Scoliosis is a lateral curvature of the spine.

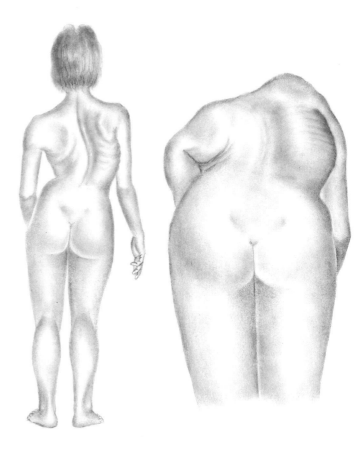

Scoliosis may be noted in infants, young children, and adolescents. In most patients with scoliosis, the cause is unknown; thus this is called idiopathic scoliosis. A familial genetic factor, as yet undetermined, is believed to play a role in scoliosis, as do hormonal and metabolic factors, which affect general skeletal growth and lead to asymmetry in the upper body and trunk. The scoliosis becomes more noticeable in the early teenage years because of the more pronounced laterality and rotatory curvatures and uneven shoulder and hip levels.

The prevalence of scoliosis is difficult to determine, because smaller curves may not be recorded in treatment protocols. Statistically, the number of cases in the United States is approximately 1.5 per 1,000 population; girls are affected more often than boys. By defining scoliosis as only curves greater than 10 degrees on the standing posteroanterior x-ray, overreferral and overtreatment is controlled. Generally curvatures greater than 20 degrees require treatment.

PATHOPHYSIOLOGY

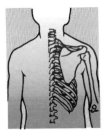

Although scoliosis has been studied intensively, the etiologic agent or agents or other causes have yet to be determined for most cases. Some connective tissue diseases have a high incidence of scoliosis, yet no collagen cross-link defect has been seen.[8] Some patients show changes in the amount of glycosaminoglycans (protein-carbohydrate complexes) in the nuclei pulposi, and Benson and colleagues propose that scoliosis could be related to excessive degradation of these proteoglycans,[8] which could affect the viscoelastic properties of the disk. Mechanical and equilibrium factors have also been studied as possible causes.

Scoliosis is a three-dimensional deformity involving concave curvature on the anterior vertebral bodies, convex posterior curves, and lateral rotation of the thoracic spine on bending or forward flexion. The normal kyphotic thoracic curve is not present in scoliosis, being replaced by lordosis in the thoracic vertebrae. As a person with scoliosis bends forward, the lordosis causes rotation and lateral flexion of the affected thoracic vertebrae, making the lateral curvature secondary to the primary lordosis in the thoracic vertebrae. The Scoliosis Study Group of Leeds, England, has stated that "lordo-

sis is the essential lesion in every structural scoliosis, no matter where it occurs in the spine and no matter what its etiology, and the larger the lordosis, the greater the rotation and lateral curvature on flexion."[72,24]

Curvatures in scoliosis become more severe or progress in deformity during the rapid growth periods of adolescence and may even continue to grow after skeletal maturity. The adolescent type makes up 70% to 90% of all curves.[95] The Scoliosis Research Study has determined that curves of 20 degrees represent the lowest limit of clinically important scoliosis[95]; curves up to 30 degrees are considered benign even though they will progress more than 5 degrees in adult years; curves between 50 degrees and 75 degrees progress the most.

Scoliotic curves are classified by their location in the vertebral column as thoracic (the most common), thoracolumbar, and lumbar. Double curves are right thoracic curve with left lumbar curve, left thoracic curve with right lumbar curve, and variations of these. Torticollis (wryneck) is scoliosis of the cervical spine.

COMPLICATIONS

Degenerative joint disease
Respiratory compromise

DIAGNOSTIC STUDIES AND FINDINGS

Diagnostic test	Findings
X-rays	Three-dimensional evidence: rotation of vertebrae in the axial plane, lordosis of vertebrae in the sagittal plane, and lateral inclination of vertebrae in the frontal plane[79]; may be wedging of posterior vertebral bodies; Schmorl's nodules may be seen in vertebral bodies; may have hemivertebrae and rib asymmetry

MEDICAL MANAGEMENT

GENERAL MANAGEMENT

Application of a Milwaukee, Boston, or other brace or orthotic device.
Application of distraction cast to gradually straighten curve (used infrequently).
Application of Cotrel's traction or halo-femoral traction before surgery.
Neuromuscular stimulator applied at nighttime (used infrequently).

SURGERY

Straightening and stabilization of curvature with Harrington or Luque rods with bone grafts to fuse spine; wires and a metallic rectangle help hold rods in place.
Cotrel-Dubousset posterior system of derotation: Several hooks are placed at specific vertebral levels connected to long rods bent to correct the sagittal curve; the rods are positioned bilaterally and locked together (see Figure 13-11, page 229).
Dwyer anterior fusion and osteotomy: Screws with holes are implanted in the vertebral bodies, and a cable is passed through the holes; tension is placed on the cable to correct the deformity (the patient may need to be placed in an external immobilizer until fusion occurs to maintain the reduction).
Modified Dwyer procedure, called ventral derotation spondylodesis: Screws are slotted, with a hole on the top or side to hold a flexible, solid, threaded rod; nuts are used to lock the rod into the screw heads and to provide compression to the system.[8]
Epiphysiodesis: The growth plate (epiphysis) is removed and bone is fused across the area (used more often in individuals with little growth potential remaining).[8]

1 ASSESS

ASSESSMENT	OBSERVATIONS
History	Parents or others may have noted uneven shoulder and hip heights, uneven skirt or pant lengths, and lateral curve with forward flexion (if curve is greater than 10-15 degrees); screening may indicate lateral curve and uneven hips or shoulders; patient may note prominent ribs on one side
Physical examination	Lateral curvature of vertebrae with or without rotation when standing; shoulder heights uneven and hips also uneven; on flexion, thoracic vertebrae rotate to left or right side of back; may have lumbar lateral curve of vertebrae also; laterality may be barely noticeable or very prominent on forward flexion; may have leg length difference with disappearance of lateral curvature when stepping forward or sitting; ribs may be more prominent on one side in anterior lower chest; one shoulder may be more prominent

2 DIAGNOSE

NURSING DIAGNOSIS	SUBJECTIVE FINDINGS	OBJECTIVE FINDINGS
Body image disturbance related to scoliosis	States likes to face people rather than be seen from back (where curvature can be seen); states curve has become more noticeable over past year and dislikes the progression; states has difficulty keeping shoulders straight and that one drops lower than the other	**From front:** Head and neck in midline; left shoulder only slightly higher than right; ribs more prominent on left lower rib cage; hip heights even; leg lengths appear even **From side:** Ears in midline over shoulder; curvature of thoracic spine shows slight increased kyphosis; lordotic curve more pronounced than normal **From posterior side and standing:** Noticeable deviation of thoracic spine to right side and deviation of lumbar vertebrae to left (double curve); left shoulder slightly higher than right; hip heights (with examiner's hands on hips) show left hip slightly higher than right; leg lengths appear equal when standing **Patient bending forward:** Noticeable increase in lateral curvature to right thorax above and to left hip area in lumbar area (S curve); rib prominence on left side; arm hangs lower on right than left **Lying on abdomen:** Tenderness over thoracic vertebrae from T4 to T10; lumbar area not tender to palpation; vertebral muscles more prominent on right side than left; patient hesitant to bend over to have curve checked
Impaired physical mobility related to scoliosis	Reports difficulty hitting ball in softball games; states back muscles seem weaker on left side than right; states back tires quickly when carrying items but feels no pain	Muscles more prominent in right thoracic area and less muscle mass in left thoracic area; grip strength, push, pull strength appear equal in both hands
Impaired gas exchange related to pulmonary compromise	States gets slightly short of breath when participating in sports (e.g., baseball, basketball, running); states has to rest going up stairs	Vital capacity slightly decreased; can hold breath for 1 min; breath sounds heard equally in all quadrants

3 PLAN

Patient goals

1. The patient's scoliosis will not progress, and patient will have a positive body image.
2. The patient will have improved physical mobility.
3. The patient will experience no pulmonary compromise.

4 IMPLEMENT

NURSING DIAGNOSIS	NURSING INTERVENTIONS	RATIONALE
Body image disturbance related to scoliosis	Assess condition's effect on body image and self-concept (see "Assessment" under "Diagnose" section).	Helps individualize nursing care.
	Encourage patient to talk about concerns related to scoliosis.	Ventilation of concerns helps individual focus those concerns.
	Discuss clothing to cover brace or make it less noticeable; Discuss adjustments to pants, skirts, or other hemlines.	Being able to cover brace adds to patient's self-confidence and freedom; equal hemlines make curvature less noticeable.
	Discuss need to wear brace as prescribed and for length of time prescribed.	Brace does not correct deformity but should help maintain degree of curvature.
	Discuss care of brace and skin under it.	Keep skin clean and using emollients helps maintain intact skin surface under brace; brace should be kept clean and free of moisture to lessen skin reactions.
	Encourage participation in usual peer activities, sports, and hobbies.	Participation in peer relationships and other activities aids psychosocial relationships and development.
Impaired physical mobility related to scoliosis	Assess effect of curvatures on muscle strength.	Helps in planning nursing care.
	Discuss use of Cotrel's traction before surgical correction, if proposed.	Traction may be used to stretch affected muscles.
	Change patient's position q 2 h if in traction, as permitted by traction.	Change of position helps perfusion to skin and other tissues to maintain integrity.
	Arrange for physical therapy according to physician's order.	Special therapy may be needed to maintain muscle-joint function.
	If surgery is performed, discuss need for bed rest for brief postoperative period (see pages 233-243 for nursing care after spinal fusion).	Bed rest is needed to permit stabilization of the patient after traumatic surgery.
	Arrange for postoperative physical and occupational therapy as ordered.	Traumatized tissues must be exercised to help them regain strength and functions; special techniques aid recovery.
	Provide postoperative care (as per spinal fusion) as needed according to specific procedure done.	Specialized care according to individual need aids recovery and discharge and prevents complications.

→ › ›

NURSING DIAGNOSIS	NURSING INTERVENTIONS	RATIONALE
	Monitor recovery process over time.	Close monitoring aids early noting of possible complications.
	Provide well-balanced diet.	Appropriate intake of needed vitamins, minerals, and other nutrients helps restore strength to tissues.
	Explain postoperative healing processes over next months.	See page 265 for bone healing over time.
Impaired gas exchange related to pulmonary compromise	Assess pulmonary functions; monitor breath sounds in all quadrants; measure vital capacity.	Breath sounds and vital capacity indicate status of pulmonary functions.
	Teach deep-breathing exercises.	Exercises help increase oxygenation and aid perfusion.
Knowledge deficit	See Patient Teaching.	

5 EVALUATE

PATIENT OUTCOME	DATA INDICATING THAT OUTCOME IS REACHED
Patient's scoliosis has not progressed.	Measurements of angles of curvatures have remained static with use of brace; x-rays show growth plates have closed and curvature has been reducedto 12 degrees. Patient expresses satisfaction with new look, and patient stands with vertebral collumn nearly straight on visual inspection.
Patient has no pulmonary compromise.	Patient has no trouble breathing. Vital capacity is within normal limits.
Patient has improved physical mobility.	Participates in routine physical activities at school or work.

PATIENT TEACHING

1. Explain the progression of scoliosis over time, if feasible, according to the patient's age and condition.
2. Explain the purposes of treatments involving a brace, traction, or surgical correction if proposed.
3. Explain the purposes of exercise regimens to maintain or retain muscle strength.
4. Explain the requirements of compliance in the treatment regimen.

Lordosis

Lordosis is a normal curvature of the lumbar spine.

Lordosis is the normal curvature in the lumbar spine; if present in other spinal areas, it can cause secondary problems such as those discussed previously (e.g., it is the primary cause of the laterality and vertebral rotation of scoliosis).

Lordosis may become exaggerated during pregnancy, with obesity, or in cases of large abdominal tumors, when overcorrection may be needed to help an individual maintain balance when upright. Structural changes do not occur, and the condition is resolved with delivery, weight loss, or removal of the tumor.

Hyperlordosis, or swayback, is fairly common in young children, especially girls, before puberty. It is thought to be caused by rapid skeletal growth without appropriate stretching of the posterior soft tissues, such as the lumbar fascia and paraspinal muscles. Permanent hyperlordosis, which is very rare, can occur as a result of degenerative conditions (e.g., osteoporosis) of the lumbosacral vertebral bodies or intervertebral disks. Treatments for hyperlordosis include use of a brace or lumbar belt, spinal fusion, or osteotomy.

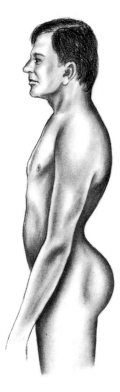

CHAPTER 10

Musculoskeletal Tumors

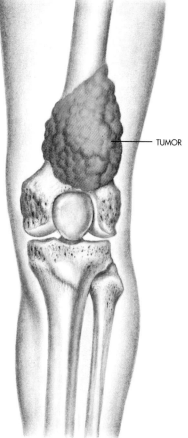

TUMOR

GJW

Most tumors of musculoskeletal tissues affect cartilage, muscles and, most frequently, bones. Synovial tumors are rare. Table 10-1 lists the various sites and types of benign and malignant tumors of musculoskeletal tissues. Because many musculoskeletal tumors are aggressive in nature, their presence causes concern, even though malignant tumors in musculoskeletal tissues constitute only 1% to 3% of all malignant tumors. It has been estimated that approximately 6,000 new bone and soft tissue sarcomas develop each year in the United States. Secondary, or metastatic, tumors in bones occur more frequently than do primary tumors but are difficult to estimate accurately.

A tumor is a new growth, or neoplasm, in a tissue. Primary tumors are those that arise in a particular tissue; secondary tumors are those that spread to another tissue from their original site. Tumors are classified as benign or malignant, depending on their growth characteristics. Benign tumors usually are not life-threatening, except when they develop in a confined space (e.g., brain tumors); malignant tumors, however, are always life-threatening because of their uncontrolled growth and metastatic nature.

Enneking[27] has stated that "the natural progression from the most benign to the most malignant connective tissue tumor is the same, lesion for lesion, whether the tumor arises in bone or somatic soft tissue." For example, a fibrosarcoma develops the same way in all tis-

10

Table 10-1

CLASSIFICATION OF TUMORS WITH TISSUE OF ORIGIN*

Tissue of origin	Benign	Malignant
Bone	Osteoma	Primary osteosarcoma
		Central osteosarcoma
		Low-grade medullary osteosarcoma
		Telangiectatic osteosarcoma
		Multicentric osteosarcoma
		Secondary osteosarcoma
		Paget's disease
		Juxtacortical osteosarcoma
		Parosteal osteosarcoma
Cartilage	Osteochondroma	Chondrosarcoma
	Chondroma	
	Enchondroma	
	Periosteal chondroma	
	Chondroblastoma	
Muscle	Leiomyoma	Leiomyosarcoma
	Rhabdomyoma	Rhabdomyosarcoma
Fibrous tissue	Fibroma	Fibrosarcoma
	Periosteal desmoid	Malignant fibrous histiocytoma
Adipose connective tissue	Lipoma	Liposarcoma
Bone marrow		Ewing's sarcoma
		Plasma cell myeloma (multiple myeloma)
Uncertain cell	Giant cell	Malignant giant cell
	Unicameral bone cyst	
	Aneurysmal bone cyst	
Vascular tissue	Hemangioma	Hemangioendothelioma
Neural	Neurofibroma	

*Not all tumors listed in this table are discussed in this chapter, because some are quite rare.

sues. Enneking's system for studying and determining the growth factors of lesions that originate in connective tissue is summarized in Table 10-2.

Enneking[27] has also devised a system for staging connective tissue tumors on the basis of (1) their grade of benignity or malignancy (G); (2) their location or site (T); and (3) whether there are metastases (M). This system which can be used for other types of tumors, is summarized in the box on page 159. Grade, site, and metastasis are further subdivided as follows:

1. Grade (G)
   G_0 Benign; low cell-to-matrix ratio; clearly differentiated cellular elements
   G_1 Low-grade malignancy; moderate differentiations; occasional distant metastasis
   G_2 High-grade malignancy; poorly differentiated cells with frequent mitoses; sparse matrix with marked anaplasia (malignant cells; frequent distant metastases; "skip" tumor sites

2. Site (T)
   T_1 Localized, encapsulated, and intracompartmental (contained entirely within antatomic confines of tissue of origin)
   T_2 Extracompartmental (has spread outside its tissue of origin)

3. Metastasis (M)
   M_0 No lymph node or distant metastasis
   M_1 Lymph node or distant metastasis

Careful, accurate staging of connective-tissue tumors helps determine optimum treatment for the specific tumor, as will be discussed later under medical treatments. Knowing before surgery the characteristics of the tumor, its stage, location, and whether it has metastasized give the surgeon and patient the information they need to decide on the medical and surgical procedures that would be most beneficial for the particular patient and tumor. Since many malignant bone tumors arise in young people, and radical resection or even

Table 10-2

ENNEKING'S SYSTEM OF LESIONS

Lesion	Growth pattern	Symptoms
1	Localized Latent Static or active Benign	Asymptomatic; accidentally noted Seldom leads to pathologic fracture or mechanical destruction (doesn't deform bone) Can become large but reaches a steady state with no additional growth Encapsulated; intracompartmental Small, movable; nontender
2	Localized Active Benign	Mild symptoms of discomfort, which lead to discovery Occasional pathologic fracture; occasional mechanical destruction Growth steady, continues to enlarge; can deform bones Encapsulated with thin reactive zone around tumor Palpable, movable; moderately tender nodule or mass
3	Aggressive Invasive Usually still benign	Symptomatic with tender, enlarging mass; sometimes grows rapidly Readily penetrates cortical bone, fascia, and even joint capsule with fingerlike projections into other compartments Firm, fixed, with thick reactive zone that is edematous and inflamed Low-grade malignant with occasional pulmonary metastasis
4	Indolent Invasive Malignant Low risk of regional, lymphatic, or distant metastasis	Slow-growing, painless, enlarging mass, indolent rate of evolution to malignancy Can differentiate into high grade and show distant metastasis with time and repeated attempts to remove Gradual growth into other compartments, seldom into joint Has late pulmonary metastasis
5	Rapidly growing Invasive Destructive Malignant High risk of lymphatic or distant metastasis	Rapidly growing sarcoma noted by an expanding mass into adjacent bone and soft tissues Destroys bone and fascial septae and grows into joint and blood vessels Tender, soft, and edematous with inflammatory reactive zone around tumor with necrotic cells Destroys normal cells and can "skip" to other areas nearby with isolated tumor in normal tissues Extracapsular
6	Rapidly growing Destructive Malignant Regional and distant metastasis	Rapidly growing; only 10% are still intracompartmental at time of diagnosis; 10% show distant metastasis Begin intracompartmentally and growth extracompartmentally and distantly Destructive with low- or high-grade malignancy

SURGICAL STAGING SYSTEM FOR BONE TUMORS			
Stage	Grade (G)	Site (T)	Metastasis (M)
IA	Low (G_1)	Intracompartmental (T_1)	None (M_0)
IB	Low (G_1)	Extracompartmental (T_2)	None (M_0)
IIA	High (G_2)	Intracompartmental (T_1)	None (M_0)
IIB	High (G_2)	Extracompartmental (T_2)	None (M_0)
IIIA	Low (G_1)	Intracompartmental or extra-compartmental (T_1 or T_2)	Regional or distant (M_1)
IIIB	High (G_2)	Intracompartmental or extra-compartmental (T_1 or T_2)	Regional or distant (M_1)

amputation might be considered, the value of such cautious diagnostic work-up systems can be readily appreciated.

Some musculoskeletal tumors are composed of more than one type of cell; this makes their diagnosis more difficult. Their rarity also makes diagnosis difficult, because many physicians see very few children or young adults with these tumors. In some cases the patient's symptoms are not diagnosed as a bone tumor for some time, and more time may pass before the best plan for treating the specific tumor is determined. Consultation with an orthopedic specialist is a necessity to ensure agreement that the diagnosis and treatment plans are accurate or correct for the particular tumor and the patient. Accurate diagnosis is critical because of the na-ture of growth of malignant bone tumors and because of the variety of treatments available. If the tumor is determined to be benign, it may not even be removed but just monitored closely for growth increases and symptom changes. Treatment for malignant bone tumors requires wide excision with removal of surrounding soft tissues and resection or amputation of a part, the entire limb, or a larger area of the body. Treatments for malignant bone tumors must take into consideration the person's life-style, quality of life, ambitions, and life goals when decisions on amputation or limb-salvage operations must be made. The surgery and follow-up treatments, if needed, must be individualized, with all factors carefully and thoroughly discussed and satisfactory to all concerned as is discussed later.

Bone and Cartilage Tumors

BENIGN TUMORS OF BONES AND CARTILAGE

Osteoma. An osteoma is a small, benign tumor of childhood and young adulthood (10 to 20 years of age) found in the bones of the skull and face. Osteomas make up 20% of benign bone tumors. Usually osteomas are external tumors, but at times they may be found intracranially, intranasally, intraorbitally, or within a sinus area. The tumor makes a hard, immovable, nontender swelling over the contiguous soft tissues. Except for the tumor mass, external osteomas have no symptoms; internally located osteomas produce symptoms referable to the site, such as headache or seizures with intracranial osteomas or pressure and pain from osteomas within a sinus. Generally this tumor grows slowly, although occasionally one will grow more rapidly until it reaches a certain size; then it stops growing. An osteoma is diagnosed by its size and site through radiologic scans (x-ray or computed tomography [CT]) or bone scan, which may show increased radioisotope uptake. Medical management is discussed in Table 10-3; recurrence is rare.

Osteochondroma. Osteochondromas constitute the largest group of benign bone tumors. They are made of spongy bone covered by a cartilaginous cap. These tumors develop during growth periods, growing in the metaphyses of bones, especially near the knee. They

Table 10-3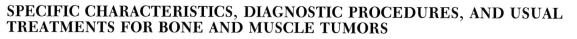

SPECIFIC CHARACTERISTICS, DIAGNOSTIC PROCEDURES, AND USUAL TREATMENTS FOR BONE AND MUSCLE TUMORS

Type of tumor	Characteristics	Diagnostic procedures	Usual treatments
Tumors of bone			
Osteoma	Benign	Physical examination for site and size; bone scan may show increased uptake of radioisotope	Excision for relief of symptoms if needed; may be left untouched
Osteochondroma	Benign	X-ray or CT scan shows outpouching of trabecular bone at metaphyseal area of bone	Excision of tumor and resection of tendon to above its point of attachment to prevent recurrence (removes all precartilaginous connective tissues)
Chondroma or enchondroma	About 75% are benign; about 25% are malignant	X-ray or CT scan shows thinned bone cortex	En bloc wide excision if malignant; if malignant and in large long bone, amputation may be required
Chondroblastoma	Benign	X-ray or CT scan shows osteolytic lesion with dots or points of calcification	Excision with curettage and packing with bone chips; about one third of these tumors recur
Giant cell tumor (osteoclastoma)	Benign	X-ray or CT scan shows bone-destroying (osteolytic) lesion with large, multilobular cells often resembling soap bubbles; radioisotope scan shows increased uptake	Careful, thorough excision in attempt to remove all tumor (has strong predilection for recurrence); if recurs, wide excision with bone grafts into defect is done; may be followed by radiation therapy
Giant cell tumor (osteoclastoma)	Malignant	X-ray, CT scan, or magnetic resonance imaging (MRI) study	En bloc wide excision with bone grafts or allograft if near joint; may amputate if there are repeated recurrences with malignant transformation
Aneurysmal bone cyst	Benign	X-rays show cystic lesion; arteriogram should demonstrate aneurysmic nature of cyst; MRI shows data similar to arteriograms	Curettage plus phenol to destroy bed or with cryosurgery (liquid nitrogen); radiation therapy is used only for inoperable lesions but is not used in areas of active cartilage growth
Unicameral bone cyst	Benign	X-rays show multiloculated cyst	Excision with bone grafts to defect; steroid injection into cyst; can recur
Osteosarcoma	Malignant	X-rays, CT scan, or MRI study show "sunburst" appearance characteristic of this tumor; may do tomogram x-rays; radionuclide scan helps determine tumor size and possible metastases, as does chest x-ray; serum alkaline phosphatase is elevated; arteriogram shows vascularity of tumor plus its relationship to contiguous tissues	Limb salvage with wide excision of tumor and surrounding tissues; may need joint replacement; excision of pulmonary metastatic lesions; both preoperative and postoperative chemotherapy and radiation therapy are also used; at times, limb amputation may be done
Parosteal osteosarcoma	Malignant, low grade	X-ray or CT scan shows tumor in metaphyseal area firmly attached to cortex of bone but nearly totally outside bone (hence name of tumor); radionuclide scan shows increased uptake in tumor	Excision of tumor
Ewing's sarcoma	Malignant	X-ray, CT scan, or MRI study greatly aids diagnosis	Radiation therapy used, since tumor is radiosensitive; chemotherapy also used

Table 10-3

SPECIFIC CHARACTERISTICS, DIAGNOSTIC PROCEDURES, AND USUAL TREATMENTS FOR BONE AND MUSCLE TUMORS—cont'd

Type of tumor	Characteristics	Diagnostic procedures	Usual treatments
Tumors of bone—cont'd			
Fibrosarcoma	Malignant	X-ray, CT scan, or MRI study should outline lesion—may be in bone or soft tissues	En bloc wide excision
Tumors of muscles			
Leiomyoma	Benign	Ultrasound studies of tumor mass (tumor develops in smooth muscle, commonly the uterus)	Surgical removal
Rhabdomyoma	Benign	Physical examination of mass in skeletal (striated) muscle	Surgical removal
Leiomyosarcoma	Malignant	Ultrasound (smooth muscle tumor)	Removal with wide resection
Rhabdomyosarcoma	Malignant	Arteriogram	Radiation therapy (tumor is radiosensitive); surgical excision; chemotherapy may be used

also grow in the tendons of large muscles and are felt as a firm, hard swelling fixed to the bone. The underlying bursa may be inflamed and tender, and there may be some limitation of joint motion if the tumor impinges on adjacent structures. The diagnosis is made from the symptoms, the patient's age, and the radiologic studies listed in Table 10-3.

Chondroma. A chondroma may also be called an enchondroma or a chondromyxoma. It is a benign tumor found most often in a central location in a finger or humerus in a young adult. Its growth destroys the cancellous portions of the involved bone. This tumor can undergo malignant transformation, particularly when located in the pelvis or a large long bone. It grows slowly during childhood, then remains stationary unless it undergoes malignant changes. There are few symptoms, with only slight soreness noted unless the person experiences a pathologic fracture, which is accompanied by severe, acute pain. Pressure of an enlarging malignant tumor may also cause severe pain. The diagnosis is made from the patient's history, a physical examination that reveals the mass, and radiologic studies (see Table 10-3 for findings and treatment).

Chondroblastoma. A chondroblastoma is a rare benign tumor of cartilage. It usually involves a primary or secondary epiphysis and may extend into the joint, epiphyseal plate, or metaphysis, primarily of long bones. Ninety percent of these tumors occur between 5 and 25 years of age; most of those affected are males. Symptoms include mild, intermittent pain for months or

years—at times as long as 2 years—before the person seeks medical care. There may be some edema and tenderness and, if the tumor involves a joint, some limitation of motion. The diagnosis is made from the patient's history, physical examination, and radiologic studies (see Table 10-3 for findings and treatments).

Giant cell tumor. A giant cell tumor is a benign tumor of young adults; approximately 70% occur between 20 and 40 years of age.[23A] It has almost equal male-female distribution; some studies show more males affected, some more females.[23A] Giant cell tumors account for 4% to 5% of benign bone tumors in the United States. The tumor is most often found in the distal femur at the epiphyseal area after the epiphyseal plate has calcified and the longitudinal bone growth has been completed. It is also found in the proximal tibia, distal radius, sacrum, and proximal humerus. The tumor is composed of large giant cells that expand from one side of the bone, causing stretching of the overlying skin. The tumor grows slowly over months to years, eventually producing dull, constant pain, worse at night, which increases with activity. Limitation of joint movement is a late symptom of the expanding tumor, and the joint is not directly involved in the tumor mass. The diagnosis is made from the patient's history, physical examination, and radiologic studies (see Table 10-3 for findings and treatment).

Aneurysmal bone cyst. An aneurysmal bone cyst is a benign lesion consisting of a mass of vascular spaces enclosed in a shell of new bone growing outward from the bone and displacing the soft tissues. It occurs predominantly in males between 10 and 30 years of age. It is found most frequently in the metaphyseal area of long bones. Symptoms include a history of trauma, bony swelling, limitation of joint motion, and pain increased by movement. If the cyst is in the vertebra, there may be signs of nerve root compression. The diagnosis is made from the patient's history, physical examination, and radiologic studies (see Table 10-3 for diagnosis and treatments).

Unicameral bone cyst. A unicameral bone cyst is a rare, benign bone growth that develops in the metaphysis of a long bone close to the epiphysis and growing away from the epiphysis as it develops. It has a thin-walled cavity containing yellow fluid. It occurs most frequently between 5 and 15 years of age and rarely after age 20. More than half of these cysts are located in the proximal humerus. Symptoms are nonexistent until it is discovered on x-ray after a fracture at the site. A limp may be noted with a unicameral bone cyst in the leg. If the cyst is adjacent to the epiphyseal plate, it may cause growth disturbances.

MALIGNANT TUMORS OF BONE AND CARTILAGE

Osteosarcoma. Osteosarcoma is the most commonly occurring tumor of bone, making up about 35% of malignant tumors. It is a highly malignant tumor that grows rapidly. It has components of fibrous, cartilaginous, and bone tissues within its stroma, and the bone cells can be traced back to primitive mesenchymal cells. Its peak incidence is between 10 and 20 years of age, with slightly more males than females affected. There is a second peak incidence in people 50 to 60 years of age from Paget's disease.

There are a variety of osteosarcomas, as listed in Table 10-1. More than half of osteosarcomas are localized around the knee, being found in the distal femur or proximal tibia, although others may be in the jaw (mandible) or humerus.

Because of its rapid growth, this tumor rather quickly destroys the inner cortex of the bone as it expands into the soft tissues. Patients complain of dull, aching, almost constant pain, which often is worse at night. The person stops using the part comfortably. Occasionally, the person may have anorexia, weight loss, and malaise. The tumor may cause edema, and the overlying skin may be stretched and shiny.

Physicians seeing patients with the above symptoms should have a high index of suspicion about the possible presence of a malignant tumor. The diagnosis must be made carefully to differentiate this tumor from other bone tumors. Diagnosis and treatment regimes are listed in Table 10-3.

Parosteal osteosarcoma. A parosteal osteosarcoma grows outside the periosteum of bone; hence the name "parosteal," meaning abnormal site or disease. It has a low grade of malignancy, and a benign form of this tumor also occurs, although it currently is thought of as malignant with differences only in degree. These tumors have a strong tendency to recur even with radical resection and removal. Parosteal osteosarcomas occur in people between 14 and 40 years of age, with no sexual predilection. The tumor grows in the metaphyseal area of long bones, primarily the distal femur and proximal humerus. It makes a hard mass firmly attached to the underlying cortex, closely adjacent to but nearly outside the bone. At times the tumor may encircle a bone. Symptoms include local pain, sometimes of several years' duration, with some swelling at the site. There may be some limitation of joint motion. The diagnosis is made from the patient's history, physical examination, and radiologic studies, shown in Table 10-3, along with treatments.

Ewing's sarcoma. Ewing's sarcoma is a tumor of uncertain cell origin. It may arise from the supportive marrow structure of bone, from the reticulum cell or stem cell, or from the bone marrow. It occurs in patients between 5 and 25 years of age. The tumor occurs in the diaphysis of the affected bone. Symptoms include pain that is intermittent and worse at night; a palpable, hard, tender tumor that is fixed to the underlying bone; reddened, edematous skin over the tumor area with noticeably dilated veins; and systemic symptoms of fever, anemia, and weight loss. The diagnosis is made from the patient's age, history, physical examination, and radiologic findings. Table 10-3 lists findings and treatments.

Fibrosarcoma. A fibrosarcoma is a tumor of the fibroblasts that make up bone fibrous tissues. Although bone fibrosarcoma is a tumor of bone, it is identical with a fibrosarcoma that arises in soft tissues (e.g., fascia). The tumor appears in the femur primarily but also can develop in the mandible, skull, or vertebrae. It grows in the metaphysis or diaphysis of the long bone or in the medullary area of other bones. It occurs in individuals over 30 years of age, with no sex predilection. Symptoms include gradual onset of continuous pain that is worse at night and gradual swelling at the tumor site with a firm, smooth, soft mass firmly fixed to the underlying bone. The diagnosis is made from the patient's history, physical examination, and biopsy findings. Treatments are listed in Table 10-3.

METASTATIC TUMORS OF BONE

Metastatic tumors are spread to bones from their primary sites. Common primary sites are the breast, lungs, prostate, thyroid, kidneys, adrenal and other sites. Metastatic spread is to bones of the pelvis, vertebral column, ribs, hip and the rest of the femur, and to the humerus. The metastatic tumor cells replace normal cells, leading to weakening in the area. Frequently a pathologic fracture is one of the first indications of the presence of metastatic disease; other symptoms are soreness and pain with limitation of joint motion and use. The diagnosis is made from the patient's history, physical examination, and from additional studies. Laboratory tests may show elevated alkaline or acid phosphatase levels. X-rays may show the metastatic tumor and additional metastatic sites. A radionuclide bone scan may indicate several sites of metastasis. A biopsy may be necessary to determine the primary tumor site, especially if the patient had no previous treatments for a tumor. Treatments may include radiation therapy to the specific metastatic site or sites and surgical repair of the pathologic fracture, with a compression plate and screws or insertion of a hip nail if the fracture is in the proximal femur. Efforts to determine the primary tumor are also made, with appropriate treatments following such as chemotherapy, radiation therapy, and hormone therapy to alter the hormonal milieu of the primary tumor if appropriate.

Muscle Tumors

BENIGN TUMORS OF MUSCLE

Leiomyoma. A leiomyoma is a benign tumor of smooth muscle. It can occur in any muscle but develops most often in the smooth muscles of the uterus. It may be present for long periods without causing any symptoms. Symptoms may include soreness, tenderness or pain in the involved muscle, and palpation of a mass. The diagnosis is made from the patient's history, physical examination, and ultrasound studies that show the mass. The tumor may be left undisturbed or may be removed if it leads to excessive uterine bleeding or discomfort. Leiomyomas in other muscles may be removed if they limit muscle action. A biopsy of the tumor is needed to determine its benignity.

Rhabdomyoma. A rhabdomyoma is a tumor of striated muscles. It is a rare tumor with few symptoms other than local tenderness and pain. It is diagnosed by its mass in a muscle and by the patient's history. It should be biopsied to determine its benignity.

MALIGNANT TUMORS OF MUSCLE

Leiomyosarcoma. A leiomyosarcoma is a malignant tumor of smooth muscle, the counterpart of leiomyoma. It occurs in the same areas as leiomyomas and has similar symptoms. It can also occur in the stomach, bladder, small bowel, esophagus, and prostate. It grows more radically, shows areas of necrosis, and has bizarre cellular patterns. These tumors must be removed, with wide resection. Radiation therapy and chemotherapy also are used.

Rhabdomyosarcoma. A rhabdomyosarcoma is the malignant correlate of rhabdomyoma. It occurs in all ages with no predominance in a specific age group; there is a slight predilection for males. The tumor occurs most often in the popliteal, gluteal, inguinal, and interscapular regions. It is a soft tumor with some hemorrhagic tendencies. Symptoms include a soft, enlarging mass with tenderness and pain from use or pressure. It may ulcerate and hemorrhage into surrounding tissues. It is diagnosed from the patient's history and physical examination (the tumor often takes the shape of the muscle from which it arises) and by cellular biopsy. Arteriograms also aid in making a diagnosis, since the vessels are large and run in different angles, and arteriovenous shunts are likely. Treatments include radiation therapy, since these tumors are radiosensitive and radioresponsive. Surgical removal plus radiotherapy may also be part of the treatment. The prognosis depends on the adequacy of the treatments and whether metastatic disease is present.

Surgical options. Surgical resection or removal of the malignant tumor by means of amputation is undertaken primarily to eradicate the primary tumor by hav-

Table 10-4

SURGICAL TREATMENT OPTIONS FOR MALIGNANT BONE TUMORS

Margin	Limb salvage	Amputation
Intracapsular	Intracapsular, piece-meal extraction of tumor	Intracapsular amputation
Marginal	Marginal en bloc excision of tumor	Marginal amputation
Wide	Wide en bloc excision	Wide through-the-bone amputation
Radical	Radical en bloc resection	Radical disarticulation (e.g., hemipelvectomy)

REPLACEMENT OPTIONS: Prosthesis; allograft with banked bone; autograft with patient's own bone; and metallic implants. Another option is "turnabout" plasty: The middle (intercalary) portion of the bone is resected with proximal and distal portions remaining, along with neurovascular bundles; bone from the tibia below is rotated 160 to 180 degrees and plated to the remaining bone portions of the femur, and the neurovascular tissues are repaired.

ing wide or radical margins, then reconstructing the resulting defect. Margins of tumor-free tissue should be at least 7 to 10 cm of normal bone[28] in the thigh if the tumor is in the distal femur. Tumors in other sites must have similar wide margins of tumor-free bone and soft tissues. Amputation is still a major option for high-grade malignant bone tumors.

In the past 15 to 20 years, limb-sparing procedures have been undertaken in many major centers. Limb-sparing resections require that the tumor be resected through normal tissue planes while preserving the neurovascular structures and the ability to reconstruct a functional extremity.[28] As with other surgical resections, limb-sparing procedures must be considered in light of the patient's age, the site of the tumor (where and in which bone), and the histologic grade of the tumor. Recurrence rates with limb-sparing procedures are 5% to 10% after local resection, compared with 2% to 5% recurrence after cross-bone amputation.[28] Recurrence is a severe complication that markedly increases patient mortality.

Table 10-4 lists the many options for replacement or reconstruction after limb-sparing surgery. These options must be discussed with the patient and family members to obtain an informed consent to the surgery.

Nursing considerations in the care of patients with bone or muscle tumors, whether benign or malignant, may be intense and uncertain because of the nature of these tumors. Nursing care must be specific for the particular patient and tumor during the patient's hospitalization and follow-up.

1 ASSESS

ASSESSMENT	OBSERVATIONS
Obvious or palpable mass	Mass may be easily seen or may be subcutaneous; may or may not be palpable
ROM of joints in area contiguous to tumor	ROM may be unimpaired or may be limited by tumor or pain

ASSESSMENT	OBSERVATIONS
Ambulation	May walk easily without limp or hesitation or may limp, hesitate, and use support of ambulatory aid, person, or furniture
Pain (type, severity, site, time)	No pain or slight to moderate tenderness at site; may have dull ache deeper below skin; may have pain only at night that wakes patient up; pain may be around knee (most commonly), in pelvis, or in upper arm
Effect of position changes on comfort	Weight bearing may increase or decrease pain; use of upper extremity may be limited; may move restlessly because of pain or pressure if pelvic or lower extremity is involved
Neurovascular functions	May have skin color changes (redder) and slight edema; skin hotter over site; may have varying motor or sensory changes; pain varies with site and tumor
Following surgical removal of tumor: neurovascular functions	Same as above, plus pain in operative site; decreased function or use of muscles and joints in operative area
Pain	Phantom pain may develop if limb is amputated
Wound and surrounding tissues	Inflammatory signs, including redness, edema, sanguineous to serosanguineous drainage; pain and presence of sutures, clips, or subcutaneous skin closure; may have split- or full-thickness skin graft
Responses or reactions to diagnosis	If benign tumor, will appear relieved; if malignant tumor, may be sad, depressed, frightened, anxious, angry, hostile, or have other emotional response; may be withdrawn, restless, sleepless; may cry easily, and be demanding or passive; may be questioning all nursing activities

2   DIAGNOSE

NURSING DIAGNOSIS	SUBJECTIVE FINDINGS	OBJECTIVE FINDINGS
Impaired physical mobility related to mass or pain	Expresses reluctance to bear weight	May limp; may use ambulatory aid or lean on another person or furniture when moving; may hold arm close to body or use sling; may move restlessly or hesitantly
Pain related to pressure of enlarging mass on bone, nerve, or other tissues	Reports pain that may be sharp, dull, or referred to another site at different times; pain may be intermittent; it may occur mainly at night and wake patient; patient may have some numbness at times	Restless and attempts to find a position of comfort; mass felt on palpation
Potential for injury related to pathologic fracture	States has noted change in strength of affected tissues	Examination may elicit crepitus, deformity, or hematoma if bone has fractured
Ineffective individual coping related to diagnosis	States has become anxious, restless, questioning, fearful, or sad	May cry or pace (if able); may be hostile or angry if diagnosis is delayed

→ › ›

NURSING DIAGNOSIS	SUBJECTIVE FINDINGS	OBJECTIVE FINDINGS
After surgery: **Impaired physical mobility** related to loss of tissues, insertion of prosthesis, internal fixation device, or amputation		Affected limb may be ordered held in abduction, adduction, neutral, or other rotation; may need immobilizer for joint; patient may have balance difficulties or hesitate to stand upright; may need ambulatory aid; may need orthotic device (prosthesis) following amputation
Impaired gas exchange related to anesthesia, procedure (e.g., thoracotomy or forequarter amputation), bed rest		May hypoventilate, be dyspneic, or use splint breathing to lessen pain; may have weak cough, productive or nonproductive, yellow or blood-tinged sputum; may have tachypnea, tachycardia; may have decreased breath sounds, rales, or rhonchi
Potential for infection related to surgical wound, fixation device, or amputation		Wound on upper or lower extremity, lateral chest (thoracotomy), or pelvis; sutures or skin clips close wound; drain in wound; WBC counts drop with radiation or chemotherapy; fixation devices are sources of infection; chest tubes may be present
Impaired skin integrity related to surgical wound or skin graft		In addition to assessments above under potential for infection, may have donor site or split-thickness graft covering donor site; may have dressing tied over skin graft (stent); may have medicated gauze over donor site, which may be very painful

3 PLAN

Patient goals

1. The patient will regain satisfactory physical mobility after surgery.
2. The patient's pain will be relieved.
3. The patient will not have a pathologic fracture.
4. The patient will cope satisfactorily with diagnosis.

5. The patient will not develop an infection.
6. The patient will have adequate gas exchange.
7. The patient will regain skin integrity after treatments.

4 IMPLEMENT

NURSING DIAGNOSIS	NURSING INTERVENTIONS	RATIONALE
Impaired physical mobility related to mass or pain	Observe patient's efforts to use affected limb or specific tissues.	Helps determine types of limitations if present.
	Assist with ROM to all joints; use caution with joints contiguous to tumor site.	ROM maintains full strength and functions of unaffected tissues and prevents muscles or joint atrophy; caution is necessary to avoid a pathologic fracture.

NURSING DIAGNOSIS	NURSING INTERVENTIONS	RATIONALE
	Assist patient while ambulating if needed; note presence of limp, hesitation, or pain with use or weight bearing.	Assistance eases strain and prevents over-tiring; noting symptoms helps aid diagnosis and care.
	Teach proper use of ambulatory aid if needed; observe use of aid.	Teaching use of aid reduces anxiety, increases confidence, and provides for safe care.
	Teach isometric exercises.	Exercises help maintain muscle and joint functions.
	Help therapist transfer patient to chair as needed if limb has been amputated or after hemipelvectomy.	Loss of balance and posture are common if part or all of a limb has been amputated.
	Maintain proper abduction, adduction, flexion, or extension position of affected limb; rotation may be internal, external, or neutral.	One or more specific positions may be dictated by insertion of prosthesis, muscle or bone transplants, allograft or skin graft.
	Remind patient about weight-bearing restrictions, if needed.	Limited weight bearing may be required after internal fixation devices have been inserted until bone has healed sufficiently to support weight bearing.
Pain related to pressure of enlarging mass on bone, nerve, or other tissues	Determine amount, type, character, duration, and severity of pain.	Helps assure proper nursing interventions.
	Reposition patient, splint, joint immobilizer, or pillows as needed.	Promotes circulation to remove wastes and ease tired or aching muscles or joints; relieves pain.
	Administer analgesics (or have patient use Patient-controlled analgesic device) as ordered q 3-4 h "around the clock" initially.	Continuous therapeutic blood levels of analgesics enhance pain relief.
	Check mass to see that there is no pressure on affected tissues.	Internal pressure from expanding mass combined with external pressure from dressings, pillows, immobilizer, or other sources "pinch" tissues between immovable objects, adding to patient's pain.
	Perform neurovascular checks to determine if pain is commensurate with patient's condition.	Severe, unrelenting pain may signify development of hematoma or abscess; patients with low pain threshold must be monitored carefully to note extent or relief of pain.
	Remove and reapply abduction pillow, joint immobilizer, or splint to see if pain is eased.	Postoperative edema may make appliances or dressings too tight; loosening lessens pressure and pain.
	Massage tired muscles and joints q 4-6 h; encourage ROM exercises as able.	Massage and ROM exercises stimulate removal of wastes through increased circulation, thereby relieving pain.

➔ ❯ ❯ ❯

NURSING DIAGNOSIS	NURSING INTERVENTIONS	RATIONALE
	Teach deep-breathing and relaxation techniques.	Pain is relieved by removal of wastes and reoxygenation.
	Listen to patient express feelings about diagnosis.	Emotional concerns may aggravate physical pain.
Potential for injury related to pathologic fracture	Gently move affected part by supporting at two joints; position part as comfortably as possible.	Supporting at two joints (above and below affected site) prevents "lever" action, which could cause further injury and increase pain.
	Apply skin traction, if used, to affected part or apply joint immobilizer if ordered.	Skin traction helps maintain immobility of affected tissues to prevent further injury.
	Prepare patient for diagnostic studies or for therapy for primary or metastatic lesion.	Pathologic fracture may be a new finding, which may require additional diagnostic studies or therapy for primary or metastatic lesion.
	Listen to patient's concerns about pathologic fracture or primary condition.	Pathologic fracture may be initial indication of metastatic or primary tumor; adjusting to diagnosis may take time.
Ineffective individual coping related to diagnosis	Listen to patient's expressions of concern over diagnosis of malignant tumor or need for radical resection or amputation; allow ample time.	Providing time for patient to express concerns lends assurance that cooperative or pertinent solutions will be undertaken; expressing concerns is calming and reassuring.
	Reflect observations to patient with appropriate communication technique (e.g., "You seem upset—or nervous" or "You look sad," or whatever is appropriate to nurse's observation).	Seeking validation helps assure correctness of observation so that subsequent care can be pertinent.
	Allow time for patient to be alone with thoughts and feelings.	Having time for reflection helps patient sort out thoughts and feelings.
	If appropriate, have a well-rehabilitated amputee visit patient.	Learning that recovery is possible can be reassuring.
	Seek consultation with mental health professional if needed.	Specialist provides knowledge and skills generally not within purview of some nurses.
	Help patient with self-care while he is grieving.	Giving temporary assistance helps move patient forward.

NURSING DIAGNOSIS	NURSING INTERVENTIONS	RATIONALE
After surgery: Impaired physical mobility related to loss of tissues, insertion of prosthesis, internal fixation device, or amputation	Interventions for impaired physical mobility, pages 166-167, remain with the additions below.	
	Seek consultation with physical therapist and orthotist as appropriate.	Specialists have specific knowledge and skills for optimum patient care.
	Turn patient to side or abdomen as appropriate for surgical procedure or amputation; use appropriate abduction pillow, splint, or joint immobilizer if ordered.	Repositioning permits optimum circulation and promotes muscle strength; turning to abdomen allows extension to prevent flexion contractures.
	Help patient do adduction, extension, or other appropriate exercises q 4 hr after amputation of limb.	Flexor and abductor muscles are stronger than extensor and adductor muscles; specific exercises help prevent flexion or abduction contractures.
Impaired gas exchange related to anesthesia, procedure (e.g., thoracotomy or forequarter amputation), bed rest	Observe respiratory patterns along with other vital signs; listen to breath sounds in all lobes q 4 h.	Tachypnea and tachycardia indicate oxygen need; breath sounds indicate ventilation (inability to hear breath sounds indicates secretions in airway).
	Teach patient deep-breathing and coughing exercises to perform q 2-3 h.	Deep breathing aids peripheral pulmonary perfusion; coughing clears secretions that could impair ventilation.
	Have patient use respiratory aid q 2-3 h.	Respiratory aids increase resistance to inhalation, enhance lowering of diaphragm, and increase oxygenation and perfusion.
	Percuss lobes of lungs q 4 h; may also use cupping, clapping, or vibration.	Helps loosen and mobilize secretions so that they can be coughed up more easily.
Potential for infection related to surgical wound, fixation device, or amputation.	Check wound closely for signs of inflammation, healing, or infection.	Signs of inflammation include redness, edema, pain or soreness, and serosanguineous drainage; healing is indicated by lessening of above signs; infection may be indicated by enlarging hematoma or abscess, increased purulent drainage, increased pain or soreness, heat in wound area, or systemic fever.
	Assess vital signs for elevated temperature, tachycardia, flushing, malaise, or headache.	Infection causes fever and/or chills; increased pulse rate, vasodilation or flushing to cool blood, malaise, and general discomfort.
	Check laboratory data for WBC counts and changes in differential counts.	Bacterial infections are noted by elevations in total WBC counts (normal: 3,000-9,000 mm^3); changes in polymorphonuclear neutrophils, lymphocytes, and other differential cells also occur with systemic infections.

→ › ›

NURSING DIAGNOSIS	NURSING INTERVENTIONS	RATIONALE
	Use strict aseptic technique for wound dressings.	Surgery lowers resistance to infection; incision lowers skin's first line of defense.
	Check drainage from all orifices for signs of infection (e.g., green sputum, cloudy urine, increased vaginal drainage).	Infection may be pulmonary, urinary, or peritoneal or may be found in sites other than the surgical incision.
Impaired skin integrity related to surgical wound or skin graft	Check skin graft for adherence to recipient bed; roll graft with applicators if ordered.	New blood vessels must develop and permeate skin graft to nourish it and maintain its integrity; rolling the graft moves edema fluid, if present, to lessen interference with "take" of graft.
	Check donor site, if present, for amount of drainage, pain, and signs of granulation or infection; change medicated gauze and cleanse donor site of secretions as needed (donor site may be covered with transparent sterile dressing instead of medicated gauze).	Donor site for split-thickness graft heals by granulation, and healing requires 4-6 wk; donor site is quite painful, since dermis, with nerve endings, is exposed; vapor-permeable barrier dressing prevents air current from coming into contact with donor site but allows gas to move out of site.
	If patient has amputation: Monitor suture line for healing or signs of infection as listed previously.	Scar tissue forms without excessive scarring if incision heals by primary intention without infection.
	Use strict aseptic technique for wound care.	Aseptic technique lessens possibility of infection.
	Teach stump wrapping techniques (see Figure 13-1, page 210).	Instruction ensures proper technique and increases patient's confidence in self-care.
	Use bed pads, heel and elbow pads, protective mattresses, special beds, and pillows as needed.	Protective mattresses and such distribute pressure over larger areas to maintain skin integrity.
	Help patient change positions q 3-4 h.	Position changes relieve pressure and increase circulation to enhance skin integrity.
	(See amputation, pages 205-211 for additional nursing interventions.)	

5 EVALUATE

PATIENT OUTCOME	DATA INDICATING THAT OUTCOME IS REACHED
Patient has regained satisfactory physical mobility and ROM of unaffected joints and muscles.	Patient walks easily (with ambulatory aid, if needed); ROM of joints in normal ranges; strength of affected muscles and joints (muscles involved in tumor or surgery) has improved.

PATIENT OUTCOME	DATA INDICATING THAT OUTCOME IS REACHED
Patient's pain has been relieved.	Patient needs no medications for pain after removal of tumor and recovery from surgery.
Patient did not have a pathologic fracture.	Surgical plating has strengthened bone to prevent fracture.
Patient has coped satisfactorily with diagnosis.	Patient reports that physicians have stated that all tumor was removed; bone scans are negative; patient states that he feels very positive about the future.
Patient did not develop an infection.	Patient's vital signs are normal; wound healing is progressing at normal rate; there is no drainage; wound edges are well approximated.
Patient has adequate gas exchange.	Breath sounds are clear in all lobes; patient has no cough; skin color is pink.
Patient has regained skin integrity following treatments (skin grafts).	Donor site is granulating in well; skin graft has adhered to recipient bed; there are no decubiti.

PATIENT TEACHING

Include family and significant others in discussions.

1. Teach the patient the specifics of the particular tumor, or reiterate the physician's explanations; use pictures and charts as needed.
2. Discuss the diagnostic regimen, explain all proposed tests, and answer questions as they arise.
3. Repeat explanations as appropriate (anxiety may prevent the patient from understanding initial explanations).
4. Discuss the proposed therapies as appropriate. Depending on whether the tumor is benign or malignant, (1) surgical resection or removal with wide excision of contiguous tissues, or amputation, (2) preoperative and/or postoperative radiation or chemotherapy (discuss side effects if appropriate), and (3) repeated follow-up visits to the physician.
5. Schedule time for the patient to ask further questions or to clarify upcoming events.
6. Discuss rehabilitative exercises as needed; include repetitive and resistive factors as appropriate.
7. Teach the patient stump wrapping techniques if an amputation was performed.
8. Reiterate the orthotist's instructions about use of the prosthesis.

CHAPTER 11

Congenital Musculoskeletal Conditions

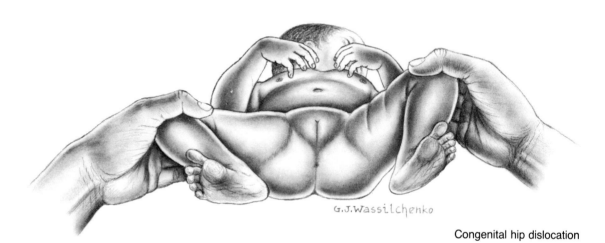

G.J.Wassilchenko

Congenital hip dislocation

Congenital anomalies are malformations or deviations in an organ or structure that an infant is born with or that become evident soon after birth. Such anomalies may be inherited, may have developed during the gestational period, or may be incurred during birth. Congenital anomalies may involve one organ, part of an organ, or a number of organs or tissues; they may be evident as absence of a part, extra members or parts, or malformed or malfunctioning organs or tissues.

Congenital anomalies generally affect the infant's movements, muscle tone, posture, ambulation at the proper or usual time, activities of daily living, and livelihood and associated activities of circulation, neural integration, nutrition, respiratory functions and, at times, gastrointestinal functions. Body image and self-concept perceptions may be involved for a short period, or the condition may have lifelong social or interpersonal repercussions.

Many factors have been suggested as possible causes of congenital anomalies. Some anomalies are associated with intrauterine positions (e.g., congenital hip dysplasia and clubfoot).

Congenital Hip Dysplasia

The term **congenital hip dysplasia (CHD)** covers a spectrum of conditions arising from abnormal development of the hip joint. These conditions range from minimum instability or congruence of the femoral head with the acetabulum to irreducible femoral head dislocation with associated adaptive changes.

Abnormal signs may not be detectable initially but become apparent as the baby becomes more mobile through crawling and walking.

PATHOPHYSIOLOGY

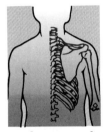

As with clubfoot, the exact cause of CHD is unknown. Currently it is thought to be caused by three major factors: lack of acetabular depth, ligamentous laxity, and intrauterine breech position.[85] At birth the acetabulum has less depth than later as the child grows; this shallowness predisposes to hip instability. Ligament and muscle laxity, common in some families, also contributes to hip instability, as does the breech position. Approximately 17% of all CDH occurs in babies born after breech presentations. The incidence among whites is 1 in 60. For unknown reasons, black and Oriental babies are less likely to develop congenital hip dysplasia.[85] Girl babies are more prone to the condition than are boys.

COMPLICATIONS

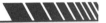

> Hip instability
> Complete hip dislocation

ASSESSMENT

Because of the hips' position in the body, it is important to check carefully for congenital hip dysplasia in the initial physical examinations of newborns and during later examinations as the baby crawls or walks. The longer the dysplasia continues, the more difficult it is to regain normal hip anatomy and functioning. Therefore early diagnosis and treatments appropriate to the specific anomaly are vital for the long-term prognosis (Figure 11-1).

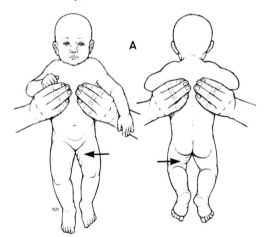

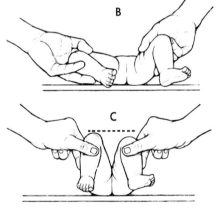

FIGURE 11-1
Signs of congenital hip dislocation. **A,** Asymmetry of gluteal and thigh folds. **B,** Limited hip abduction, as seen in flexion. **C,** Apparent shortening of the femur, as indicated by the level of the knees in flexion. **D,** Ortolani's click (if infant is under 4 weeks of age). **E,** Trendelenburg sign or gait (if child is weight bearing). (From Whaley LF and Wong DL: Nursing care of infants and children, ed 4, St Louis, 1991, Mosby–Year Book, Inc.)

DIAGNOSTIC STUDIES AND FINDINGS

Diagnostic test	Findings
X-rays	May not be definitive for newborn; older child may show increased obliquity of acetabular roof and displacement of femoral ossific nucleus[85] Lines drawn on x-ray across each acetabular roof show lower or superior placement of dysplastic hip

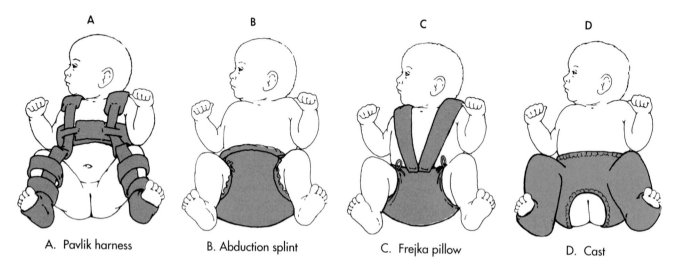

FIGURE 11-2
Various devices used to reduce a congenitally dislocated hip.
A, Pavlik harness. **B,** Abduction splint. **C,** Frejka pillow splint.
D, Plaster cast.

MEDICAL MANAGEMENT

GENERAL MANAGEMENT

Meticulous skin care around immobilized tissues; ROM exercises to unaffected tissues; orthosis (shoe lift).
Immobilization of hips in less than 60-degrees abduction per hip
Pavlik harness (Figure 11-2, *A*)
Abduction splint (Figure 11-2, *B*)
Frejka pillow splint (Figure 11-2, *C*)
Plaster cast (Figure 11-2, *D*)
Triple diapering: Imprecise for definitive treatment but may be used to help determine precise nature of hip disease.
Application of skin traction: Bryant's or split Russell traction (see Figure 12-6, *A*, page 194 and Figure 12-6, *C*, page 195)

SURGERY

Closed or open reduction; osteotomy; adductor tenotomy; arthroplasty.

The child should be examined for Allis' sign, Barlow's maneuver, Ortolani's maneuver, and Trendelenburg's sign (see inside back cover). Specific findings include uneven knee heights, an uneven number of thigh skin folds, shortened thigh length, fullness of the buttocks from posterior displacement of the femoral head, and asymmetric position of the greater trochanter. In addition, the mobility triad can be assessed: hip flexion contracture, hip adduction contracture, and knee flexion contracture (a normal newborn has 20 to 40 degrees of hip flexion contracture, no or minimum hip adduction contracture, and some degree of knee contracture).

NURSING CARE

Nursing diagnoses and interventions are very similar to those for clubfoot (see page 177). The pelvic and hip areas may be substituted for ankle and foot assesments and interventions. Nursing interventions for patients in traction or casts or after surgery are discussed in appropriate chapters.

Talipes Equinovarus (Clubfoot)

Talipes equinovarus is a condition of adduction of the forefoot, inversion (varus) of the foot, and downward pointing of the foot and toes (equinus) (Figure 11-3).

Clubfoot is one of the most common congenital anomalies, occurring at a rate of one to three cases per 1,000 live births; boys are affected twice as often as girls.

True clubfoot has all three of the components mentioned above. In addition, the Achilles tendon is shortened, the foot and talus may not be in their normal positions, and there may be subluxation of the talonavicular joint. The neck of the talus may be short and rotated abnormally. If the condition is unilateral, the affected foot is smaller, as are the calf tissues on that side. Joint tissues in the ankle and foot are contracted and thickened, inhibiting their functions.

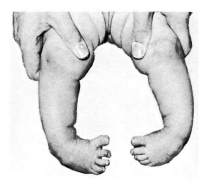

FIGURE 11-3
Bilateral congenital talipes equinovarus in a 2-month-old infant. (From Brashear HR Jr and Raney RB: Handbook of orthopaedic surgery, ed 10, St Louis, 1986, The CV Mosby Co.)

PATHOPHYSIOLOGY

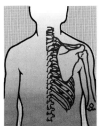

The cause of clubfoot is a matter of controversy. Theories include genetic and chromosomal variations with some hereditary correlations, intrauterine position or compression of developing tissues, interruption of development during the first trimester, and maternal use of certain medications such as abortifacients and drugs containing curare.

COMPLICATIONS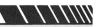

Degenerative joint disease
Abnormal ambulation

DIAGNOSTIC STUDIES AND FINDINGS

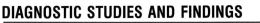

Diagnostic test	Findings
X-rays	Abnormal positions; subluxations of tissues and bones; varus of metatarsal bones

FIGURE 11-4
Feet casted for correction of bilateral congenital talipes equinovarus. (From Brashear HR Jr and Raney RB: Handbook of orthopaedic surgery, ed 10, St Louis, 1986, The CV Mosby Co.)

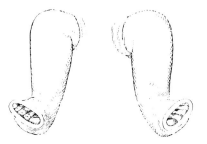

MEDICAL MANAGEMENT

GENERAL MANAGEMENT

Gentle massage of both feet before and between casts; repositioning infant q 2 hr.
Application of plaster or fiberglass cast to affected foot or feet (Figure 11-4); cast changes q 2-3 wk for 3-5 mo.
Application of Denis Browne splint to feet.
Orthosis or special shoe(s); leg orthosis to aid foot dorsiflexion and correct varus.

DRUG THERAPY

Acetaminophen: Dosage determined by infant's age; phenobarbital: Dosage determined by infant's age.

SURGERY

Corrective procedures (most are done at 3-18 mo of age or older); release of Achilles tendon; osteotomy or resection of metatarsal bones to correct metatarsal varus; arthrodesis of tarsal and subtalar joints; osteotomy of tibia and fibula to correct persistent deformities.

---

1   ASSESS

ASSESSMENT	OBSERVATIONS
Size, shape, and position of each foot and ankle	One or both feet deformed; ankle in equinus; heel (hindfoot) varus or valgus; forefoot everted or inverted and adducted; foot in equinus
Calf of each leg	Equal or smaller on affected foot
Achilles tendon of each foot	Tighter and shorter on affected foot
Possible other anomalies	Flatfoot or flatfeet; congenital dislocation of talus; genu varus or valgus; other upper extremity anomalies

2 DIAGNOSE

NURSING DIAGNOSIS	SUPPORTIVE ASSESSMENT FINDINGS
Impaired physical mobility related to casts, splints, or braces	Infant cries or frets when unable to lift or move casts; infant in Denis Browne splint stays in position in which placed; parent moves infant's feet and legs and changes infant's position
Potential body image disturbance related to residual deformity or need for surgical repair	Baby or child cries when bearing weight and sits down quickly; shoes don't fit well; heel and ankle remain in some degree of equinus; parents express concern for child's deformity even after treatment; forefoot remains adducted and in varus position

3 PLAN

Patient goals

1. The infant will eventually be able to walk satisfactorily and will gain satisfactory anatomy of foot and ankle.

2. The infant or toddler will develop a positive body image regardless of residual deformities or sugical repair.

4 IMPLEMENT

NURSING DIAGNOSIS	NURSING INTERVENTIONS	RATIONALE
Impaired physical mobility related to casts, splints, or braces	Assess feet and ankles for positions, size, and shape.	Determines extent of anomalies for proper treatment.
	Help infant change positions as needed q 2 h; provide ROM to all joints as able.	Keeps circulation and strength in muscles, joints, and all tissues.
	After casts or splints are applied: provide skin care to areas around casts or splints.	Casts and splints can irritate the child's tender skin.
	Help parents aid infant's mobility (e.g., take infant about in carriage, cart, wagon, or carrying vest).	Maintains activity and interactions to stimulate infant's interest, growth, and development; aids parent-infant interaction.
	Measure infant's growth and development, using accepted norms.	Determines if additional services are needed.
	Explain serial cast changes (to accommodate child's growth) or application of splint.	Understanding increases parents' full participation in care.
Potential body image disturbance related to residual deformity or need for surgical repair	Encourage discussion of concerns and feelings regarding child's appearance.	Discussion eases anxiety and aids understanding.
	Discuss methods to improve body image with clothing, shoes, stockings, or socks and through personal interactions.	Helps improve self-acceptance and parents' positive feelings toward infant or child.

5   EVALUATE

PATIENT OUTCOME	DATA INDICATING THAT OUTCOME IS REACHED
Patient walks satisfactorily and has satisfactory anatomy of feet and ankles.	Infant holds foot and ankle in nearly normal positions; infant stands with feet and ankles in satisfactory positions. Infant crawls at appropriate age; stands and uses table or chairs for support while standing.
Patient is developing a positive body image regardless of residual deformities or surgical repairs.	Child smiles, has happy expression after bringing self to standing position; grips parent's fingers to walk about.

PATIENT TEACHING

1. Explain or repeat explanation about infant's clubfoot.
2. Clarify specific treatments for infant's condition.
3. Discuss the parents' feelings and reactions to infant's anomaly.
4. Discuss and explain serial use of casts, splints, or orthoses for their infant.
5. Teach the parents how to apply the splint or orthoses, and discuss how to care for the equipment to maintain its integrity.
6. Teach the parents how to perform neurovascular checks.
7. Teach the parents how to care for the skin to maintain its integrity.
8. If surgery is to be done, discuss with the parents its purposes and probable schedule or recovery program.
9. Discuss with the parents (and child, if old enough) ways to improve body image with clothing, shoes, stockings, or socks.
10. Explain to the parents the importance of parent-child interactions to maintain bonding and normal psychological development.

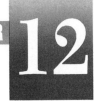
Casts, Traction, and External Fixation Devices

Casts

A **cast** is a means to provide immobilization to permit healing of a fractured bone, to stabilize an unstable fracture, to relieve pain by resting a part through immobilization, and to aid or assist in realigning deformed or malpositioned tissues such as club foot or congenital hip dislocation or dysplasia.

The firmness of the cast helps overcome the forces of rotation or distraction for the time needed for bone union, for changing alignment of bones and soft tissues, and to aid joint stability. The length of time required for immobilization in a cast varies with its purpose, the specific condition being treated, and the evidence of healing, realignment, or joint stability. Names given to casts are related to their length and part or parts encased in the cast (see box on page 180 and Figure 12-1).

APPLICATION OF CASTS

The majority of casts are still applied with plaster because of its strength. Other materials used for casts are fiberglass, thermoplast, or various types of cast tapes of polyester/cotton blends.

Prior to application of a cast, the physician discusses with the patient, significant others, or parents (if the patient is a child or baby) the purposes of the cast, area to be encased, probable length of time in the cast, and any special concerns or care required during the time the cast is being applied, while it is drying, and long-term care factors.

The cast may be applied in a room specially equipped with a cast table, cart with needed supplies which can be moved into various sites or positions, and other necessary supplies and equipment such as rolls of various sizes of Stockinette, felt, sheet wadding, Spandex or Webril, cast cutter, scissors, and sink and pail for dampening the plaster rolls. Supplies may also be kept in a room in the emergency department or in the surgical suite for applying casts in those settings.

Nursing preparations and observations of the patient and the site to be encased are vital for the safety and comfort of the patient. Observations are made of the neurovascular status of the tissues, skin integrity, open areas, rash, bruises, edema, deformity, and dirt or foreign material. Skin surfaces are cleansed as needed. Signs of nervousness or anxiety are assessed

NAMES OF CASTS ACCORDING TO ANATOMIC AREA

Short arm cast   Forearm and wrist
Long arm, or hanging, cast   Upper, arm, forearm, and wrist
Body cast   Chest and abdomen, front and back
Minerva jacket   Head, neck, and chest to hip area
Body spica* cast   Hip, abdomen, and back, thigh, and leg (one or both legs)
Thumb spica* cast   Thumb and wrist
Shoulder spica* cast   Shoulder, chest, back, and arm
Long leg cast   Thigh, leg, and foot
Short leg cast   Leg and foot

*The word *spica* comes from the Latin word for spear of grain, which has overlapping parts making up the grain heads. The rolls of plaster in a spica cast overlap and form a **V** similar to the kernels in the grain heads.

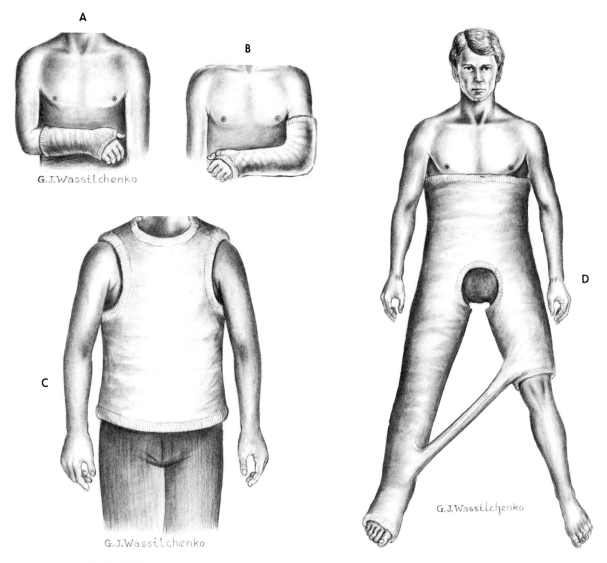

FIGURE 12-1
Types of casts. **A,** Short arm cast. **B,** Long arm cast. **C,** Plaster body jacket cast. **D,** One and one-half hip spica cast. (From Thompson JM et al: Mosby's manual of clinical nursing, ed 2, St Louis, 1989, The CV Mosby Co.)

and, if indicated, an order for a sedative, muscle relaxant or analgesic should be sought and the proper medication administered, especially if a fracture will be reduced prior to application of the cast. The nurse may assist radiology technicians to position the patient as comfortably as possible for x-rays to be obtained, both before and after the reduction is done. If the cast is being applied for deformity such as club foot, the assessments will include measuring the present position or condition of the tissues in relation to each other so that changes can be noted when the casts are removed and reapplied at later times. Muscle strength and reflexes may also be assessed prior to application of a cast.

Plaster Casts

The specific techniques used while applying a cast vary with the materials used for the cast. When applying a plaster cast, the physician usually covers the skin surfaces with pieces of Stockinette, felt, sheet wadding, or Spandex to protect them, and then wraps the area to be encased with the wet plaster rolls. The water reacts with the plaster (calcium sulfate) to liberate heat that can be felt by the patient and physician as the cast is applied. The plaster is molded into the desired shape or position by the physician by using the free hand to smooth the plaster as it is unrolled and by making small tucks in the edges of the plaster to provide an even, smooth contour to the finished cast. At times, the physician may apply small amounts of water to aid in molding or shaping the cast. The physician overlaps each succeeding turn of the plaster by one-half for strength and durability in the cast. Plaster rolls of widths of 4, 6, or 8 inches are most commonly used for casts. If used, a walking heel is incorporated into the sole of the cast, being placed under the center of the foot, usually placed midway between the posterior tip of the calcaneus and the distal end of the "ball" of the foot. The cast is trimmed and the edges of the plaster rolls at both ends of the cast are covered by turned-down pieces of the Stockinette around the cast. The stockinette is then covered by the damp plaster that will hold the stockinette in place and protect the skin from the rough plaster edges. Usually the toes are left free of a cast and the fingers and thumb are left free (the cast is ended at the metacarpal heads dorsally and the proximal flexor creases of the palm volarly) to permit normal finger movements.

Fiberglass Casts

When applying a fiberglass cast, the person applying it wears gloves as fiberglass is irritating to the skin. The patient's skin is covered with Stockinette, then wrapped with sheet wadding for padding. Just prior to applying the cast, the person applying it immerses the

---

EQUIPMENT NEEDED FOR APPLICATION OF A CAST

For plaster cast

Rolls of plaster: Sizes 3, 4, or 6 inch rolls
Skin protective materials: Sheet wadding, Webril, Spandex, or Stockinette in various widths
Gloves and apron or protective cover
Scissors with blunt end
Plastic-lined pail
Water, warmed at time of application
Fracture table, gurney, or chair for patient
Walking heel (various shapes and sizes)
Weights, weight holder or Stockinette to hold weights and finger traps on intravenous pole or ring

For fiberglass cast:

Fiberglass rolls: 2, 3 or 4 inch
Pail with water to dampen rolls
Skin protective materials: Stockinette, sheet wadding, Webril or spandex
Gloves and protective cover, apron, or towels
Elastic bandages or cream
Cast cutter to trim edges, if needed

---

fiberglass roll in water, squeezing out the excess. Water activates the fiberglass polyurethane material to help it adhere to the previous turn of the roll. The edges of the Stockinette are turned back over the fiberglass to create a smooth edge. The fiberglass cast is molded to the part with smooth strokes. Rough edges of the fiberglass are smoothed either with small amounts of a cream or with elastic bandages rolled around the cast that are left in place for several minutes and then removed. As the fiberglass "sets," it feels warm to the skin for about 5 minutes, after which the cast is hard and firm. It can be trimmed with a cast cutter if needed to assure joint freedom as desired.

CARE FOLLOWING APPLICATION OF A CAST

Depending on the amount of plaster used, it may take 2 to 3 days or longer for a cast to dry. During the period the cast is damp, it must be supported well on firm surfaces or it may become deformed by molding into soft surfaces. The cast is placed on firm pillows, without plastic covers, and the casted area may be elevated to lessen edema formation. The cast is lifted by supporting under two joints to avoid stress in the soft tissues at the injury site, and to lessen stress on the damp cast. Personnel also lift using the palms of their hands and avoid pressing their fingers into the cast as pressure could be reflected inward to body tissues that would lead to pressure sores.

The damp cast is left uncovered to facilitate drying. The patient is turned every 2 to 4 hours to permit drying of all surfaces of the cast. Fans may be used to aid drying except following an open reduction because the increased air currents could blow pathogens under the cast, which could lead to an infection. Heat lamps should not be used to help dry the cast because the light beam of an infrared lamp could burn the skin under the cast because of its directed beam. Low-wattage bulbs of 40 watts can be used if necessary to dry a very large, thick cast. The cast must be thoroughly dry inside and out to prevent its developing a musty odor.

At times a person will have a cast applied and, following a "setting" period, will be discharged. This is commonly done for babies with club foot who have cast changes every 10 to 14 days. Written home care instructions must be given to the parents (see page 272) for safety and continuity of care.

COMPLICATIONS

Neurovascular compromise
Compartment syndrome
Cast syndrome
Posttraumatic arthritis

Generally patients in casts have no major complications resulting from being in a cast. However, a small minority of persons may have one or more complications that may necessitate removal of the cast or cutting the cast off the tissues. Some of these complications include neurovascular compromise, cast syndrome and muscle atrophy, joint stiffness, and posttraumatic arthritis.

Neurovascular Compromise

This severe complication is usually detected by one or more changes in the neurovascular checks made both before and after the cast is applied. *All* eight observations must be made each time the neurovascular checks are done, and care must be taken to detect subtle changes (see inside back cover).

When one or more of the neurovascular checks indicate that changes are becoming "negative," the physician may elect to bivalve the cast or to, at least, cut the cast from one end to the other. Cutting the cast relieves compression to allow more return of arterial circulation and to allow edema to increase or lessen. Bivalving the cast permits one entire surface, either the anterior or posterior shell, to be removed completely to relieve compression or anxiety. Two signs that indicate unhealthy increase in venous pressure are marked in-

crease in edema and increased pain on passive movement of the digits. Venous pressure increases above normal (normal pressure being 15 to 25 mm Hg) are indicative of **compartment syndrome,** a very serious complication that could lead to ischemic contracture if the pressure is not relieved.

Compartment syndrome is a condition of marked increase in venous pressure brought about because of constriction of edematous tissues within a muscle compartment (Figure 12-2). The constriction is caused by unyielding fascial coverings over muscles. With trauma, bleeding and inflammatory changes in injured tissues, venous pressure rises as venous return is compromised by the trauma and decreased arterial inflow. Venous pressures above 30 mm Hg compromise arterial inflow leading to ischemia. Ischemia longer than 6 hours can lead to permanent tissue damage, and the venous pressure *must* be relieved to lessen ischemia. Venous pressure can be lessened by elevation, by cutting the cast, or by surgical fasciotomy, which permits the edematous muscle to expand thereby lowering venous pressure. Release of the constricting fascia also permits arterial inflow to lessen ischemia and restore circulation.

Some words of caution are needed regarding elevation of an injured limb. Injured tissues affect both the venous and arterial circulation. Elevating an injured limb *to* heart level increases venous return (usually) through gravity because low venous interstitial pressures need the "push" of elevation to flow faster toward the heart. Elevating an *injured* limb *too* high impedes venous return; in fact, may *increase* venous pressure because for venous blood to flow from a limb, there must be sufficient arterial inflow to help "push" the venous blood out of the limb. When a limb is injured, the artery or arteries may also be injured, causing arterial vasoconstriction, which decreases arterial inflow. The heart beats faster to get more blood into the injured tissues, but the arterial vasoconstriction and the soft tissue injury block full arterial and capillary perfusion. Decreased capillary oxygenation causes a build up of carbon dioxide which is a potent vasodilator. Vasodilation allows increased capillary permeability and blood flows into the interstitial tissues raising the interstitial pressures, inhibiting arterial inflow and venous outflow. If a limb is elevated above the patient's central venous pressure (normal central venous pressure is 5 to 13 cm water pressure), the heart must increase its cardiac output (tachycardia) and the arterial pressure must increase to force blood up the elevated limb to overcome the venous pressure. Therefore an injured limb should not be elevated more than 5 inches about the heart;* elevation to heart level is usually ordered and can be

*1 cm = 2.5 inches; 13 cm = 5.2 inches

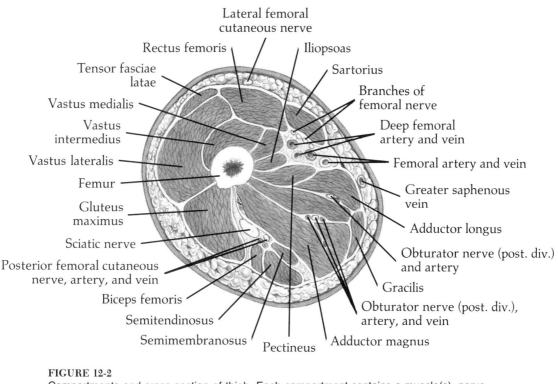

FIGURE 12-2
Compartments and cross section of thigh. Each compartment contains a muscle(s), nerve, artery, and vein. (From Thompson JM et al: Mosby's manual of clinical nursing, ed 2, St Louis, 1989, The CV Mosby Co.)

accomplished by elevating the entire limb on 1 or 2 pillows. In addition, the foot or hand must be higher than the knee or elbow for the force of gravity to effectively aid venous return and to prevent pooling in the foot and toes or hand and fingers.

Interstitial venous pressures can be measured through a catheter, or connected to a transducer, into the affected compartment (Figure 12-3). Saline is inserted into the compartment and readings are made. Readings above 25 to 30 mm Hg indicate compartment syndrome may be developing.

The second sign of compartment syndrome is increased pain on passive movement. When the part distal to the injury is flexed, there is increased stretch on an already ischemic muscle, causing increased pain.

Compartment syndrome is a serious complication that can lead to ischemic contracture of the extremity, if the pressure is not reduced. Therefore, performing careful and thorough neurovascular checks is a vital nursing behavior.

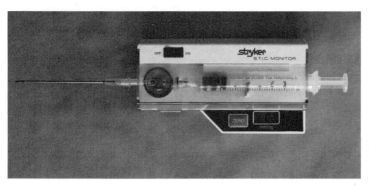

FIGURE 12-3
Equipment for measurement of interstitial venous pressure. (Courtesy Stryker, Inc.)

Cast Syndrome

This condition is a series of events caused by loss of blood flow through the superior mesenteric artery, resulting in severe small intestinal ileus and at times, small bowel ischemia or small bowel obstruction. The decreased blood supply through the mesenteric artery results from excessive bending or kinking of the artery because of the patient's position in a body or hip spica cast, although it can also occur in persons in other casts. The decreased blood supply leads to stasis, increased intestinal putrefaction, and ileus. Ileus alone can also be caused by excessive air swallowing, (*aerophagia*) in an anxious or nervous patient. Gastric or intestinal ileus can thus lead to decreased blood flow. In this second situation the patient need not be in a body or spica cast.

Signs or symptoms of cast syndrome include the patient's complaints of a feeling of being bloated, having fullness in the stomach or intestine, feeling as if the cast is too tight and that they cannot take a deep breath. The patient also may be nauseated. If the syndrome continues, the nausea and ileus become more severe and may cause vomiting. The vital signs become elevated and the patient becomes more dyspneic and frightened. Treatments should be undertaken to relieve the condition. Treatments include bivalving the cast to reduce the pressure of the ileus, inserting a nasogastric tube to relieve the gastric ileus, administration of intravenous fluids, administration of a sedative, often diazepam, and, at times, surgical resection of the ischemic bowel. The cast may need to be entirely replaced or the bivalved shells may be taped together so that they may be removed for assessments or dressing changes if necessary.

Posttraumatic Arthritis

This condition can arise from the injury itself or, at times, from the treatment or treatments used for the injury. Posttraumatic arthritis from the injury can occur if the joint tissues themselves were involved in the injury, as, for example, meniscal damage in a knee, or a fracture of the acetabulum. Both can lead to posttraumatic arthritic changes.

When the condition arises secondary to treatment, it can occur secondary to joint immobilization and nonuse, as, for example, a knee joint that is not used when a patient has balanced suspension skeletal traction to treat a fracture of the femur. Cartilage must have the pressure of active movement and weight-bearing to maintain its nourishment and health since cartilage has no intrinsic blood supply. Therefore non–weight bearing deprives cartilage of nutrients needed to maintain its integrity, and can lead to posttraumatic arthritis, or, at least, to joint stiffness.

Muscle atrophy can be secondary to ischemic conditions, to the severity of the injury itself, or to lack of muscle use and exercise. The atrophy can be so severe that the limb is nonfunctional, or it can be milder and respond to active exercises and use. Therefore, again to prevent the milder degrees of atrophy, it is vital that the patient perform active ROM exercises to all unaffected muscles, and isometric, muscle-sitting exercises to the muscles inside a cast or in traction.

CAST REMOVAL

Nurses caring for patients in casts should understand the principles and techniques for removal of a cast although casts are usually removed by physicians, specially prepared nurses, or orthopedic technicians.

The only equipment needed to remove a cast is the cast cutter and a pair of blunt-end scissors. Prior to the removal, explanations should be given about the noise of the saw cutting the plaster or fiberglass, and about the saw's not cutting the skin because the blade is removed as soon as it breaks through the plaster to the skin coverings that protect the skin (Figure 12-4). The cutter blade cuts through the plaster from end to end of the cast. When completed, scissors are used to wedge the cut edges open wider and to cut through the Stockinette, sheet wadding, or Spandex. The cast can then be removed by sliding it off the area. Spica casts, minerva jackets, and body casts may be bivalved for ease of removal.

Post-removal Care

Following removal of a cast, the patient may experience increased tenderness or even pain, edema, and muscle weakness or soreness.

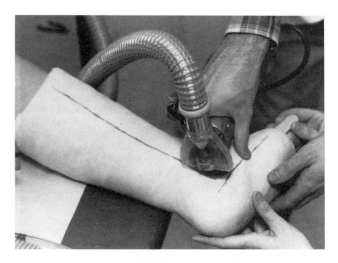

FIGURE 12-4
Removal of a cast.

SKIN CARE

Instructions on skin care and strategies to relieve the pain, edema, and muscle weakness should be given in writing prior to discharge.

Instructions related to skin care

- Wash the areas with full-strength cold-water wash solution with enzymes such as Woolite or Delicare. Apply the solution liberally and leave in place for at least 20 minutes. The enzymes in the solution loosen dead cells and help emulsify fatty or crusty lesions but cause no skin irritation.
- After 20 minutes, immerse the area in warm water and gently wash away all the debris. Caution the patient not to rub or scrub the skin areas but to gently rinse off the areas with a soft cloth.
- Rinse with clear warm water and **pat** dry.
- Apply a moisturizing skin lotion, gently massaging it in to help maintain the integrity of the cells.
- Instruct the patient to repeat the above steps in 24 hours, after which the area should need no special care.

Instructions for relieving edema

- Apply ice bags if the edema is marked
- Wrap (or have the edematous tissues wrapped) from distal to proximal areas with elastic bandages
- Elevate the affected tissues for the next 24 hours

Instructions for tenderness, soreness or pain

- Take prescribed nonnarcotic analgesic every 3 to 4 hours to build a therapeutic blood level, and to continue the medication for 24 to 48 hours.
- Immerse the part or entire body in warm water and gently exercise muscles under water.
- Begin to re-use affected tissues and muscles slowly to avoid frank pain. Explain that usually it takes twice as long to regain full function as the part was in the cast. Thus, it would take 8 weeks to regain full function of a part that was in a cast for 4 weeks.
- Perform prescribed muscle exercises with 5 to 10 repetitions every 4 hours to aid in regaining muscle strength. If muscle soreness persists, continue intake of prescribed nonnarcotic analgesic and preexercise soaking in warm water. Soreness should lessen as the muscle regains strength.

1 ASSESS

ASSESSMENT	OBSERVATIONS
Prior to application of cast: **Skin surfaces and tissues to be placed in cast**	Observe condition of skin; look for integrity, cleanliness, bruising or hematoma areas, and, at times, presence of deformity
Neurovascular condition of tissues to be placed in cast	Observe color, temperature, edema, motor and sensory functions, pain, and capillary refill and compare with contralateral tissues

ASSESSMENT	OBSERVATIONS
Patient's level of anxiety and ability to cooperate	Observe patient's ability to listen, answer questions correctly and ability to maintain desired position; if baby or child, observe crying, fearful expressions or looks and ability of parent to interact with patient
Need for sedation or analgesics	Observe verbal and nonverbal expressions of pain or discomfort
After cast application: Position of tissues in cast and extent of cast	Observe extent of cast, which tissues are in cast and whether joints are flexed, extended, internally or externally rotated
Condition and type of cast	Plaster casts will be damp; fiberglass and cast tape casts will be "set," firm and dry (fiberglass will have a "lotion-like" substance noted for approximately 4 hours, then cast will be hard and dry
Neurovascular tissues in and around cast	As above
Patient's ability to move about and ambulate with cast	Observe ability to maintain normal or proper upright posture, or hyperextended position of body cast if that is desired post-cast position
Need for sling for upper extremity cast or need for ambulatory aid if lower extremity	Observe size and shape of cast to determine weight and if sling would help patient maintain proper position such as flexion or elevation; if lower extremity, observe position of walking heel, patient's ability to bear weight (if permitted) and ability to move with cast and ambulatory aid
ROM of unaffected joints and muscle strength	Observe patient's movements before and after cast is applied
Patient's ability to do own ADL	Observe patient's ability to feed self, open cartons and prepare foods for eating; groom or bathe self; perform personal toileting or hygiene care and dress self

2 | DIAGNOSE

NURSING DIAGNOSIS	SUBJECTIVE FINDINGS	OBJECTIVE FINDINGS
Impaired physical mobility related to cast	States cast is so restricting that can't use fingers to help self (short arm cast); must learn to use crutches (long leg cast); states cast is heavier than expected	May be unable to use fingers in and around cast normally; may have sling to entire arm and forearm; may be unable to ambulate with short or long leg cast without use of ambulatory aid; may be required to remain in bed or in certain position while plaster cast is very damp (immediately after application and 24-48 h or longer, depending on type and size of cast)

NURSING DIAGNOSIS	SUBJECTIVE FINDINGS	OBJECTIVE FINDINGS
Pain (acute) related to trauma or cast	States injured area is very painful but cast gives more support to part; pain is sharp and movement increases pain	Has grimace and frown on face; holds area gingerly but carefully; doesn't want others to touch area; area very edematous and discolored; has good peripheral pulses and color of nail beds pink
Altered patterns of urinary elimination related to cast and bed rest	States has difficulty voiding while lying down; feels can't empty bladder	24 h urinary output <intake; no edema noted in feet or uninvolved leg or around eyelids; no burning or urgency in voiding; temperature may be slightly elevated
Constipation related to bed rest or decreased fluid and food intake	States has been unable to have bowel movement for 2 days; feels bloated and uncomfortable in abdomen; isn't hungry at mealtimes	No recording of bowel movement for 2 days; bowel sounds active in all quadrants; eructating occasionally
After cast removal: Impaired physical mobility related to post-removal pain, edema, or muscle/ joint weakness	States area is sore, tender, and very weak; states joints feel stiff	Skin dry, crusted, and wrinkled; some muscle atrophy compared with opposite side; joints can be moved with assistance; no edema noted

3 PLAN

Patient goals

1. The patient will regain full physical mobility following rehabilitation after cast removal.
2. The patient will experience complete relief of pain.
3. The patient will regain normal urinary and bowel elimination.

4 IMPLEMENT

NURSING DIAGNOSIS	NURSING INTERVENTION	RATIONALE
Impaired physical mobility related to cast	Assess areas above and below cast.	Vital to detect early signs of pressure.
	Assist patient with ROM exercises q 3-4 h.	Active muscle movements are needed to maintain strength, to maintain joint functions, and prevent atrophy or stiffness.
	Teach isometric exercises as needed, including muscles in or around cast; exercises such as quadriceps, buttocks, and triceps setting should be performed q 4 h.	Muscles must be actively moved to prevent weakness or atrophy. Joints must be moved actively or by isometric movements of muscles to force synovial fluid and nutrients into cartilage to prevent cartilage degradation. Cartilage will degrade without circulation or weight bearing as it has no intrinsic blood supply. Isometric exercises force nutrients into joint cartilage, and through muscles.

➔ ❯ ❯

NURSING DIAGNOSIS	NURSING INTERVENTION	RATIONALE
	Assist and encourage patient ambulation as able; use gait belt if needed until stable.	Ambulation maintains or improves circulation, maintains joint nutrition and functions and enhances sense of well being and positive steps toward regaining health.
	Teach and observe the patient's use of cane, crutches or walker, if needed (Figure 12-5).	Knowledge and proper techniques for use are absolutely vital for patient safety and to prevent additional injury.
	If upper arm is in sling, encourage patient to hunch shoulder, raise and lower it; do triceps and biceps exercises to maintain elbow circulation; remove arm from sling for exercises if permitted.	Active ROM, passive or isometric exercises are necessary to prevent shoulder joint atrophy (degradation of joint cartilage can cause the development of a "frozen" shoulder), muscle atrophy or elbow stiffness.
	Encourage or assist with flexion and extension exercises q 4 h, especially to feet and ankles, elbow, shoulder and knee.	Active exercises help prevent foot or wrist drop, joint weakness or stiffness and post-traumatic arthritis (usually develops secondary to cartilage degradation).

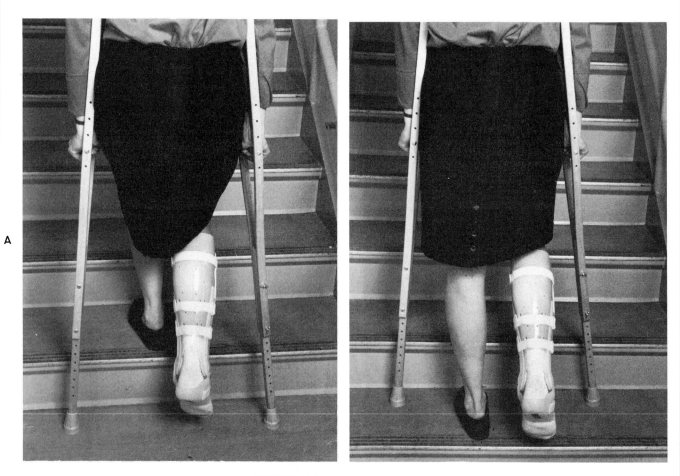

A

FIGURE 12-5
Crutch walking. **A,** Ascending stairs.

NURSING DIAGNOSIS	NURSING INTERVENTION	RATIONALE
	Support cast under two joints when moving cast; avoid lifting between joints (or of soft tissues).	Support at two joints provides greatest stability to injured tissues. Lifting between joints or lifting only one joint can cause disruption at the fracture site and can cause severe pain.
	Secure services of physical or occupational therapists as needed.	Specialized professionals offer care and insights usually not available to nurses to enhance the patient's recovery.
	If patient is on enforced bed rest, turn to abdomen q 2 h while cast is drying, then q 4 h; position pillows to provide comfort when on abdomen; if in spica cast, be sure toes are off end of mattress; place side rails in up position as needed.	Turning helps dry cast to aid evaporation. Turning aids circulation, relieves tired muscles and prevents pressure areas by increasing circulation. Pillows ease pressure of hard cast on soft tissues. Placing toes off mattress lessens pressure on soft tissues and prevents abnormal position of toes and foot in cast. Side rails up provide a safer environment for the patient in a cumbersome cast.

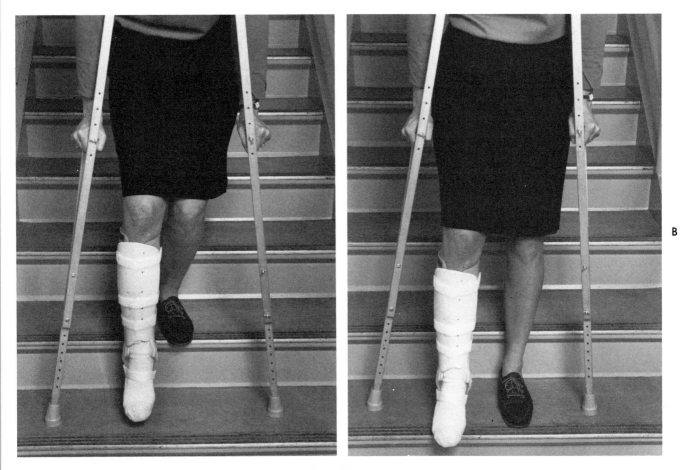

B

FIGURE 12-5, cont'd
Crutch walking. **B,** Descending stairs.

NURSING DIAGNOSIS	NURSING INTERVENTION	RATIONALE
	Periodically observe patient while moving, turning or ambulation; note whether patient is using casted tissues as a lever; note use of ambulatory aid.	As patient becomes comfortable with cast, he/she may use cast unsafely (injured tissues may not tolerate pressure from levering). Careless use of ambulatory aid can lead to further injury.
	Teach patient how to ascend and descend stairs with ambulatory aid.	Use of unfamiliar ambulatory aid is frightening; safe practice is anxiety-reducing and is vital for safety.
Pain (acute) related to trauma or cast	Assess patient's complaints and descriptions of pain amount, severity, type and length of time of pain; note site of pain and ask if pain is increasing or abating.	Knowledge of the specificity of the patient's complaints helps assure that proper care will be provided.
	Reposition patient or cast; adjust elevation or positions of pillows.	Repositioning eases sore or tired muscles and increases circulation to remove wastes thereby lessening pain.
	Apply ice bags as needed.	Ice causes vasoconstriction, which decreases edema; edema may cause pressure on nerves causing pain.
	Administer narcotics or non-narcotic analgesics q 3-4 h initially after trauma; administer "around the clock"; utilize patient-controlled analgesia (PCA) methods if ordered or indicated.	Trauma and/or bone disruption as with a fracture may cause acute pain from pressure on nerve endings. Around the clock administration helps maintain therapeutic blood levels for adequate pain relief. PCA methods help pain control to be maintained by the patient as needed without necessity to ask for and wait for administration of analgesics.
	Perform neurovascular checks to determine source of pain if pain is more severe than expected from injury.	Severe or increasing amounts of pain may indicate that a compartment syndrome is developing (see pages 182-183). Increased pain on passive movement is a major indicator of compartment syndrome—stretch of muscle by movement increases ischemia and thereby pain.
	Check amount of tightness of cast by running finger around cast ends; ask patient how cast feels (avoid asking if cast feels too tight; let patient say what he/she feels); prepare to bivalve cast, or to assist with bivalving if it is deemed necessary by physician.	A cast is firm and inflexible and does not allow space for marked increases in edema. Because edema may become more extensive after the cast is applied, the cast may need to be cut from end to end or on both sides (bivalved) to relieve the pressure of the edema.
	Massage the patient's back and other tissues q 4-6 h.	Massage increases circulation to enhance removal of wastes and thereby relief of soreness, tiredness or pain.
	Encourage the patient to learn or practice relaxation techniques.	Relaxed muscles permit optimal circulation to remove wastes and relieve pain.

NURSING DIAGNOSIS	NURSING INTERVENTIONS	RATIONALE
Altered patterns of urinary elimination related to cast and bed rest	Assess intake and output.	Intake and output should be approximately equal.
	Provide privacy for patient for use of bed pan and allow sufficient time for voiding.	Privacy and time permit maximal muscle relaxation to promote emptying of bladder.
	Offer fluids frequently; use a variety of fluids of patient's liking; increase intake to 3000 ml/24 h.	Increase in fluid intake helps maintain proper function of all cells and fosters increased urinary output.
	Listen to patient's statements of burning, urgency or frequency when voiding.	Such statements indicate possibility of urinary tract infection.
	Measure intake and output every shift.	Measuring at intervals allows time for changes in following shifts.
	Note temperature elevations if present; listen for complaints of chills or fever.	Such patterns are indications of urinary tract infection.
Constipation related to bed rest or decreased fluid and food intake	Provide privacy for use of bed pan; allow sufficient time for toileting; position comfortably on bed pan.	Privacy, time, and comfort permit the patient to relax so bowel can be emptied.
	Ask if patient has any straining or soreness while having bowel movement.	Such patterns may indicate constipation.
	Check characteristics of stool, such as hardness, quantity, and color.	Hard stool of small pieces or small amount may indicate constipation; bloody streaks may indicate hemorrhoids or more serious bowel condition.
	Discuss need to increase fluids, fiber, and high-residue foods.	Fiber and high-residue foods increase amount and bulk in stool; fluids help soften stool.
	If constipation persists, seek physician's order for stool softener, laxative, or suppository.	Medications may ease straining, aid bowel emptying, and ease patient's concerns.

5 EVALUATE

PATIENT OUTCOME	DATA INDICATING THAT OUTCOME IS REACHED
Patient regains full physical mobility after cast removal and rehabilitation.	Patient uses affected part as previously, without edema, pain, or limitation.
Patient experiences relief of pain.	Patient uses no analgesics and reports absence of pain.
Patient regains normal urinary and bowel elimination.	Patient has no urinary problems or complaints; no fever or chills; has daily (or every other day) soft, formed bowel movement.

→ → →

PATIENT TEACHING

1. Explain the purpose of cast, areas covered, and materials used.
2. Provide written instructions to patient and family to help them dry the cast, maintain the cast clean and intact, and correctly position the cast and contiguous tissues.
   a. If the cast is plaster, explain the drying time needed and the positioning and turning required. Plaster must dry from inside out and takes 48 to 72 hours, depending on the size of the cast and the amount of plaster used. The cast should be kept uncovered while drying. Explain that the drying of plaster can be helped with exposure to heat and increased air movement from low-wattage bulbs and fans (if no incisional areas are under the cast). All surfaces of the cast must be dry; therefore the patient must be turned to permit drying of all surfaces.
   b. Explain the care required to maintain cast cleanliness and integrity. Covering a dry cast helps keep it clean. Plaster must not become wet after drying or it might become weak.
3. Explain and have the patient practice proper use of a cane, walker, or crutches, including ascending and descending stairs.
4. Explain and have the patient practice ROM or isometric exercises.
5. Explain bone healing stages and the need for intake of well-balanced meals, high vitamin A and C intake, and adequate fiber and fluid intake.
6. Explain the symptoms the patient should report to the physician: increased severity of pain, persistent or increased numbness or tingling, lessened ability to move tissues, burning pain under cast, or marked edema.
7. Provide written appointment for return to physician.
8. Provide written instructions for post-cast removal care (see page 272).
9. Provide physician's or other appropriate phone numbers for continuity or emergency care.

Traction

Traction is the use of force or pull applied to a body part either directly or indirectly to bones to restore alignment following a fracture, to overcome deformity to relieve muscle spasms or pain, and to maintain alignment while a fractured bone heals.

Traction is applied to the distal fragment or distal to the deformity or injury because the distal tissues are "more manageable" than the proximal ones. For traction to be most effective, the pull or stretching forces must be relatively constant in amount and direction with respect to each of the involved tissues until the bones unite, the deformity is reduced or corrected, and the muscle spasms or pain are relieved. In addition, countertraction provided by the patient's body and position in bed increases the effectiveness of the over-all traction. Some movement of the patient is encouraged to maintain the health of all body tissues while the traction is in place; the specifics of movements are discussed later in this chapter.

Traction applied indirectly to bones is skin traction, where the pull in directly on the skin and subcutaneous tissues and indirectly to bones. Skeletal traction is direct traction to the bone initiated by a pin or wire through the bone, with the pin attached to the traction weights through ropes and pulleys. The principles associated with skin and skeletal tractions are listed in Table 12-1. Table 12-2 lists common uses for each type of traction.

COMPLICATIONS

Increased muscle spasms
Numbness, tingling
Decreased ROM, joint laxity
Decreased muscle strength
Decubiti
Headache
Pin necrosis
Infection, osteomyelitis
Delayed union or nonunion

Table 12-1

PRINCIPLES OF SKIN AND SKELETAL TRACTIONS

	Skin	**Skeletal**
Time of application	Relatively short periods; may be from several hours to a week	Longer periods; may be from 7 days to 10 or more weeks
Amount of weight used	Varies from 2-10 lbs (1-4.5 kg); less weight for very young and elderly persons	Varies from 10-30 or more lbs (4-13.6 kg)
Continuity of application	May be intermittent; can be removed for rest and to check skin tissues	Must be maintained continuously until removal
Conditions used for	Relatively less severe injuries with less associated soft tissue trauma	More severe injuries with associated soft-tissue trauma

Table 12-2

USES OF SKIN AND SKELETAL TRACTIONS

Type	**Uses**
Skin traction	
Bryant	Fracture of the femur; congenital hip dislocation in children under 3 years of age and under 30 lbs
Buck extension	Reduce muscle spasms in back of hip; fractured hip prior to surgical repair; contractures of joints such as elbow, hip or knee; hip dislocation
Russell	Hip contracture or hip fracture; fracture of femur.
Cervical head halter	Temporarily prior to insertion of skull tongs for fracture of cervical vertebra; arthritic conditions of cervical vertebrae; torticollis
Pelvic sling	Fracture of one or more pelvic bones; "open book" separation of symphysis pubis and fracture of innominate bones
Pelvic belt	Low back pain; muscle spasms of lumbosacral area; herniated intervertebral disk
Cotrel	Scoliosis
Dunlop	Fracture of distal humerus; supracondylar fracture of humerus
Skeletal traction	
Skull tongs (Crutchfield, Vinke, Gardner Wells or Barton)	Fractures of cervical or thoracic vertebrae
Skeletal Dunlop	Supracondylar fractures of humerus
Balanced suspension to femur	Fractures of femur
Halo	Fractures of cervical vertebrae
Halo-femoral or halo-pelvic	Scoliosis
90-90	Fractures of femur in children

TYPES OF TRACTION

Bryant traction. This traction is used only for young children under 18 kg (70 lb) in weight (Figure 12-6, *A*). It is applied bilaterally with the legs vertically at right angles to the buttocks. Strips of moleskin are placed on both sides of each leg; the strips are wrapped with elastic bandages; and ropes and weights are applied to foot plates buckled to the moleskin strips. The amount of weight should be sufficient to lift the buttocks slightly off the bed to provide the traction and countertraction.

Buck extension. This traction may be applied unilaterally or bilaterally, depending upon the purposes of its use (Figure 12-6, *B*). It may be applied with use of a foam boot or with adhesive strips on the sides of one or both legs held in place by wrapping with elastic bandages. A foot plate or spreader bar is attached to the distal ends of the adhesive strips or the foam boot, to which the ropes and weights are attached. The foot of the mattress/bed may be slightly raised with the knee gatch raised also to prevent hyperextension of the knee if the foot of the bed is elevated. A pillow should *not* be placed under the leg or legs in Buck extension because friction caused by the leg-pillow or pillow-bed interaction lessens the effectiveness of the traction.

Russell traction. This traction begins with Buck extension with the addition of a sling under the knee and

two more pulleys to the traction frame (Figure 12-6, *C*). Through the arrangement of the knee sling, pulleys, and rope the amount of pull is doubled and the weight is more effectively distributed under and throughout the entire limb. The pull is doubled because of Newton's law of thermodynamics, which states that for every force in one direction there is an equal force in the opposite direction. Because of the distribution of pull through greater skin surfaces and areas, this traction is less injurious to the skin tissues. Split Russell is a variation of classic Russell traction.

Cervical head halter. In this traction, a soft cotton halter is fitted around the head and chin. Side straps on each side of the halter are attached to a spreader bar, a rope is tied to the spreader and weights are applied. Head halter traction is not to be used for fractures of the cervical vertebrae except to maintain immobility prior to insertion of skull tongs.

Pelvic sling. This treatment is less used now with the advent of external fixation devices. It involves placement of a sling under the lower back and buttocks. Metallic bars are slid into sewn areas at each end of the sling. The bars are fitted into grooves of a specially made spreader bar. Ropes, a spring, and weights are then hooked to the spreader. Sufficient weight is applied to lift the buttocks slightly off the bed. The pelvic sling is beneficial for patients with marked bruising, ec-

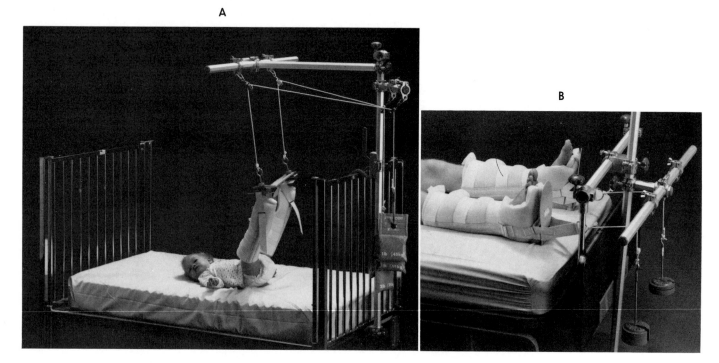

A

B

FIGURE 12-6
Skin traction. **A,** Bryant traction. **B,** Buck extension traction.

chymosis, and tenderness associated with fractures of one or more pelvic bones and with specific types to pelvic injuries, as listed in Table 12-2.

Pelvic belt. In this traction, a wide belt is fitted around the pelvis with the top of the belt closed snugly above the iliac crests (Figure 12-6, *D*). Hooks on the ends of long straps on each side of the belt are hooked to a large spreader bar with rope and weight applied. The amount of weight varies with the size and weight of the patient and the specific injury being treated, with 20 to 30 pounds commonly used.

Cotrel traction. This traction is a combination of head halter and pelvic belt tractions used simultaneously to treat or overcome muscle actions in persons with scoliosis prior to surgical correction.

Dunlop. This traction is basically Buck extension applied horizontally to the humerus and vertically to the forearm (Figure 12-6, *E*). The forearm traction is primarily to maintain the forearm upwardly to provide the proper direction for the traction to the injured humerus. Skeletal Dunlop traction replaces the humeral traction with a pin or wire through the distal humerus, with the forearm traction remaining the same.

Skull tongs. The skull tongs are placed into small drilled holes in the skull, or they may be "sprung" and impinged into the skull through the skin. The specific tongs used depends on the person's injury and the physician's choice. After the tongs are in place in the skull, ropes and weights are attached. The patient may be placed on a Circ O lectric bed or Stryker frame to facilitate care.

Balanced suspension to the femur. In this traction a pin or wire is drilled through the upper tibia (Figure 12-7). A spreader is attached to the protruding ends of the pin or wire and ropes and weights are applied to the spreader to initiate the traction. The thigh is sus-

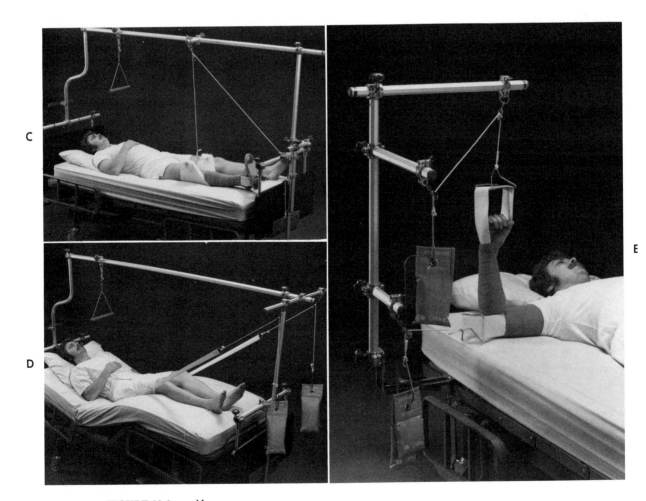

FIGURE 12-6, cont'd
C, Russell traction. **D,** Pelvic belt. **E,** Dunlop traction. (**B, C, D** from Thompson JM et al: Mosby's manual of clinical nursing, ed 2, St Louis, 1989, The CV Mosby Co.)

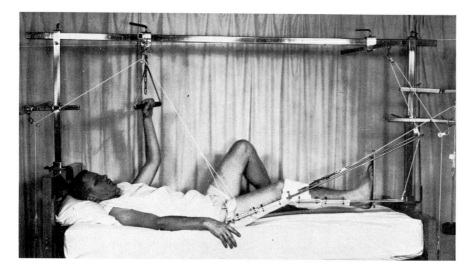

FIGURE 12-7
Balanced suspension skeletal traction to the femur. (From Brashear RH Jr and Raney RB Sr.: Shands' handbook of orthopaedic surgery, ed 20, St Louis, 1986, Mosby–Year Book.)

pended in a Thomas or Harris splint and the leg is suspended in an attachment (Pearson) which is clamped to the thigh splint at the knee area. The thigh and leg splints are suspended above the bed by ropes and weights. Countertraction is applied by ropes and weights usually going to pulleys over the head of the bed frame, thus the name—balanced suspension skeletal traction—as the suspension is balanced by equal amounts of weight used for countertraction.

Halo. In this traction, four holes or more are drilled into the skull bones above the forehead. Short pins are placed in the holes; each pin is then tightened into a curved frame or halo that holds the pins tightly. The halo frame is then tightly attached to 4 vertical metallic bars that are threaded into a metal shoulder support or harness, or the vertical bars may be held in a plaster cast instead of the metal shoulder support. The halo pins and the vertical pins are tightened equally to avoid twisting (torque) that could alter the effectiveness of the halo traction.

Halo-femoral or halo-pelvic. This traction is a combination of halo traction and skeletal traction to the iliac bones or femurs used simultaneously to correct severe scoliosis prior to corrective surgery.

90-90. This traction combines skeletal traction to the femur with the skeletal pin or wire placed in the lower femur or upper tibia. The thigh is held at a 90-degree angle to the hip. The leg is encased in a plaster cast for weight, and the cast and leg are suspended in a sling at a right angle to the thigh, hence the name 90-90. This traction is used for children between the ages of 5 and 15 years who have particular fractures of the femur with displacement and marked muscle spasms.

Preparation Prior to Establishing Traction

The patient must be prepared both physically and emotionally for the traction. The need for a specific traction is determined by the patient's history, the physical examination, and x-ray results. The skin surfaces involved in the specific traction are examined carefully for open areas, bruises, rashes, and scars. The injury or deformity is assessed and all parts of the neurovascular assessment are done. The chest, abdomen, and head are examined, percussed, palpated, or auscultated appropriately if one of these areas is to be placed in traction. The physician discusses the benefits and risks of the proposed traction with the patient and significant others for informed consent and to relieve anxiety or concerns. A sedative may be administered if ordered. The traction may be applied in the patient's room, in the surgical suite, or in the recovery room, depending on the type of traction and the condition it is treating. Skin traction may be applied by the physician, nurse or orthopedic technician; if applied by the nurse or technician, the traction is to be checked by the physician as soon as possible for the patient's safety and to ascertain the accuracy of the traction set-up and direction of pull. The physician must order the amount of weight applied, whether or not the traction can be intermittent (only for skin traction), whether or not the traction can be off at night (orders may be "in 2 hours, out 2 hours, out at night"), and other special considerations that are to be followed while the patient is in the specific traction.

1 ASSESS

ASSESSMENT	OBSERVATIONS
Assess skin tissues	Observe color, temperature, edema, wrinkles, creases or other signs of pressure Listen for complaints of pain or discomfort of part or parts in traction; complaints of numbness, burning or pins and needles of part(s) in traction; complaints of itching of tissues in traction (may be allergic reaction to moleskin, if used); assess motor function of joints distal to traction Check capillary refill of fingers or toes in traction; compare with contralateral tissues
Assess traction set-up and equipment	Check entire set-up by beginning at one end of set-up and check all parts to other end of traction; complaints of being pulled to end of bed by traction; complaints of pressure and soreness in temporomandibular joint if in head halter; direction of pull of traction ropes, pulleys and weights; condition of bed linens, wrinkles, dampness or loose linens; position of head halter, pelvic belt, splints or spreaders
Assess patient's response to traction	Observe bed position and if patient appears "comfortable" or tolerant in traction; listen to complaints of feeling "tied up," restricted, or claustrophobic in set-up; complaints of traction adding to pain or causing more muscle spasms; observe for crying, writhing, or other complaints from traction
If permitted, remove traction (e.g., head halter, pelvic belt, or Buck extension) and assess skin tissues in the traction areas. Assess patient's understanding of traction purposes and set-up.	Observe skin tissues for color, edema, or open or pressured areas, and for rash, pimples or blisters; statements of feelings of tightness, itching or relief of soreness; complaints of muscle spasms when traction released; responses when traction is reapplied. Observe reactions to being in traction; to questions, concerns, or feelings of anxiety about traction; Observe ROM exercises; listen to complaints of muscle weakness

2 DIAGNOSE

NURSING DIAGNOSIS	SUBJECTIVE FINDINGS	OBJECTIVE FINDINGS
Impaired physical mobility related to bed rest and traction		Traction completely or partially restricts movement by patient
Pain related to muscle spasms and/or pull of traction	Complains of frequent muscle spasms, muscle and joint soreness, and pull of traction on skin; states pain is almost always present, is sharp and distressing; says is somewhat less since in specific traction	Grabs back at times; has frown and pinched look on face and forehead; sighs frequently; moves around in bed within restrictions of traction; appears more comfortable after pain medication administered; able to move more freely after physical therapy, or diathermy treatments
Potential impaired gas exchange related to bed rest and traction	Complains of difficulty taking deep breaths and in coughing deeply; states isn't used to being in bed all the time	Respirations are short and rapid; occasionally takes deeper breaths; coughs shallowly, nonproductive; breath sounds clearly heard in all lobes; nail and skin color normal; normal temperatures

→ > >

NURSING DIAGNOSIS	SUBJECTIVE FINDINGS	OBJECTIVE FINDINGS
Altered peripheral tissue perfusion related to traction and patient's specific condition	Complains of swelling of feet and lower legs; has numbness and tingling in toes and sides of feet; has radiating soreness in back and buttocks	Normal capillary refill; numbness to touch; motor functions intact; slight edema of toes and ankles; oriented to time, place, and person; no external bruised or pressure areas noticeable
Potential impaired skin integrity related to bed rest and traction	Complains of soreness and some numbness of "tail bone" and heels when on back	Skin tissues around bony prominences appear pink and intact; no dryness; some complaint of soreness when coccyx and heels are pressed or massaged; no temperature changes around bony prominences; no rash or itching; no drainage from pin sites (if skeletal traction in use)
Altered nutrition: less than body requirements related to inactivity, bed rest, pain and/or medications	Reports loss of appetite, nausea after narcotics given; states pain makes him/her not want to eat, states isn't hungry because hasn't done anything but lie in bed	Intake < half of food served; 24 h intake and output less than desirable for age and sex; hematocrit 30%; hemoglobin 12 g; nursing notes state complaints of loss of appetite and nausea in several notations
Constipation related to bed rest and traction	Complains of being unable to have usual daily bowel movement since hospitalized; states feels bloated and "full of gas"	No notation of BM on chart; bowel sounds active; abdomen slightly distended
Altered patterns of urinary elimination related to bed rest, traction, and decreased intake	States hasn't used urinal much since admission; doesn't need urinal at night	24 h urinary output only 1200 ml; no color changes in urine except appears more concentrated (yellower than straw-colored); no complaints of burning or dysuria

3   PLAN

Patient goals

1. The patient will regain mobility and have relief of muscle spasms or pressure on nerves through use of traction.
2. The patient will have relief of pain through treatments.
3. The patient will regain satisfactory gas exchange.
4. The patient will regain satisfactory peripheral perfusion and retain skin integrity.
5. The patient will have necessary nutritional intake to meet healing needs.
6. The patient will regain usual bowel and bladder functions.

4   IMPLEMENT

NURSING DIAGNOSIS	NURSING INTERVENTION	RATIONALE
Impaired physical mobility related to bed rest and traction	Assess patient's traction and bed position.	Skin traction can usually be on 2 h, off 2 h and not on at night so patient can rest; recumbent position is most efficient for most traction; side-lying only permitted for brief periods to relax tired muscles; time periods in traction vary according to purpose.

NURSING DIAGNOSIS	NURSING INTERVENTION	RATIONALE
	Assist patient with ADL as needed.	Assistance may be required because of specific traction set-up; also conserves energy.
	Teach strengthening exercises to quadriceps, gluteus, triceps, and biceps; have patient do 10 repetitions q 2-4 h.	Helps maintain muscle strength, joint functions, and peripheral circulation. Repetitions are necessary to strengthen weak muscles over time.
	Have patient do ROM exercises to unaffected muscles and joints.	Maintains muscle strength and helps cartilage be perfused. Cartilage has no intrinsic blood supply, joint action required to force synovial fluid and nutrients into its layers to maintain its integrity when patient is on bed rest. ROM exercises help maintain strength of cartilage and prevent atrophy or degeneration.
	Teach patient to use trapeze and side rails to reposition self when necessary.	Repositioning self aids independence and rests tired or sore muscles.
	Secure consultation with physical or occupational therapy.	PT or OT programs help maintain strength and independence and provide outlets for boredom and imposed restrictions of bed rest or traction.
	When permitted, assist patient to sit at bedside or to ambulate with or without ambulatory aid as needed.	Bed rest may lead to orthostatic pressure changes, causing dizziness or weakness temporarily. Assistance is needed for safety.
Pain related to muscle spasms and/or pull of traction	Assess patient's complaints of pain, its character, duration, site, associated symptoms such as muscle spasms, crying, wincing, moaning.	Pain is an indicator of pressure on nerve endings.
	Discuss effects of traction on relief of or increases in pain or muscle spasms.	Helps determine the effects of traction.
	Reposition within limits of traction or remove from traction if pain is markedly increased.	Traction may temporarily increase pain or spasms in acutely traumatized tissues. Skin traction can be administered intermittently.
	Administer ordered analgesics every q 3-4 h or non-narcotic analgesics, if ordered.	Acute pain may require use of narcotics or other analgesics for relief due to presence of bradykinins and other substances in interstitial tissue, as well as pressure on nerve endings of edematous, traumatized tissues.
	Apply ice applications in first 48-72 h after acute trauma; heat as diathermy or ultrasound may be used for chronic pain or after 72 h with acute trauma.	Ice constricts vessels to lessen edema and bleeding, thereby lessening pain on nerve endings. Heat causes vasodilation to relax muscles and remove wastes to ease pain.

→ > >

NURSING DIAGNOSIS	NURSING INTERVENTION	RATIONALE
	Teach methods to ease pain e.g., deep breathing exercises, relaxation techniques, and visualization; monitor effects of each technique to determine most effective measures.	Muscle relaxation techniques and deep breathing increase oxygenation to tissues to help relieve ischemic pain. Various techniques are successful for pain relief for different patients.
	Use diversion such as music or television.	Takes mind off pain by substituting other things to occupy consciousness.
Potential impaired gas exchange related to bed rest and traction	Assess respiratory rates, depth, character of breathing, cough and sputum. Monitor vital signs and temperature.	Assessment secures data for on-going care. Changes in vital signs give indication of inflammation or infection.
	Observe skin for color and capillary refill.	Pink color of tissues and a capillary refill of 2-4 seconds are indicators of satisfactory peripheral perfusion.
	Auscultate breath sounds in all lobes q 4 h; listen for rales or rhonchi.	Hearing clear breath sounds in all lobes gives assurance of adequate gas exchange.
	Encourage deep breathing and coughing exercises q 2 h.	Deep breathing and coughing help maintain maximum breathing competence. Coughing keeps respiratory passages clear of secretions.
	Teach patient to use respiratory aid or incentive spirometer q 2 to 4 h.	Respiratory aids provide resistance to maintain respiratory competence.
	Encourage or assist patient to change positions (or turn to side if permitted by traction).	Exertion and changing positions enhances deep breathing and helps clear respiratory passages.
Altered peripheral tissue perfusion related to traction and patient's specific condition	Perform neurovascular checks q 1-2 h initially.	Neurovascular checks help ensure that potential complications will be determined as early as possible.
	Apply ice to traumatized tissues.	Ice constricts bleeding vessels and lessens edema.
	Check traction set-up q 4 h.	Improperly placed or maintained traction may increase trauma.
	Monitor traumatized tissues for increases or resolution of trauma.	Bruises, ecchymosis, edema and pain should resolve over time with ice, rest, elevation and traction. Return of a pink color and relief of edema are signs of resolution of trauma.
	Monitor level of consciousness and orientation q 1-2 h in acutely injured persons.	Changes in consciousness or orientation may indicate decreased peripheral perfusion.

NURSING DIAGNOSIS	NURSING INTERVENTION	RATIONALE
Potential impaired skin integrity related to bed rest and traction	Assess all skin tissues for signs of pressure such as color changes, edema, or tenderness.	Color changes indicate circulatory adequacy—white tissues indicate lack of circulation; blue indicates stasis; increased redness may indicate capillary injury or inflammation.
	Listen for complaints of numbness, burning or tingling in dependent body tissues, elbows, heels, or back.	Numbness, tingling, or burning are indications of pressure on nerve endings and lack of oxygenation leading to ischemia.
	Monitor for complaints of itching, rash, or open areas of tissues in traction.	Such complaints are indicative of skin reaction or allergic reaction to traction materials.
	If in skeletal traction, clean pin sites of drainage, if present, by pin-site care: cleanse around pin entrance and exit sites with hydrogen peroxide soaked sterile applicators; remove drainage with dry swabs; leave sites uncovered; or, clean sites with hydrogen peroxide, dry clear of secretions, and wrap sites with small amounts of stretch gauze (Kerlex); change gauze wrappings q 3 days; if sites are clean and drainage-free, replace only the gauze wrap; if drainage is present, cleanse free with hydrogen peroxide and replace gauze wrap.	Pin sites may have scant amounts of serosanguineous drainage for 1-3 days after pain insertion because of the inflammatory response to the drilling of the bone. Drainage that becomes more or that is cloudy may signify pin necrosis, a condition of a ring of necrotic cells around the pin channel through the bone (pin necrosis is less common recently because of higher speed drills). Drainage from pin sites should be minimal to none by 4 to 5 days after pin insertion.
Altered nutrition: less than body requirements related to inactivity, bed rest, pain, and/or medication	Assess food likes and dislikes.	Provides data for dietary adjustment.
	Monitor 24 h nutrient intake.	Data of nutritional adequacy.
	Weigh patient daily, if possible.	Data as basis for adjustment of intake.
	Monitor hematocrit, hemoglobin and total proteins.	Data give evidence of protein balances.
	Listen for complaints of anorexia, nausea or vomiting; if present, determine frequency and times of occurrence.	May be side effects of medications.
	Secure assistance of dietitian to assist in helping increase intake of vital nutrients.	A patient in traction for a bone fracture needs additional intake of vitamins B and C and required daily allowances of vitamins A and D, plus high-biologic value (contains all essential amino acids) foods to aid bone healing.

➜ ❯ ❯

NURSING DIAGNOSIS	NURSING INTERVENTION	RATIONALE
Constipation related to bed rest and traction	Assess for daily bowel movements or usual evacuation pattern.	Normally, a person has a bowel movement daily or every other day.
	Monitor the amount, color, and consistency of the bowel movement.	Normal bowel movements should be brown, soft, formed and of varying amounts. Constipated stool is hard and difficult to evacuate.
	Listen to complaints of difficult evacuation or straining to evacuate stool.	Signs of constipation.
	Monitor fluid and dietary intake for roughage and fiber.	Fluids soften stools; roughage and fiber increase stool bulk and quantity.
	Monitor bowel sounds and flatulence every shift.	Bowel sounds should be active and low-pitched (high-pitched sounds are indicative of ischemia); peristaltic rush should be heard q 30 seconds. Flatulence may be a sign of decreased bowel peristalsis and constipation, although high roughage or high fiber foods may also cause flatulence.
	Secure order for stool softener or laxative if constipation is pronounced or uncomfortable.	Medications that soften stool decrease the surface tension of the stool so it can absorb water more easily. Laxatives increase peristaltic motion to increase bowel evacuation.
	Increase fluid intake to 3000-3500 ml if there are no contraindications. Record every bowel movement.	Increased fluid intake aids in softening stool for easier evacuation. Maintaining accurate records avoids possibility of developing fecal impaction or diarrhea.
Altered patterns of urinary elimination related to bed rest, traction, and decreased intake	Assess intake and output q 8 h.	Accurate records supply data for care.
	Monitor urinary output for color, odor, burning, dysuria, frequency or hesitance, or feeling that bladder doesn't empty when voiding.	Normally, urine is clear and straw-colored; may have a slight odor that is not pungent (some foods may cause temporary pungent odors to urine); markedly odorous urine, along with burning, dysuria, frequency or hesitancy may indicate a urinary tract infection; feeling that the bladder doesn't empty may be related to urinary retention, bladder flaccidity, or enlargement of the prostate.
	Increase fluid intake if output <1500 ml urine q 24 h, if patient has no contraindications.	Normal urine output for adults is 1500 ml q 24 h. Increased fluid intake should increase urinary output.
	Report signs of urinary tract infection, including elevated temperature to physician.	Medications may need to be administered to clear infection.

5 EVALUATE

PATIENT OUTCOME	DATA INDICATING THAT OUTCOME IS REACHED
The patient regains mobility and has relief of muscle spasms or pressure on nerves.	Following use of traction, patient expresses relief of all muscle spasms, was able to walk unaided, and had no numbness or tingling. X-rays reveal bone fragments in good alignment with no angulation or overriding.
The patient has relief of pain with treatments.	Patient needs only occasional nonnarcotic analgesic medications for soreness or discomfort.
The patient regains satisfactory gas exchange.	Breath sounds clear in all lobes; no dyspnea; no cough or production of sputum; respiratory rate 16/min.
Patient regains satisfactory peripheral tissue perfusion and retains skin integrity.	Capillary refill is normal (2-4 seconds); skin color is pink and warm; no skin openings or sores.
The patient had necessary nutritional intake for healing needs.	Patient selected foods with all essential amino acids and from all food groups from menu; appetite returned; ate all foods served.
Patient regains usual bowel and bladder functions.	Has daily or every other day bowel movement; intake and output are equal; no urinary tract infection or complaints.

PATIENT TEACHING

1. Explain purposes of specific traction to patient and family members, and probable therapeutic regimen.
2. Explain traction set-up and individual pieces of equipment.
3. Explain application and removal techniques of traction.
4. Explain necessary positions for effective traction.
5. Explain effects of bed rest on body.
6. Explain need to increase intake of high–biologic value nutrients and fluid intake.
7. Explain ROM exercises, deep breathing, relaxation, and other exercises as appropriate to patient and traction.

External Fixation Devices

External fixators are used for maintaining bones and surrounding tissues for limb lengthening such as the Ilizarov procedure (see pages 248 to 255) or for treating other musculoskeletal conditions such as osteomyelitis and fractures.

External fixators are of various sizes and shapes that consist of transfixing pins inserted at oblique or right angles to the long axis of bones in which they are inserted, with the pins then firmly held in the fixator frame as shown in Figure 12-8. The number of transfixing pins inserted varies with the injury but the same number of pins are inserted above and below the injured area for equality of immobilization. The physician carefully tightens the pins to prevent torque which could alter the relationship of the fracture fragments to each other, or torque could delay bone union. The transfixing pins are inserted aseptically following thorough skin cleansing with soap, water, and antiseptic application, and injection of a local anesthetic at insertion and exit sites to lessen the client's discomfort.

The use of external fixators has the advantages of maintaining the patient's overall mobility while the injured part remains immobilized; permits care at home; allows more freedom to continue some normal activities while the treatment is continuing; and, helps maintain self-esteem, roles and family relationships. Fixators do have disadvantages of having increased sources of infection because of the multiple skin openings; torque or twist which could delay healing; and, the possibility of refracture after the pins are removed because of the multiple bone incursions from the transfixing pins. Benefits outweigh the risks, however, and the use of external fixators has increased in these days of cost containment for health care.

The nursing aspects of care are related to teaching patient pin site care and safe handling of the fixator. Nursing factors have been incorporated in the section on traction (pages 192 to 203).

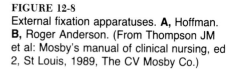

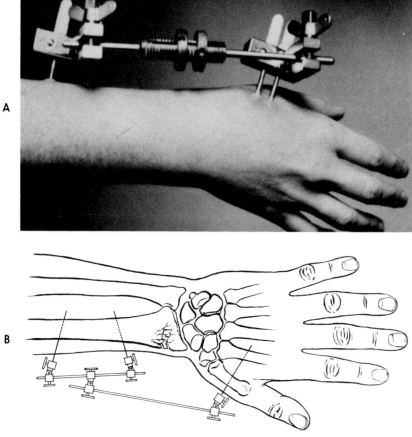

A

B

FIGURE 12-8
External fixation apparatuses. **A,** Hoffman. **B,** Roger Anderson. (From Thompson JM et al: Mosby's manual of clinical nursing, ed 2, St Louis, 1989, The CV Mosby Co.)

CHAPTER 13

Surgery for Musculoskeletal Conditions

Amputation

Amputation is removal of part or all of a body tissue or organ.

Amputation of musculoskeletal tissues is frequently required after severe trauma, crush injuries, or severe sepsis (such as gas gangrene) or for gangrene due to loss of arterial or venous circulation. Formerly, amputations were also done for musculoskeletal tumors; however, because of advances in adjunctive therapies, amputations are less frequently done now. They are also less frequently done now for treatment of intractable pain or to rid the person of chronically draining sinus tracts and infection of osteomyelitis because of advances in care and treatments.

The type of amputation (see box on page 207), site, and type of closure will be determined preoperatively by the patient's condition and the surgeon's recommendations. The wound or incisional closure also is determined related to whether or not weight bearing is to be borne on the stump or if infection is present. Sufficient tissue should be available to cover the stump if use of a prosthesis is planned for the patient. Gangrenous or necrotic tissues require that the amputation be sufficiently proximal to ensure arterial circulatory adequacy.

During the surgical procedure, bleeding is controlled with application of a tourniquet unless there is arterial insufficiency. Skin flaps are made, usually of equal length for upper limb or above-knee amputations and with a longer posterior flap for below-knee amputations. The muscles are divided distal to the intended site of bone resection, and later opposing muscle groups are sutured over the bone end to each other and to the periosteum to provide better muscle control and circulation. Nerves are divided proximal to the bone end. After the bone is cut, all vessels and bleeders are ligated, the skin flaps are sutured closed (unless tissues are infected), drains are inserted, and the stump is firmly dressed.

CONTRAINDICATIONS AND CAUTIONS

Metastasis of the primary tumor to distant sites is usually a contraindication to an amputation.

PREPROCEDURAL CARE

1. Cleanse skin meticulously with antiseptic solutions to remove transient and some resident microorganisms.
2. Determine presence of peripheral pulses (may be absent in "dry" gangrene related to arterial blockage).
3. Compare affected tissues with those on opposite side for color, temperature, skin condition, pain (if present), and edema. Edema may be pronounced in venous obstruction.
4. Observe the skin for open or draining area.
5. Monitor patient's general condition and monitor vital signs for possible systemic infections.
6. With crush injuries, monitor the patient for hemorrhage, shock or renal shutdown.
7. Determine factors related to age, developmental or educational level that could affect recovery and self-care postoperatively.
8. When feasible, have a rehabilitated person with a similar amputation visit the patient preoperatively for psychosocial support.

MEDICAL MANAGEMENT

GENERAL MANAGEMENT

Stump elevated for 24 h, then kept flat and extended (order for elevation depends on presence or amount of edema in stump)

Adduction exercises of amputated extremity, 10 times per hour after 24 h

For lower extremity amputation, turning to prone position four times daily

Thigh (hamstring) tightening exercises in prone position begun after 24 h (10 times every 4 h)

Up with crutches three times daily as condition permits

Physical therapy consultation for exercise regimen and to assist with ambulation

Regular diet as desired

Stump wrapping after fifth postoperative day (or after sutures are removed)

Orthotic technician (prosthetist) to measure stump for prosthesis, if one is to be worn

Stump check every hour for first 24 h to note color, drainage, edema, bleeding, sutures (wound), and pulses proximal to incision site

Tourniquet always present at bedside

Up in chair after 12-24 h

Pulmonary deep breathing and coughing q 4 h

NOTE: Some patients may return from surgery with a prosthesis already in place, held to the stump with plaster (an immediate postsurgical fitting). It is usually left in place up to 10 days, after which it is removed, the sutures are removed, and a new cast is applied. This fitting lessens edema and pain, although the rigidity of the plaster delays the shaping of the stump into a conical shape. However, the immediate postsurgical prosthesis does permit earlier ambulation and discharge, particularly in younger patients.

SURGERY (see box on page 207 for types of amputations and wound closures).

Continuous wound suction, if wound closed; change dressings as needed.

DRUG THERAPY

Anti-infective agents: Cephalothin (Keflin), 500-1000 mg IV q 4-6 h for 48-72 h or longer, then Keflex, 500 mg PO q 6 h × 72 h.

Narcotic analgesic agents: Meperidine (Demerol), 50-100 (or more) mg, IM q 3 h.

Intravenous fluid replacement: 5% dextrose in 0.45 normal saline, 2000-3000 ml for 24 h.

1 ASSESS

ASSESSMENT	OBSERVATIONS
Stump area and dressing	Assess for drainage, bleeding, edema in stump area, or pain (acute) related to surgical procedure; pulses proximal to stump; temperature of stump area
Operative extremity	If below proximal joint: assess for extension of joint, ROM of proximal joints, limitations or stiffness; phantom pain
Patient area	Tourniquet at bedside; trapeze, side rails, walker, or crutches
Wound or incision	Sutures, drains, drainage, edema, redness
General patient data	Vital signs and temperature; breath sounds, cough; bowel sounds, passage of flatus; intake and output; bed position and physical strength; psychosocial concerns; age and developmental status

2 DIAGNOSE

NURSING DIAGNOSIS	SUPPORTIVE FINDINGS
Impaired physical mobility related to loss of limb or part of limb	Patient has amputation of extremity; on bed rest for 24 h, then to be up with walker or crutches; patient expresses concern about ability to walk with only one leg (or ability to dress self with only one arm)
Body image disturbance related to loss of limb	Appears withdrawn and sad; gets upset quickly; wants to stay in bed and not have other patients see him; asks questions about why this happened

➔ ➔ ❯

NURSING DIAGNOSIS	SUPPORTIVE
Pain related to surgical trauma	Patient complains of pain around incision and asks for "pain shot"; asks questions about phantom pain; incisional area is edematous and slightly reddened; area is very tender to touch; narcotic analgesic relieves pain for 2½-3 h
Potential for injury related to wound dehiscence or infection	Temperature ranges from 99°-101° F (37-38.33° C); redness and edema along lateral half of incision

3 PLAN

Patient goals

1. The patient will regain mobility with a prosthesis or ambulatory aid, if required.
2. The patient will regain a positive body image.
3. The patient will not have lingering phantom or surgical pain.
4. The patient's incisional area will heal without dehiscence or infection.

4 IMPLEMENT

NURSING DIAGNOSIS	NURSING INTERVENTIONS	RATIONALE
Impaired physical mobility related to loss of all or part of limb	Assess ROM of all limbs.	Sufficient movement of all musculoskeletal tissues needed for mobility.
	Maintain elevation of stump for 24 h on pillow; then place stump flat on bed with knee extended (if BKA); maintain bed in low Fowler's position.	Elevation lessens edema formation. Placing limb flat lessens chance of development of contracture of hip or knee.
	Turn, and place on side, abdomen or back (after 24 hrs); allow to remain 15-30 min in prone or flat position; reposition q 2-3 h; explain purposes of various positions.	Lying flat (dorsal recumbent) or prone extends joints, lessening chance of development of contractures. Explanations and understanding aid compliance.
	Assist patient to be up in chair with thigh level and knee extended 4-6 h, as required; assist to ambulate with walker or crutches as able; teach stair climbing techniques.	Keeping thigh level (hip at right angle when in chair) and knee extended lessens development of edema and contracture of knee. When ambulating, leg (remaining limb) should be straight and perpendicular to floor.
	Secure consultation with physical therapists for ambulation techniques, and for adduction, extension exercises; assist patient to do exercises q 4 h	Specialists provide optimal care to aid recovery. Adduction and extension exercises prevent abduction or flexion contractures. Repetition of exercises helps muscles develop or maintain strength.
Body image disturbance related to loss of limb	Encourage patient to wear personal clothing and to interact with other patients and family members.	Personal items and clothing help patient feel more positive and outward-looking.

NURSING DIAGNOSIS	NURSING INTERVENTIONS	RATIONALE
	Arrange for social service consultation if needed.	Social services may be able to arrange for financial assistance for prosthesis.
	Ask patient if would like a visit from a fellow amputee; discuss purposes of such a visit; honor patient's refusal if visit not wanted.	Usually, a visit from a person with a similar amputation is received positively by patient and positively influences patient's recovery.
Pain related to surgical trauma	Assess for type, duration, severity, and site of pain.	May elicit evidence of acute pain related to surgical trauma or of chronic pain related to long-standing pain experiences.
	Reposition patient q 2 h: turn to side or abdomen as permitted or ordered.	Changing positions relieves tired, sore, or aching muscles to relieve pain. Turning to abdomen lessens chance of development of flexion contractures of hip or knee.
	Administer analgesic medications q 3-4 h PRN.	Analgesics help relieve acute pain related to severing or sectioning of nerves, and relieve the edema related to surgical trauma.
	Explain causes of phantom pain, if thought to be present, and discuss steps to relieve.	Phantom pain is the sensation of burning, aching, tingling, or itching in the amputated portions of limb as if part(s) still present; may be related to trauma to nerve endings at surgery or to pathologic process existing before surgery; may last briefly or may linger for several months after amputation; may be more likely to develop if person experienced pain in limb before amputation.
Potential for injury related to wound dehiscence or infection	Assess wound healing after amputation: assess for edema, redness or heat, amount and type of drainage, or type and amount of pain; assess sutures or skin clips for drainage around sutures or clips.	Assessment of healing should be done daily to detect early signs of dehiscence or infection. The first three postoperative days show the inflammatory processes of mild edema, redness, acute pain, and tenderness in incisional area that should markedly decrease over the next 3-5 days. Persistent tenderness or pain, with edema, redness and increased temperature in and around incisional area, with or without drainage may indicate the presence of hematoma, abscess, or other wound infection.
	Monitor vital signs q 4 h initially (first 24 h postoperatively), then q 8 h × 3, or as ordered.	Changes such as increases in pulse readings and elevations in temperature may indicate wound infection or infection elsewhere in the body.
	Change wound dressings as needed using aseptic technique.	To lessen chance of infection, which could cause dehiscence.

NURSING DIAGNOSIS	NURSING INTERVENTIONS	RATIONALE
	Teach patient and family members wound care techniques.	Self-care increases patient's self-confidence and independence.
	Teach stump-wrapping techniques to patient and family members (see Fig. 13-1).	Proper wrapping techniques aid venous return to lessen stasis which could increase chance of infection.
	Administer antibiotics q 4-6 h as ordered.	To lessen possibility of wound infection.

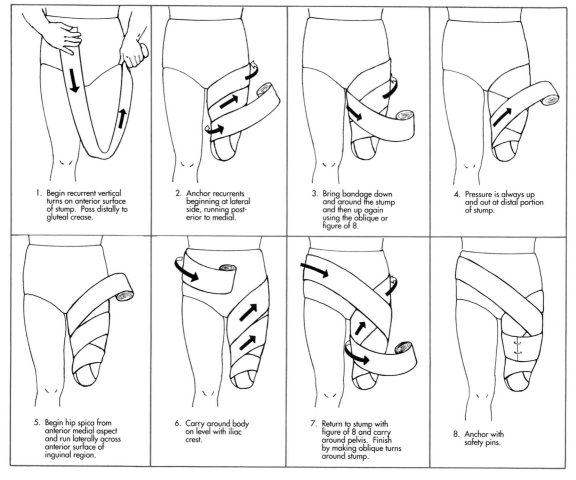

1. Begin recurrent vertical turns on anterior surface of stump. Pass distally to gluteal crease.

2. Anchor recurrents beginning at lateral side, running posterior to medial.

3. Bring bandage down and around the stump and then up again using the oblique or figure of 8.

4. Pressure is always up and out at distal portion of stump.

5. Begin hip spica from anterior medial aspect and run laterally across anterior surface of inguinal region.

6. Carry around body on level with iliac crest.

7. Return to stump with figure of 8 and carry around pelvis. Finish by making oblique turns around stump.

8. Anchor with safety pins.

FIGURE 13-1
Method of wrapping to help shape stump after above knee amputation.

5 EVALUATE

PATIENT OUTCOME	DATA INDICATING THAT OUTCOME IS REACHED
Patient is regaining mobility with a prosthesis.	Patient has been fitted with a prosthesis and is ambulating in parallel bars and with crutches without assistance.
Patient is regaining a positive body image.	Patient verbalizes meaning of loss of limb with clarity and positive statements. Can state feelings before and immediately after amputation and reasons for reactions and responses. Patient is returning to usual friends/family and activities.
Patient has no lingering phantom or surgical pain.	Patient is taking no analgesics or sedatives for pain or stump sensitivity. Can bear weight on stump without discomfort.
Patient's incisional area of stump healed without dehiscence or infection.	Suture line is well-approximated and intact; no drainage, edema, or redness present; stump is becoming conically shaped.

PATIENT TEACHING

1. Clarify purposes for amputation to ease patient's/family's concerns or anxieties.
2. Discuss recovery processes and prosthetic-fitting procedures.
3. Discuss wound healing and stump maturing stages.
4. Teach incisional care and stump wrapping techniques.
5. Teach crutch walking or use of walker, if pertinent.

Meniscectomy

Meniscectomy is removal of a part of the meniscus of the knee.

Tears in the meniscus may result from twisting or sudden turns when the knee is fully flexed or even when slightly flexed and the foot is planted.

The medial meniscus is **C**-shaped and is larger in diameter and less mobile than the lateral meniscus (Figure 13-2). The anterior horn of the medial meniscus attaches to the anterior cruciate ligament. The lateral meniscus is attached to both the anterior and posterior cruciate ligaments. The lateral meniscus is less constrained than the medial, therefore the lateral meniscus is less frequently injured than the medial meniscus. Cruciate ligament tears may accompany meniscal tears.

The majority of meniscal tears are related to sports, particularly basketball, soccer, and football. The mechanism of injury is valgus stress and external rotation of the lower extremity with the knee in flexion.

Repair of the torn areas of the meniscus is usually done arthroscopically, unless there has been severe and associated ligament tears, which require more extensive surgical exposure and repair. The repair may be done as either an in-patient or out-patient procedure, usually under local anesthesia.

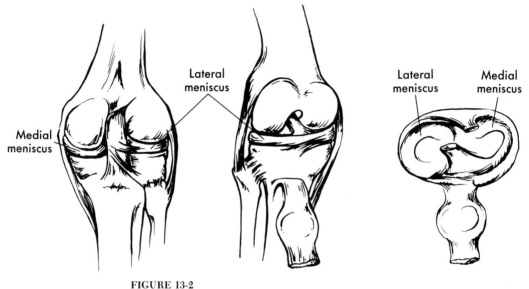

FIGURE 13-2
Medial and lateral menisci of knee. (From Thompson.)

CONTRAINDICATIONS AND CAUTIONS

The injured person should not continue to use the knee but should have it immediately immobilized and ice applied to the area to lessen bleeding and edema.

Examination and repair by an orthopedic surgeon should be made as promptly as possible.

Small tears may be overlooked if only one arthroscopic port is used because they may be hidden under other joint tissues.

Scar formation may predispose to future tears of the meniscus or ligaments.

Generally, only the torn meniscal pieces are removed; total meniscectomy predisposes to development of degenerative changes, crepitus, and knee instability.

The long-term effects of partial and total meniscectomy are not fully known.

PREPROCEDURAL NURSING CARE

1. The patient should not bear weight on the affected knee and use crutches for ambulation before meniscal repair.
2. The limb should be elevated and ice bags applied to lessen bleeding and edema.
3. The patient must be kept NPO (nothing by mouth) even though local anesthesia is used because of the rare possibility that open arthroscopy may be required.
4. A knee immobilizer should be sent to the operative suite with the patient.

DIAGNOSTIC STUDIES AND FINDINGS

Diagnostic test	Findings
Arthrocentesis	Synovial fluid may be clear even with a meniscal injury; it may be red-tinged, indicating meniscal injury or other intra-articular injury, or bloody, indicating meniscal injuries, or tears of the anterior cruciate ligament or medial collateral ligament; dark venous blood may indicate dislocation of the patella
Radiologic studies	
X-rays	Include anterior-posterior (AP) and lateral (L) and "skyline" views: may or may not be positive for specific injury
MRI (procedure of choice)	Shows specific tissues and clearly indicates exact injury(ies)
Diagnostic arthroscopy	Shows meniscal and ligament injuries

MEDICAL MANAGEMENT

GENERAL MANAGEMENT (FOR MENISCAL AND LIGAMENT REPAIRS)

Initial postoperative care: Elevate operative leg on pillow (foot of bed may also be elevated); apply ice bags to operative site; do neurovascular checks q 1 h × 4, then q 2 h × 4, then q 4 h; maintain on bed rest for 8-24 h, then up with crutches, no weight bearing on operative leg; application of cast brace locked in 40 degrees flexion or sports brace; ambulation with crutches, no weight bearing on operative leg.

Exercise regimen (varies per injury)   Quadriceps strengthening exercises (initially isometric, advancing to isotonic exercises q 2-4 h); ROM exercises to unaffected joints, then to affected knee with flexion of operative knee to 90 degrees after second week; straight-leg raising exercises to operative leg q 2 h; weight bearing permitted after brace is removed (worn for 4 weeks postoperatively after partial meniscectomy); Leg press exercises after able to do straight leg raises; use of resistive exercises per machine or with weights; resumption of running in straight lines (after patient is free of pain and has no joint tenderness and no effusion, and has regained 90% of previous quadriceps strength); no rotational stress is allowed for next 4 months after running is permitted.

SURGERY

Arthroscopy: Under local anesthesia with one or more ports (number of ports is determined by patient's specific injury) to repair meniscal tears.

Partial meniscectomy: Removal of part of the torn meniscus (may involve 15% to 30% of meniscus).

Total meniscectomy: Reserved primarily for degenerative tears in older patients because of postoperative instability of joint.

Repair of ligaments may accompany meniscal repairs.

MEDICATIONS

Narcotic analgesic medications: Meperidine, 75 to 100 mg IM q 3 h for severe pain; Morphine, 10 to 15 mg IM q 4 h for severe pain; Paracetamol with codeine (Tylenol with codeine), 30 mg q 4 h prn.

Analgesic antipyretic medications: Acetaminophen 500 to 1000 mg q 4 h prn for moderate pain; aspirin, 600 to 1000 mg q 4 h (if bleeding has been controlled).

Anti-inflammatory (NSAID) medications: Naproxen sodium (Anaprox), 500 mg bid.

Antiinfective agents: Cefazolin sodium (Ancef) or cephalothin sodium (Keflex), 500-1000 mg q 6-8 h IV for 48-72 h; Cephalexin (Keflex), 250-500 mg q 6 h PO after IV antibiotic is discontinued.

1   ASSESS

ASSESSMENT	OBSERVATIONS
Preoperative assessment **Mobility and joint ROM**	Used crutches to enter examining area; unable to put full weight on leg and knee without aid; may be "locking" of the knee, sensations of "giving way," snapping or clicking on flexion or extension; full flexion of knee may be very difficult if there is marked effusion, and pain may be increased on full extension. all joints except affected knee have full ROM
Neurovascular status around knee	Marked edema in and around knee joint; slight increased in redness with lateral bluish discoloration; skin surfaces intact; peripheral pulses full in all sites; knee joint slightly warmer than other knee; winces when knee areas palpated and states is very painful when pressure put on knee to walk or move
General health	Vital signs in normal ranges; no temperature elevation
Special tests **Childress' test**	Patient attempts to walk from the squatting position; if the meniscus is torn, it will be very painful or impossible to walk
Stress testing of knee	Knee is put through varus and valgus positions
Anterior drawer test (see page 32)	Positive if movement of tibia on femur forward and backward >6-8 mm (indicates anterior cruciate tear)
Posterior drawer test (see page 32)	Positive if both tibial condyles subluxate posteriorly an equal amount without rotation (indicates posterior cruciate tear)
Lachman test (see page 295)	Positive if firm pressure applied to posterior aspect of proximal tibia moves the tibia forward (indicates tear in cruciate ligaments)
Lateral pivot shift test (MacIntosh test) (see page 295)	Positive if subluxation occurs with 30 degrees to 40 degrees flexion of the knee with the leg held by the examiner. (Indicates tear in cruciate ligament or medial or collateral ligament)
Rotational instability of knee	Measured with patient supine, knee bent at 30 degrees, then at 90 degrees, then externally rotated; rotation may elicit instability, which could be related to the posterior cruciate ligament, fibular collateral ligament, or posterolateral capsule pathologic process.
Postoperative assessment	See following sections

2   DIAGNOSE

NURSING DIAGNOSIS	SUPPORTIVE ASSESSMENT FINDINGS
Impaired physical mobility related to trauma and surgical repairs	On bed rest following surgery; knee immobilizer on operative knee
Altered peripheral tissue perfusion related to surgery and use of tourniquet during surgery	Operative limb cooler and paler than opposite limb; moderate edema at operative site; peripheral pulses weak; capillary refill delayed; possible increase in pain
Impaired skin integrity related to trauma and surgical repair	Incision on knee closed with sutures; drain in wound; moderate edema at site
Altered patterns of urinary elimination related to bed rest and decreased intake	Was NPO preoperatively; IV replacement in surgery only; blood loss during surgery; has voided approximately 200 ml highly concentrated urine
Pain (acute) related to trauma and surgical intervention	Had removal of portion of medial or lateral meniscus; may have had repair of one or more ligaments

3   PLAN

Patient goals

1. The patient will regain usual physical mobility.
2. The patient will regain full peripheral tissue perfusion after healing.
3. The patient will regain skin integrity with well-healed scar.
4. The patient will regain normal urinary functions.
5. The patient will become pain free.

4   IMPLEMENT

NURSING DIAGNOSIS	NURSING INTERVENTIONS	RATIONALE
Impaired physical mobility related to trauma and surgical repair	Assess strength and ROM in unaffected joints.	Data help determine extent of impaired mobility.
	Maintain bed rest as ordered; reposition q 2-4 h; adjust pillows as needed.	Bed rest allows recovery from surgical stress; turning increases circulation and relieves tired muscles.
	Encourage ROM exercises to unaffected muscles and joints q 2-4 h; include quadriceps setting, gluteus setting, and ROM of all joints except operative knee.	ROM exercises maintain functions of all tissues. Cartilage has no intrinsic blood supply and must be perfused through joint motion or weight bearing or it will begin to deteriorate in 6-8 h.

→ › › ›

NURSING DIAGNOSIS	NURSING INTERVENTIONS	RATIONALE
	Begin straight leg raises when ordered.	Helps maintain strength of quadriceps, hamstring, and other muscles and prevent atrophy.
	Assist to be up with crutches with no weight bearing initially; elevate leg when up in chair; check position of cast brace or knee brace when up and in bed.	Being up and out of bed helps maintain all body functions and helps maintain muscle strength. Elevation helps prevent edema formation by increasing venous return.
	Encourage being up and ambulating more often and longer distances as able.	More frequent and longer distances helps maintain or regain muscle/joint strength.
	Secure physical therapy consultation for rehabilitation exercises as ordered.	Specific patterns and types of exercises are required for full rehabilitation.
	Emphasize necessity to continue exercise program after discharge.	Exercise program is progressive over months for full rehabilitation.
Altered peripheral tissue perfusion related to surgery and use of tourniquet during surgery	Assess color and temperature of skin above and below dressing.	Assessment gives information related to adequacy of peripheral circulation.
	Perform all 8 parts of neurovascular checks q 1 h, then q 2-4 h (see inside front cover); record findings and report abnormal findings to physician.	Use of the tourniquet can predispose to development of clots in distal arteries noted by color changes, prolonged capillary refill and marked increase in pain in the operative limb.
	Observe dressing for presence of drainage or bleeding; check cast brace or brace for tightness; check wound suction drainage tubing for presence and amount of drainage; empty q 4-8 h as ordered; record amount of drainage.	Soft tissues, such as menisci, ligaments, and skin may have edema, sanguineous or serosanguineous drainage for 1 to 3 days after surgery related to resolution of trauma and inflammation.
	Elevate operative leg on pillow, and elevate foot of bed, if ordered.	Elevation enhances venous return and decreases edema formation. Care should be taken not to elevate above heart level or to a maximum 5¼ inches above the heart to avoid exceeding central venous pressure.
	Apply ice bags to knee area.	Ice constricts blood vessels to decrease edema.
	Monitor tightness of dressing or cast q 2 h; listen to complaints of increased pain and that "dressing feels too tight."	Surgical trauma may lead to more edema. Restrictive dressings may need to be loosened to relieve edema and pain.
Impaired skin integrity related to trauma and surgical repair	Assess wound and knee area for signs of inflammation and healing.	Inflammatory changes may indicate progression toward healing of trauma and incision, or need for additional interventions.

NURSING DIAGNOSIS	NURSING INTERVENTIONS	RATIONALE
	Change dressings q 12 h as needed; note presence of and amount of drainage, edema, redness, or pain in or around incisional area.	Cleansing wound areas of drainage removes organisms that could lead to infection. Drainage should be markedly decreased by third postoperative day. The incisional area should be minimally tender by fourth or fifth postoperative day.
	Report to physician if drainage has green color, is increased or has marked odor; if mass or bulge around incision, or if pain in incisional area is increased.	These are signs of wound infection and require medical attention and possibly additional interventions.
Altered patterns of urinary elimination related to bed rest and decreased intake	Monitor intake and output q 8 h; increase intake to 3000 ml/day.	Decreased urinary output may be related to insufficient intake.
	Offer bedpan or urinal q 4 h or assist to stand (if male) or to use bathroom when allowed to be up.	Privacy and usual voiding positions facilitate urination and bladder emptying. Upright positions help voiding for males.
	Monitor administration of narcotics.	Narcotic medications relieve pain so patient can relax, which should aid voiding; however, narcotics also cause constriction of sphincters, which may hamper voiding.
Pain (acute) related to trauma and surgical intervention	Assess presence of, amount, type, and severity of pain; determine if pain is increasing or decreasing over time.	Increasing pain may indicate circulatory compromise.
	If pain is increasing, check wound dressing, brace or cast brace to determine tightness; release dressing or brace as needed.	Postoperative edema may cause the dressings, cast or brace to become too constrictive causing increased amounts of pain; releasing tight bandages or brace relieves constriction.
	Adjust position of elevation or pillows or turn to side.	Position of muscles or joints may need adjusting or straightening to relieve stress or tension on sore tissues.
	Administer ordered narcotic analgesic q 3-4 h as ordered, or encourage patient to self-administer medication in PCA pump.	Continuous administration at proper intervals helps maintain therapeutic blood levels for pain relief.
	Report to physician if ordered medications do not relieve patient's pain.	Young men up to age 27 years metabolize narcotics up to 2 times as rapidly as women (meniscectomy is performed more frequently on young men).
	If ordered, administer aspirin q 4 h between narcotic analgesic administrations.	Aspirin is an antiinflammatory analgesic to enhance pain relief. It should not be used if bleeding is a concern.
	Note complaints of increasing pain, presence or absence of peripheral pulses.	Increasing pain may be a sign of developing compartment syndrome (page 182). Lack of peripheral pulses may indicate thrombus formation in artery possibly related to use of tourniquet at surgery.

5 EVALUATE

PATIENT OUTCOME	DATA INDICATING THAT OUTCOME IS REACHED
The patient is regaining physical mobility.	Patient is walking using crutches with weight bearing on operative knee; ROM in all other joints in normal limits; discharged with crutches.
The patient has regained full peripheral tissue perfusion.	Patient has normal color, temperature of knee and distal tissues; peripheral pulses all full and palpable.
The patient has regained skin integrity.	Operative incision healing well with all sutures removed; wound edges approximated; cross paper strips holding incisional area until healing completed.
Patient has regained normal urinary functions.	Patient has approximately equal intake and output; urine clear; no complaints of burning, frequency, or dysuria.
Patient is pain free.	Patient needs only occasional nonnarcotic analgesic for discomfort; no other analgesic needed.

PATIENT TEACHING

1. Teach patient purposes of neurovascular checks.
2. Teach patient use of crutches and stair walking.
3. Teach patient postoperative exercise regimen or use physical therapist for teaching.
4. Teach patient incisional healing pattern and skin care.
5. Clarify need to refrain from activities that could reinjure tissue or joint.
6. Explain purposes of slow resumption of walking and running activities.

Open Reduction with Internal Fixation

Open reduction with internal fixation is performed for many purposes: to repair a bone fracture by fixation with a compression plate held with screws; to hold a reduced fracture with one or more screws; to hold fracture fragments with an intramedullary rod; to hold a fractured femoral neck with a hip nail with or without a side plate; to replace an avascular femoral head with an endoprosthesis; to hold new bone surfaces after an osteotomy with a blade plate or staple; to hold a straightened spine with special rods and hooks; and to hold fused joints for healing with bone grafts, pins or screws.

Open reduction with internal fixation (ORIF) can be done on nearly any bone in the body except the skull and facial bones. The bones most frequently treated with this type of operative repair are the bones of the arms and legs, forearms and thighs, and the vertebral column. The operation is most frequently done to repair a fractured bone. The operation permits the patient to be up and ambulatory without weight bearing for some time, and to be discharged from the health care facility. ORIF also allows the person to return to employment, if the physician permits, and allows the person to regain independence relatively quickly.

Specific operations with internal fixation include osteotomy, arthroplasty, insertion of endoprosthesis, arthodesis, spinal fusion, hip nailing, and insertion of an intramedullary rod.

CONTRAINDICATIONS AND CAUTIONS

Open reduction is usually avoided when there is tissue loss or wound contamination present because of the high possibility of infection.

The patient undergoing an open reduction should be sufficiently competent to understand the weight-bearing restrictions and other requirements to prevent dislodging the implants.

Internal fixation devices are foreign objects that may cause severe inflammatory reactions or infections necessitating their removal.

Implants may lead to superficial or deep wound infections at the site of operation or at distant sites, leading to osteomyelitis.

Open reduction necessitates general anesthesia; therefore the patient's condition must be sufficiently stable to withstand the surgery.

Preoperative treatments for concurrent systemic diseases such as diabetes or rheumatoid arthritis may need to be changed or modified before surgery, for example, long-acting insulin may be changed to regular insulin, and corticosteroids for rheumatoid arthritis should be discontinued before surgery to prevent masking an infection.

PREPROCEDURAL NURSING CARE

1. The patient may be placed in skin or skeletal traction before surgery to lessen muscle spasms or aid in patient's comfort.
2. Careful, meticulous skin cleansing is done to remove as many organisms as possible to lessen chance of infections.
3. X-rays are done to determine exact pathologic process and exact site(s) of repair or correction.
4. Serologic and urologic studies are done and results must be on patient's charts before surgery.
5. An enema may be administered to clear lower bowel.
6. Depending on the patient's age and presence of chronic disease, an electrocardiogram and chest x-ray may be done; results should be on chart.
7. At times an indwelling catheter may be inserted into the urinary bladder.
8. Food and fluids are held for 8-10 h before surgery.
9. A full-length foam bed pad or alternating pressure mattress may be placed on mattress.
10. A knee immobilizer or abduction pillow may be sent to operative suite with the patient.

NURSING CARE

See pages 233 to 243.

MEDICAL MANAGEMENT

GENERAL MANAGEMENT

Maintain bed rest for 12-24 h, then up in chair with no weight bearing (if spinal fusion, will be on flat bed rest for 24-48 h, then up with brace at all times); IPPB q 4 h; deep breathing and cough exercises q 2 h; use respiratory aid q 2 h; reinforce dressing as needed.

Neurovascular checks q 2 h; if spinal fusion, do laminectomy checks q 2 h; keep patient NPO for 24 h, then give clear liquids for 24 h; advance to regular diet (or special diet if condition indicates) as tolerated.

Force fluids to 3000 ml/24 h after intravenous line is discontinued; keep sling, brace, or splint in place when up; may use abduction pillow, splint or sling to arm when in bed also; apply antiembolism hose to legs; remove twice daily for skin care; elevate leg or arm cast on pillows; keep uncovered until dry; secure consultation with physical and occupational therapist for ROM and isometric exercises and home management techniques.

DRUG THERAPY

Narcotic analgesic agents: Morphine, 1.0-1.5 mg q 4 h per PCA pump; dilaudid, 2-4 mg q 4 h per PCA pump; meperidine, 75-100 mg q 3 h IM or per PCA pump; oxycodone, 15-30 mg q 4 h PO (later during recovery period).

Analgesic antipyretic agents: Aspirin, 600-1000 mg, q 4 h PRN for moderate pain or for temperature over 38.3° C (101° F); acetaminophen, 600-100 mg q 4 h PRN for moderate pain or for temperature over 38.3° C (101° F)

Anti-infective agents: Cefazolin (Ancef) or cefamandole (Mandol), 500-1000 mg q 6 h IV; tetracycline, 500 to 1000 mg q 6 h PO; cefaclor (Ceclor), 250 mg q 8 h PO.

Intravenous 1000 ml 5% D/.45 N/S at 75 ml/h with 10-20 mEq KCl every other liter (total fluids 3000 ml/24 h and 40 mEq KCl).

Total Hip Replacement (THR)

Total hip replacement is the most common orthopedic operation performed on older persons, done over 200,000 times a year as the major surgical treatment for osteoarthritis.

The operation was introduced in England 1953 by Dr. John Charnley. It has been modified first with the use of various shaped prostheses, then by the addition of methyl methacrylate cement, and most recently with the use of noncemented, porous-coated prostheses that permit bioingrowth for stability and retention.

Total hip replacement (THR) differs from prosthetic replacement of the femoral head by the fact that in THR both sides of the hip joint are replaced. The femoral side is very similar to the replacement described for femoral head replacement. The acetabular side is replaced with a high-density polyethylene prosthesis.

Both sides may be cemented into place or each may have the porous-coated prostheses. To assist in keeping the acetabular component in place, several screws may be screwed into the innominate bone. The press fit of the femoral component holds it firmly in place (Figure 13-3). After the prostheses are in place, the muscles and soft tissues are replaced to eliminate dead space around the femoral prosthesis, and the incision is closed and dressed. A suction drainage system (Figure 13-4) may be placed, although all orthopedic surgeons do not use them. Additionally, the patient's operative leg may be wrapped from the foot to the thigh, or thigh-high antiembolism hose are applied to lessen venous stasis and edema formation. A knee immobilizer may be placed over the knee on the operative side to prevent knee-hip flexion. The patient is transferred to the hospital bed and an abduction pillow is placed between the legs to maintain the desired abduction position (Figure 13-5).

A   B

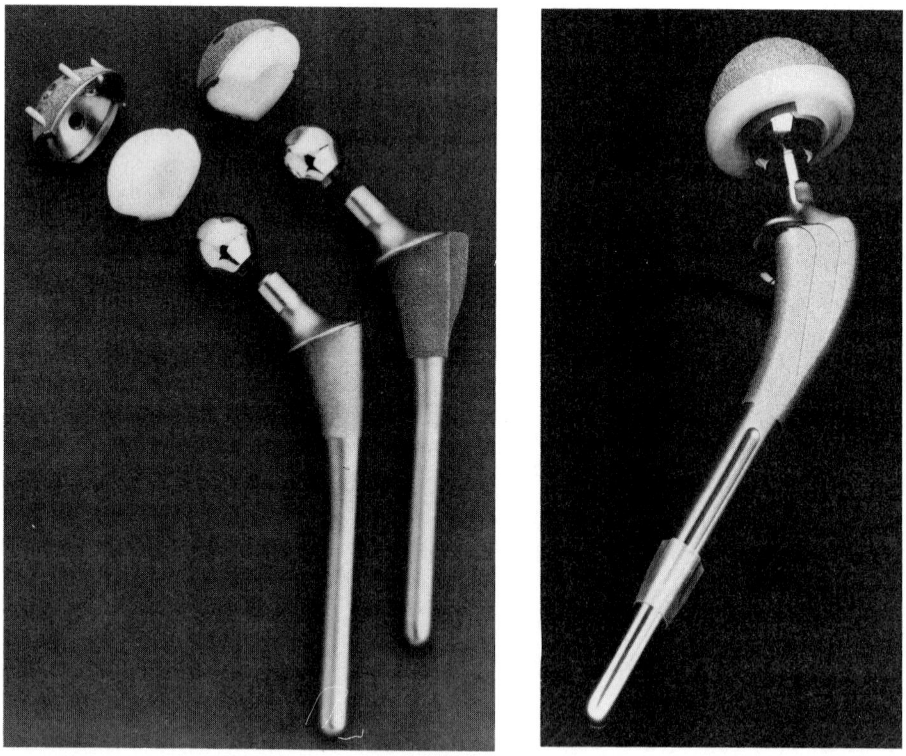

FIGURE 13-3
Several types of total hip replacement prostheses. (**A** Courtesy Zimmer, Warsaw, IN. **B** Courtesy Biomet, Warsaw, IN.)

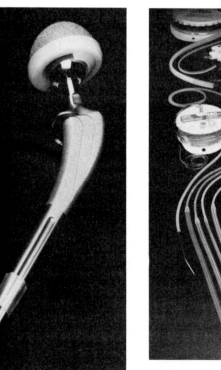

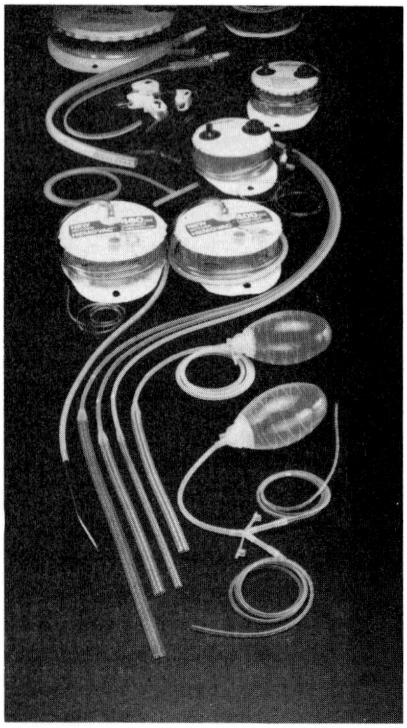

FIGURE 13-4
Several types of wound drainage systems used after total joint replacements. (Courtesy Zimmer, Warsaw, IN.)

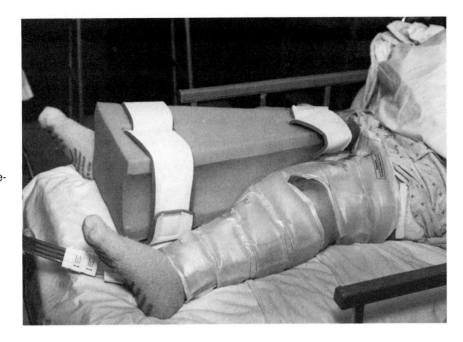

FIGURE 13-5
Abduction pillow used to help maintain postoperative abduction after total hip replacement.

CONTRAINDICATIONS AND CAUTIONS

Arterial peripheral vascular disease and venous stasis ulcers are contraindications which could cause delayed wound healing, thrombophlebitis or infections if marked disease is present.

Prior implants may leave insufficient bone stock for proper seating into the acetabulum or femoral shaft leading to instability or loosening.

Marked obesity may negate having the operation due to greater operative difficulty and postoperative weight bearing problems.

Marked debility or muscle weakness may be contraindications because of requirements for postoperative rehabilitation.

Joint infection with or without systemic infection is a major deterrent as infection predisposes to loosening, delays healing and may lead to osteomyelitis.

Acute flare-up of chronic rheumatic or other inflammatory disease is a contraindication until the flare is controlled or becomes quiescent.

Since methyl methacrylate is excreted through the lungs, the respiratory tissues must be healthy prior to surgery when cement is used.

Bleeding or clotting disorders require special medical and nursing considerations to prevent hemorrhage or excessive bleeding.

Porous-coated prostheses used without cement must be "press fit" for bioingrowth requiring sufficient femoral shaft bone stock for proper seating. Fracture of the femoral shaft can occur with weakened bone.

PREPROCEDURAL NURSING CARE

1. Serologic and urologic studies are done; results should be on chart
2. Because of the older age of patient, chest x-rays and electrocardiogram are done to determine presence of chronic diseases or condition that could require postponement of surgery.
3. Current x-rays are taken and measurements done to determine size of prostheses; x-rays are sent to surgery with the patient.
4. An enema is given to clear the lower bowel.
5. An indwelling catheter may be inserted into the urinary bladder.
6. A trapeze and foam mattress pad are placed on the patient's bed (new foam mattress may be sent to operating suite with the patient for placement after surgery).
7. Food and fluids are held 8-10 h before surgery.
8. An abduction pillow is sent to the operating suite with the patient, who usually is sent to surgery in the hospital bed.
9. Corticosteroids are discontinued before surgery to prevent infection.
10. Meticulous skin cleansing is done to prevent infections.
11. Exercises such as deep breathing and foot exercises are taught preoperatively.

NURSING CARE

See pages 233 to 243.

MEDICAL MANAGEMENT

GENERAL MANAGEMENT

Neurovascular checks q 1 h × 4, then q 2 h × 4, then q 4 h; bed rest for 24 hrs (or 48 hrs—varies per physician); May turn to unoperative side (if both hips done, patient is not turned) head of bed can be elevated to 30 degrees; abduction pillow in place (see Figure 13-5); begin ROM exercises to unaffected joints; deep breathe and cough exercises q 2 h; respirex q 2 h; apply antiembolism hose to unoperative leg; remove AM and PM; begin physical therapy exercises as ordered; keep NPO til further orders (will progress from clear liquids to regular diet in 1-3 days).

DRUG THERAPY

Narcotic analgesic medications: Meperidine, 75 to 100 mg IM q 3 h PRN; morphine 1 to 1.5 mg per PCA pump PRN with 10 min lockout interval (maximum 30 ml/4 h).

Anti-anxiety agent: Hydroxyzine (Vistaril), 25 to 50 mg q 6 h IM PRN

Analgesic antipyretic medications: Acetaminophen, 500 to 1000 mg, q 4 h PRN for moderate pain (no aspirin if on heparin or coumadin).

Anti infective agents: Cefazolin (Ancef), 1 g IVPB q 8 h × 6 doses or tobramycin (Nebcin) 60 mg IVPB q 8 h × 6 doses; or clindamycin (Cleocin) 600 mg IVPB q 6 h × 8 doses; then cephalexin (Keflex) 500 mg PO q 6 h × 5 days.

Anticoagulant medications: Heparin 3000 U sq q 12 h × 5 days Coumadin 3-5 mg q day.

Intravenous 1000 ml 5% D/0.45 N/S or 1000 ml Ringer's lactate at 75-100 ml/h; add 20-40 mEq KCl per liter.

Total Knee Replacement (TKR)

In a **total knee replacement,** the femoral condylar cartilage and the tibial condylar surfaces are replaced with metallic and high-density polyethylene prostheses, respectively.

The prostheses may be cemented in place or held with short-lug "studs" placed into holes in the recipient bones. The prostheses are porous coated, if uncemented, for bioingrowth. A variety of different prostheses are available for the knee. Because of the more complex movements and the relationship of the femur and its alignment with the tibia total knee replacement requires excellent surgical precision. There is a natural angle of valgus of the tibia in relation to the femur of approximately 6-7 degrees, therefore placement of the prostheses is more difficult requiring that the center of line of weight bearing in the tibia to be about 3 degrees off a vertical line when the person is standing. Femoral prostheses are placed parallel to the ground and the tibial components are usually set at a valgus angle 3 degrees of vertical. A patellar prosthesis may also be placed on the joint side of the patella if there has been erosion of its surface from osteoarthritis (Figure 13-6).

CONTRAINDICATIONS AND CAUTIONS

Repeated prior surgical procedures may leave insufficient remaining bone stock for proper seating leading to instability and loosening.

Severe valgus or varus deformities may prevent satisfactory placement of prostheses.

Marked obesity is a contraindication because of the pressure of weight-bearing.

The patient should have no systemic infection that could predispose him or her to a postoperative wound infection.

The patient should be physically able to participate in postoperative rehabilitation exercises.

PREPROCEDURAL NURSING CARE

1. Ice applications are usually applied to lessen edema before surgery.
2. Exercises are taught preoperatively when patient is alert and can cooperate fully; postoperatively, reteaching is easier because patient already understands purposes and principles.

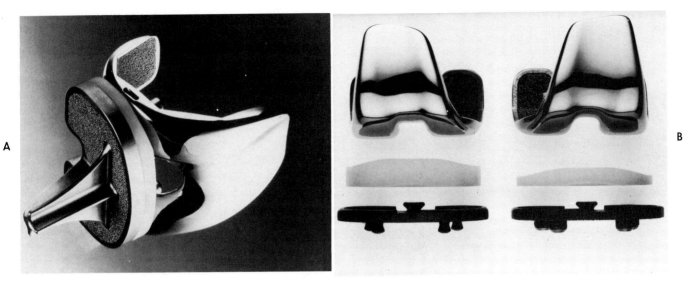

FIGURE 13-6
Several types of total knee replacement prostheses. (Courtesy Zimmer, Warsaw, IN.)

3. X-rays and measurements are done to determine extent of pathologic process; results should be on patient's chart, and roentgenograms are sent to surgery with the patient.
4. Hematologic (serologic) and urologic studies are done and results should be on patient's chart.
5. Corticosteroid medications should be discontinued before surgery to prevent masking infection.
6. Meticulous skin cleansing is done to remove organisms.
7. Food and fluids are held 8-10 h before surgery.

NURSING CARE

See pages 233 to 243.

MEDICAL MANAGEMENT

GENERAL MANAGEMENT

Bed rest for 24 h; turn to either side q 4 h PRN; elevate operative leg on pillow when recumbent; keep NPO until further orders (will progress to regular diet in 2 to 3 days); neurovascular checks q 1 h × 3, then q 2 h × 3, then q 4 h; empty Hemovac q 4 h × 24 h, then q 8 h.

DRUG THERAPY

Narcotic analgesic medications: Morphine 1.0 to 1.5 mg prn per PCA pump with 10 min lockout interval (maximum 30 ml/4 h); morphine 10-15 mg q 4 h IM; dilaudid 1-2 (or up to 4 mg) q 4 h IM.

Anti-anxiety agents: Hydroxyzine (Vistaril), 25 to 50 mg IM q 6 h PRN.

Analgesic antipyretic medications: Acetaminophen 500-1000 mg rectal suppository for moderate pain q 4 h PRN then 500-1000 mg PO when on diet and fluids; aspirin 500-1000 mg q 4 h PRN for moderate pain (no aspirin if patient is on heparin or warfarin sodium).

Antiinfective agents: Cefazolin (ancef), 1 g q 6 h IV × 6 doses; or tobramycin (Nebcin) 60 mg IV q 8 h × 6 doses; or clindamycin (Cleocin) 600 mg IV q 6 h × 8 doses, then cephalexin (Keflex) 500 mg PO q 6 h × 5 days.
Intravenous 1000 ml 5% D/0.45N/S or 1000 ml Ringer's lactate at 75-100 ml/h with 20-40 mEq KCl per liter.

Anti-coagulant medications: Heparin 3000 U sq q 12 h for 5 days; coumadin 3 to 5 mg q day.
Deep breathe and cough exercises q 2 h × 24, then q 4 h; use Respirex q 2 h; begin basic ROM exercises except for operative knee; apply antiembolism hose to unoperative leg, remove AM and PM; begin physical therapy exercises as ordered.

Total Shoulder Replacement (TSR)

Total shoulder replacement (TSR) involves placement of a metallic prosthesis into the humeral shaft following removal of the head of the humerus, and placement of a high-density polyethylene prosthesis in the glenoid area of the shoulder. Each prosthesis is usually cemented in place.

Replacement of shoulder structures is done for repair of damage related to rheumatoid arthritis or osteoarthritis, but the operation has not yet achieved the successes of those of the hip and knee. The patient may eventually achieve 70 to 90 degrees of abduction after a total shoulder replacement.

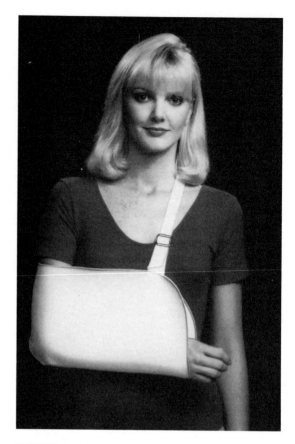

FIGURE 13-7
One type of sling used for upper arm or shoulder immobilization. (Courtesy Zimmer, Warsaw, Indiana.)

MEDICAL MANAGEMENT

GENERAL MANAGEMENT

Bed rest for 24 h; keep sling (see Figure 13-7) and swathe for 48 h, if used, or elevate arm on pillows if shoulder spica (or airplane splint) is used; turn to unoperative side q 4 h; assist to be up after 48 h; neurovascular checks q 2 h.

DRUG THERAPY

Narcotic analgesic medications: Meperidine, 75-100 mg q 3 h per PCA pump or IM; morphine, 10-15 mg, q 4 h per PCA pump or IM; dilaudid, 2-4 mg, q 4 h per PCA pump or IM; Vistaril 25 mg q 6 h IM to enhance narcotic effectiveness

Analgesic antipyretic medications: Aspirin, 600-1000 mg, rectal suppository q 4 h PRN for moderate pain; then PO after on regular diet, q 4 h for moderate pain or for temperature elevation to 38.3° C (101° F); acetaminophen, 600-1000 mg q 4 h PRN for moderate pain or for temperature elevation to 38.3° C (101° F).

Anti-infective medications: Cefazolin (Ancef) or cefamandole (Mandol), 500-1000 mg q 6 h IV
Intravenous 1000 ml 5% D/0.2N/S or 5%D/0.45N/S at 75 ml/h with 10-20 mEq KCl every other liter
Apply ice bag to shoulder q 2 h; empty Hemovac q 8 h and prn; record drainage; secure physical therapy for ROM to uninvolved joints q 4 h; encourage patient to do finger and wrist exercises of operative arm q 4 h.
Begin passive arm and shoulder exercises after 48 h; do not adduct or internally rotate operative arm; begin pendulum exercises on tenth PO day (after physician checks arm and patient); repeat pendulum exercises 5 to 10 times to tolerance; apply passive shoulder exercises on third postoperative day q 4 h or continuous rate.

CONTRAINDICATIONS AND CAUTIONS

Repeated prior procedures may have left insufficient bone stock for insertion of prostheses, leading to possibility of instability and loosening.

Corticosteroid medications for rheumatic conditions should be discontinued before surgery.

Joint infection precludes total joint replacement because the prostheses themselves predispose to development of infection.

Preoperative teaching of rehabilitative care and exercises must be understood so patient can participate actively for maximal results.

PREPROCEDURAL NURSING CARE

1. Serologic and urologic studies are done; results should be on patient's chart.
2. X-rays are done to determine exact pathologic process; previous x-rays may be secured for comparison.
3. A special splint (referred to as an airplane splint) may be sent to operative suite with the patient for postoperative application.
4. Food and fluids are withheld 8-10 h before surgery.
5. Meticulous skin cleansing is done to prevent infections.

NURSING CARE

See pages 233 to 243.

Total Joint Replacements for Wrist, Elbow or Ankle

Total joint replacements of these three areas are done to correct deformities, repair traumatic damage, or restore motion to joints partially destroyed by rheumatoid arthritis or osteoarthritis.

Wrist replacement. This operation involves insertion of a metallic implant into the radius and metacarpal bones following removal of the carpal bones. It restores motion and relieves pain in the wrist. Prostheses are undergoing modification to provide more satisfying prostheses for this operation.

Elbow replacement. Prostheses are inserted into the humerus and radius to correct degenerative changes due to rheumatoid arthritis or osteoarthritis that have destroyed joint surfaces.

Ankle replacement. The joint surfaces can be replaced with metallic and polyethylene prosthetic devices. This operation, as with wrist and elbow replacement, is still undergoing study with ongoing revisions of prosthetic materials. Therefore, each of these operations is not undertaken lightly.

CONTRAINDICATIONS AND CAUTIONS

Acute flare-up of rheumatic or other systemic disease may necessitate delaying surgery until the flare is controlled.

Surgical replacement may be delayed until the proper prosthesis is available to treat the patient's exact condition; otherwise, satisfactory results may not occur.

Total replacement of the wrist, elbow, and ankle is presently not at the same level of perfection as other joint replacements.

PREPROCEDURAL NURSING CARE

1. Meticulous skin cleansing is done to prevent infection.
2. Serologic and urologic studies are done; results should be on the patient's chart.
3. Corticosteroids should be stopped before surgery.
4. X-rays are taken and sent to surgery with the patient.
5. A splint or joint immobilizer may be sent to surgery with the patient.

MEDICAL MANAGEMENT

See page 223 following total knee replacement for medical management.

NURSING CARE

See pages 233 to 243.

Endoprosthetic Replacement of Femoral Head

Endoprosthetic replacement of femoral head is done to repair fractures of the femoral neck during which the head of the femur is replaced with a metallic endoprosthesis. It is also done as treatment for avascular necrosis of the head of the femur when the cartilage of the acetabulum is intact and healthy.

Prosthetic replacement of the femoral head is done when the fracture of the femur is of the femoral neck. The mechanism of injury resulting in the fracture disrupts the blood supply to the femoral head, which gets its blood supply through nutrient arteries within the femoral capsule and through the ligamentum teres from the center of the acetabulum to the middle of the femoral head (see Figure 13-8). Because of disruption of the blood supply, the femoral head is very subject to the development of avascular necrosis. Other causes of avascular necrosis include systemic steroid therapy, sickle cell disease and, at times, alcohol abuse.

Various types of prostheses are available for insertion (Figure 13-9). Porous coated prostheses are manufactured to provide surfaces that promote stability and bioingrowth of bone cells. Other prostheses are smooth-surfaced, with openings in the stem for placement of bone pieces horizontally to aid in holding within the femoral shaft. Correctly sized prostheses should fit snugly into the socket without any play, yet be able to move freely through the joint ranges of motion. Porous-coated prostheses are "press fit" into the femoral shaft, while smooth surfaced prostheses may be cemented into the femoral shaft with methyl methacrylate cement.

CONTRAINDICATIONS AND CAUTIONS

Since general or spinal anesthesia is required for this surgery, the patient's condition must be sufficiently stable to tolerate such surgery.

If methyl methacrylate is used to cement the endoprosthesis in place, it is excreted through the lungs; therefore respiratory tissues must be healthy to prevent pulmonary complications.

Acetabular damage or cartilage degeneration would negate replacement of only the femoral head; possibly a total joint replacement would be necessary.

If the femoral head is being replaced because of avascular necrosis, it may have been related to steroid medication administration. Steroids are discontinued before surgery to prevent masking an infection.

MEDICAL MANAGEMENT

See management for Open Reduction with Internal Fixation, page 219.

NURSING CARE

See pages 233 to 243.

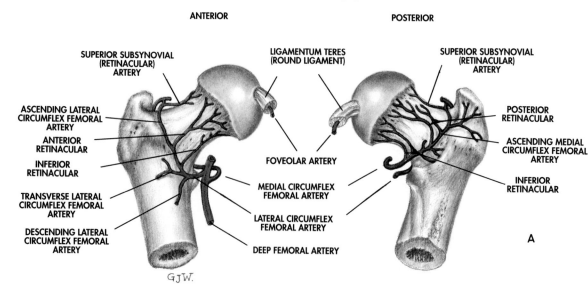

FIGURE 13-8
Blood supply to hip joint.

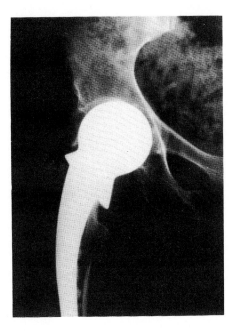

FIGURE 13-9
One type of femoral head prostheses. (From Thompson.)[98a]

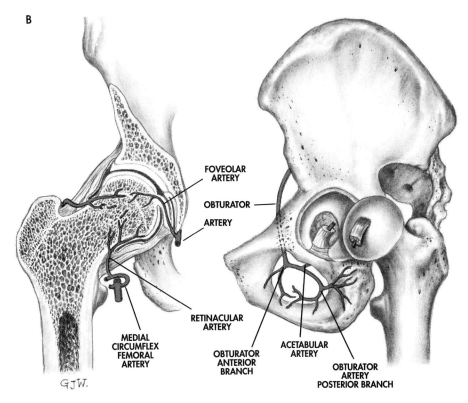

FIGURE 13-8—cont'd

Osteotomy

An **osteotomy** is done to change the weight-bearing surfaces of a bone within a joint, to straighten a part of a bone, to correct an abnormal curvature or deviation, or to provide more stability to a bone.

Osteotomy, literally cutting a bone, is done primarily to change the position of the bone for more effective weight bearing. Several kinds of osteotomies are:

Rotational: distal femur is rotated more inwardly or laterally in relation to the proximal femur; **angulation:** changes the direction of the iliac bone in relation to the acetabulum. The iliac bone is osteotomitized (cut) at the level of the greater sciatic notch or above the hip capsule so that the roof of the acetabulum will more fully cover the femoral head to make the joint more stable; **abduction:** the femoral shaft is osteotomitized below the trochanter to create a false joint high on the wing of the ilium to correct long-standing congenital dislocation of the hip with osteotomitized bones held in place with a plate and screws; **displacement:** the femur is osteotomitized below the greater trochanter at an angle with the shaft of the femur which places the distal femur more medially on the upper portion as one type of treatment for osteoarthritis of the hip.

In each of the osteotomies above, a wedge or slice of bone is removed from the medial or lateral surface of the bone according to the purpose for the specific procedure. The two cut surfaces are then brought into approximation and held in the new position by plates with screws, a compression plate with screws, or with staples.

CONTRAINDICATIONS AND CAUTIONS

The patient should be old enough to understand the restrictions on ambulation and mobility required by osteotomy. Infants or children who are too young to understand are usually placed in braces or casts to prevent improper weight bearing.

Presence of a systemic infection would preclude having an osteotomy because it could predispose to development of additional systemic or wound infection.

Insertion of metallic implants to hold the osteotomized bones predisposes to wound infection which could cause loosening.

PREPROCEDURAL NURSING CARE

1. Meticulous skin cleansing is done to prevent infection.
2. X-rays are taken and measurements are made to determine exact corrections necessary; x-rays are sent to operating suite.
3. Casts or braces are removed; a new brace or cast may be applied at the time of surgery for infants or young children.
4. Food and fluids are held for 8-10 h prior to surgery.
5. A full-length foam mattress is applied to cover mattress.
6. Serologic and urologic studies are done, and results should be on chart.

MEDICAL MANAGEMENT

See management following open reduction with internal fixation, page 219, for usual management.

NURSING CARE

See pages 233 to 243.

Spinal Fusion with Bone Grafts or Metallic Rods

Spinal fusion operation is basically an arthodesis (fusion) of the vertebral column.

It is done to straighten abnormal spinal curvatures, to strengthen joints damaged by a herniated nucleus pulposus (ruptured disc), from trauma with vertebral fracture, and for correction of spondylolisthesis, slipping forward of vertebrae from their normal anatomic positions (see Figure 13-10). A spinal fusion limits the flexion of the vertebral column as well as the rotation in the operated segments. Limiting these functions is the purpose of the surgery.

Several methods of fusing the spine are available. In one, bone chips are placed along several vertebrae that have been denuded of some periosteal segments, are roughened, and having bleeding surfaces. The bone chips are placed over the prepared vertebral segments and in the spaces between the laminae and posterior spinous processes. The bone chips have bleeding surfaces, having been secured from cancellous bone areas from the patient's iliac crests or anterior tibia. The bleeding surfaces form a hematoma, which through inflammation and bone healing processes forms fibrous and bone tissues that calcify and become fused.

Fusion may also be achieved through the use of metallic rods placed parallel on each side of 3 to 5 or more vertebral segments. Harrington and Luque rods are two types of such rods. They differ in size, shape, method of attachment to the vertebrae, and their associated instrumentation steps and materials. Use of the particular rod is dependent on the patient's specific condition. These rods are used to correct spinal curvatures, such as scoliosis or kyphosis, for crush injuries,

or for osteomyelitis of vertebral bodies. Rods may also be used if the vertebral body has been destroyed by a tumor or osteoarthritis.

When Harrington or Luque rods are used for the spinal fusion, one rod is placed on each side parallel to the posterior spinous processes. The upper end of each rod is hooked into the laminar area of each vertebral body above the injured or deformed site and the lower ends are hooked into the vertebrae below the area under repair. Cross wires may be placed at each vertebral segment that are attached to the rods, or cross wires may be placed only at selected vertebral areas. Sleeves such as Edwards sleeves may be placed in areas of the vertebral column to add pressure and stability to weakened areas. After the cross wires and/or sleeves are in their desired places, the rods are tightened on each side to bring about the correction or stability to the spinal column.

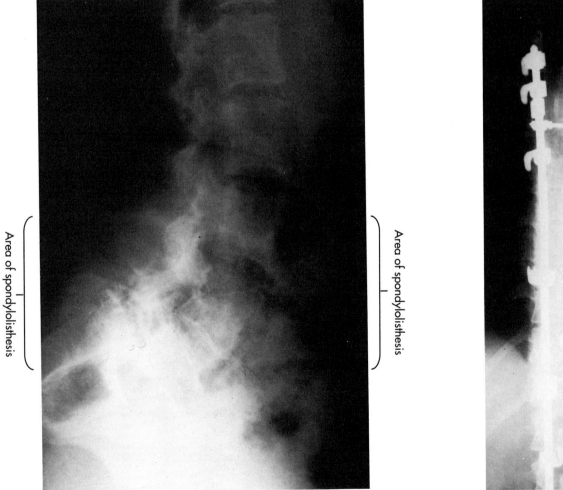

FIGURE 13-10
Grade IV spondylolisthesis.

FIGURE 13-11
Cotrel-Dubousset rod used to treat scoliosis.

Another method for spinal fusion to correct scoliosis involves the use of the Cotrel-Dubousset instrumentation (Figure 13-11). This system provides three-dimensional (frontal, sagittal and axial) correction and compares favorably with the Harrington and Luque rod systems in relation to failure rates, pseudoarthrosis, and improved cosmetic appearance. Additionally, the CDI system improves the vital capacity and voluntary ventilation in adolescent patients with scoliosis.

CONTRAINDICATIONS AND CAUTIONS

Metallic implants such as screws or rods predispose to infection and, at times, may cause severe inflammatory reactions.

Wound infections may predispose to meningeal infections.

Multiple bone grafts may be used, necessitating healing of each graft piece; lack of healing of one or more graft may lead to non-union or lack of sufficient healing for stability.

Marked respiratory compromise from severe curvature may predispose to postoperative respiratory distress, atelectasis, or pneumonia.

Spinal attachments of the metallic rods may loosen, allowing the rods to move and threatening the repair. Major movement could necessitate reoperation.

PREPROCEDURAL NURSING CARE

1. The patient may be placed in skin or skeletal traction (Cotrel's or halofemoral) or in a Risser cast to stretch contracted muscles before surgery.
2. Deep breathing exercises are taught and practiced q 4 h.
3. X-rays are taken for current condition; results should be on chart.
4. A back brace may be sent to surgery with the patient.
5. Meticulous skin care is done to prevent infections.
6. Hematologic (serologic) and urologic studies are done.
7. An enema may be given to empty the lower bowel.
8. An indwelling catheter may be inserted into the urinary bladder.
9. A full-length foam or alternating pressure mattress is placed on the patient's bed.
10. Food and fluids are held 8-10 h before surgery.

MEDICAL MANAGEMENT

See management of open reduction with internal fixation, page 219 for usual care.

NURSING CARE

See pages 233 to 243.

Rotator Cuff Tears

The **rotator cuff** muscles of the shoulder include the supraspinatus, the teres minor, and the infraspinatus, which rotate the humerus externally, and the subscapularis, which rotates the humerus internally (see Figure 13-12).

These muscles completely envelop the head of the humerus. Through their coordinated movements, they hold the humeral head in the glenoid and cause the head to descend as the humerus is abducted.

Tears in the tendons of the rotator muscles at or near their insertions into the humeral tuberosities can occur as a result of acute trauma or from deterioration with age. Degenerative changes occur over time and calcium deposits may occur in the insertion sites. Disintegration or degeneration of the tendons predisposes to tears or rupture of the tendon. At the time of rupture, a snap and acute pain are felt immediately and the patient cannot abduct the arm.

Tendon tears that are acute are repaired immediately to restore motion and preserve strength of the involved tissues. The edges of the tear are approximated and sutured. The affected arm is placed in a cast with 90 degrees abduction, 60 degrees external rotation, and 30 degrees forward flexion for 3 weeks, after which active exercises are instituted.

CONTRAINDICATIONS AND CAUTIONS

Concomitant trauma to major organs or tissues may prevent repair until the patient's condition is stabilized.

Calcium deposits may need to be removed and inflammatory changes calmed before tears are repaired.

Injection of steroids into the tendon areas may predispose to tears or ruptures; oral steroid therapy should be discontinued before surgical repair.

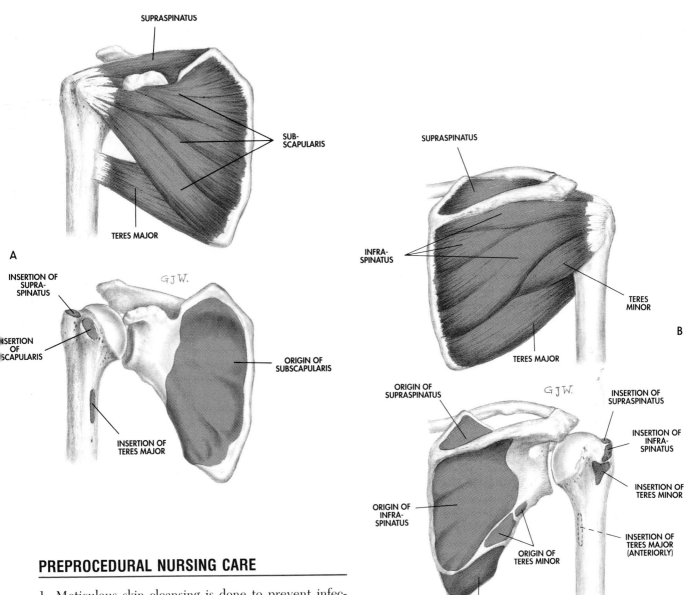

FIGURE 13-12
Shoulder muscles (rotator cuff). **A,** Anterior view. **B,** Posterior view.

PREPROCEDURAL NURSING CARE

1. Meticulous skin cleansing is done to prevent infections.
2. Serologic and urologic studies are done; results should be on patient's chart.
3. X-rays, including arthroscopic or arthrographic views, are taken; results on chart; roentgenograms are sent to the operating suite.
4. An airplane splint or sling with shoulder restraint may be sent to surgery with patient.
5. Ice applications may be applied to lessen bleeding and edema before surgery.

MEDICAL MANAGEMENT

See usual care following open reduction with internal fixation, page 219.

NURSING CARE

See pages 233 to 243.

Recurrent Shoulder Dislocations

Several operations are available to correct frequent or recurrent dislocations. These are listed below.

Bankart procedure: involves direct reattachment of the labrum and anterior capsule to the anterior rim of the glenoid. Suturing the medial flap of the capsule over the lateral flap reinforces the repair while allowing excellent range of motion in the joint.

Putti-Platt procedure: involves dividing the subscapularis tendon and the capsule one inch from their attachment to the humerus, then the cut end of the lateral portion is sutured to the anterior rim of the glenoid fossa, and the cut end of the medial portion is attached to the tendon cuff over the greater tubercle of the humerus so the medial portion of the tendon overlaps the lateral portion. This operation limits external rotation of the shoulder so subsequent dislocations are prevented.

Magnuson-Stack procedure: involves removing (cutting loose) the tendon of the subscapularis muscle and reattaching it more laterally and proximally on the humerus, thereby restricting external rotation.

Bristow-Helfet-Latarjet procedure: involves moving the terminal 1 cm end of the coracoid process (of the scapula) with its attached conjoined tendon of the biceps and coracobrachialis muscles to the neck of the scapula medial to the anteroinferior edge of the glenoid rim.

Eden-Hybbinette procedure: involves placing bone grafts against the anterior portion of the neck of the scapula and the rim of the glenoid cavity to prevent anterior dislocation or displacement of the head of the humerus.

Glenoplasty: involves bone grafts and osteotomy of the glenoid to rotate it forward plus plication (folding and ridging) of the posterior capsule to correct posterior dislocation of the humerus. The first five procedures are to treat anterior dislocations.

NURSING CARE

See pages 233 to 243.

Synovectomy

Synovectomy involves removal of the synovial lining of a joint or joints. Portions or all of the lining may be removed, depending on the purpose of the operation.

Synovectomy may be done because of overgrowth associated with rheumatoid arthritis or, rarely, because of a synovial tumor. The operation is most frequently done in the small joints of the fingers. It is less frequently done now in knees because of advances in total knee replacements, as removal of the synovium from the knee does little to retard the progression of rheumatoid destructive processes in the knee area.

Synovectomy as a treatment for RA is done when the disease has progressed despite intense medical treatment and before the joint cartilage is irreparably damaged. It is done to relieve the joint pain, correct deformity, provide stability to the joint, help restore muscle balance, and to increase the mobility in the joint(s). Along with removal of the synovium, there may also be tendon repairs, release of tendon or ligament contractures, and removal of subcutaneous nodules. Multiple synovectomies are commonly done simulta-

neously to lessen repetitive surgical trauma. The joint space, following synovial removal, is maintained with implants of silicone which help to restore joint functions. If implants are not used after synovectomy of a joint, the synovial lining usually regenerates in 2 to 3 months but is less vascular and is again subject to the destructive processes of rheumatoid arthritis.

CONTRAINDICATIONS AND CAUTIONS

Acute flare-up of rheumatoid arthritis precludes this surgery until the disease is controlled or is quiescent.

Mental incompetence or incapacity may preclude this surgery because of the postoperative exercise regimen and wound care required unless a responsible adult is available to assist and supervise the care.

Recovery time and rehabilitation require that the patient be off work for a minimal 6-week period, and possibly longer.

PREPROCEDURAL NURSING CARE

1. Corticosteroids are discontinued before surgery, but antiinflammatory NSAID medications are usually continued until 10-12 h before surgery to maintain therapeutic blood levels.
2. Serologic and urologic studies are done (if ESR is too elevated, surgery may be postponed).
3. X-rays of affected joints and chest are done to determine present condition of joints and possible chest condition which may delay surgery.
4. An electrocardiogram is done to determine the condition of the heart.
5. Meticulous skin cleansing is done as there may be multiple incisional areas if synovectomies of fingers are done.
6. Food and fluids are held 8-10 h before surgery.

NURSING CARE

See pages 233 to 243.

MEDICAL MANAGEMENT

GENERAL MANAGEMENT

Elevate both hands and forearms on pillows (or elevate using IV poles and soft restraints); ice bags to both hands continuously; neurovascular checks q 1 h × 8, q 2 h × 4, then q 4 h; begin clear liquids in 24 h, advance to regular diet as tolerated; begin physical therapy exercises in 24 h; secure consult with occupational therapy for home management.

DRUG THERAPY

Narcotic analgesic medications: Meperidine, 75-100 mg IM q 3 h PRN; morphine, 10-15 mg IM q 4 h PRN; dilaudid, 2-4 mg IM q 4 h PRN.

Anti-anxiety agent: Hydroxyzine (Vistaril), 25 to 50 mg IM q 6 h PRN.

Analgesic antipyretic medications: Acetaminophen 600-1000 mg q 4 h for moderate pain.
Restart anti-inflammatory medications (if rheumatic disease is present) when patient can tolerate oral intake.
Intravenous 1000 ml 5% D/0.45 N/S at 75 to 100 ml/h; add 20 mEq KCL to each liter.

---

1   ASSESS

ASSESSMENT	OBSERVATIONS
Physical mobility, ROM of all unaffected joints	Mobility impairments should only be related to operative limb, joint, or area except for pre-operative local or systemic involvement of one or more joints or areas; general anesthesia may temporarily limit physical mobility as will presence of cast, splint, immobilizer, or sling; bed rest may be ordered, thus limiting ambulation; ROM of all joints other than operative area should remain at preoperative levels
Neurovascular status	Operative area will be paler, cooler, more edematous, and more painful than contralateral tissues; operative tissues less functional initially and possibly for several or more days; all peripheral pulses should be felt although the posterior tibialis and dorsalis pedis (if leg operative area) and radial and ulnar (if arm operated) may be slightly weaker than preoperatively; incisional area painful and tender

→ › ›

ASSESSMENT	OBSERVATIONS
Skin integrity	Incisional area reddened, edematous, and painful; drains and drainage may be present; wound will be initially covered with dressings
Breathing and respiratory functions	Breath sounds should be heard in all lobes, although they may be heard weakly in lower lobes related to operative site (spinal area, shoulder, or ribs); cough may be weak or may be forceful and productive; sputum may be slightly bloody or frothy; respiratory excursions may be decreased due to preoperative condition, operative site, or pain
Pain	Postoperative pain is usually localized, acute, and sharp in the operative area; other body areas may be tender or sore related to positions required or bed rest; pain usually remains present in slightly decreasing amounts and duration over the first 1-5 postoperative days; persistent, sharp, or acute pain in operative area or distal to site may be indicative of developing infection or compartment syndrome
Position of operative site	Limb may be held in abduction or adduction (if required), internal or external rotation (neutral rotation is usual)
Bowel elimination	Bowel sounds may be absent on day of and first postoperative day, after which they should return in all four quadrants, although initially may be weak; may have no bowel movement for 1 or more postoperative days; may complain of feeling bloated
Urinary elimination	Indwelling catheter may be present on operative, first postoperative day or longer; urinary output less than intake in first 24-48 h
Body temperature	Usually will have elevation of 1-2° for 2-3 postoperative days; should have no chills; may have diaphoresis at times

2 DIAGNOSE

NURSING DIAGNOSIS	SUPPORTIVE ASSESSMENT FINDINGS
Impaired physical mobility related to large incision, surgical implant, internal fixation, or other device	Dressing covers 4-8 inch area at operative site; operative sheet lists type of implant (prosthesis or total joint replacement), internal fixation device (compression plate with screws, hip nail, multiple femoral pins, intramedullary or metallic rods to spinal area), or bone grafts in operative area
Altered peripheral tissue perfusion related to use of tourniquet in surgery, operative site, or preoperative condition	Limb pale and cool; peripheral pulses palpable but weak; capillary refill delayed; mild edema present; states has some throbbing in operative area
Impaired skin integrity related to drain in wound, incision, and sutures	Hemovac drainage system in incisional area; drainage is serosanguineous; has incision closed with sutures; other skin area clear

NURSING DIAGNOSIS	SUPPORTIVE ASSESSMENT FINDINGS
Impaired gas exchange related to anesthesia, bed rest, or operative site (shoulder or vertebral column)	Respiratory rates increased to 28-32/min; may be dyspnea; breath sounds weak; weak cough (productive or nonproductive); states it hurts in operative site (back) when takes deep breaths; use of Respirex weak—doesn't reach goals
Pain (acute) related to surgical trauma and incision	Complains of sharp, steady, pain, which may not be entirely relieved with narcotics
Potential for injury related to dislocation of prosthesis, internal fixation devices, or to disruption of operative repair	Keeps abduction splint or pillow in place; limb turns inward at times when unattended; knee immobilizer in place; pillows support limb; incision edematous with sutures cutting into skin
Constipation related to anesthesia, bed rest, and decreased intake	No bowel sounds heard on operative or first postop day; heard weakly and irregularly on second postoperative day; abdomen slightly distended and flatulent when percussed; no bowel movement first and second postoperative days
Altered patterns of urinary elimination related to bed rest, anesthesia, and surgical trauma	Urinary catheter may be present for 2 postoperative days; urinary output less than intake; no urgency or burning after catheter removed
Hyperthermia related to anesthesia or surgery	Temperatures may fluctuate to 101° F (38.3° C) but usually stays around 99.6° F (37.5° C); has diaphoresis when temperature falls; no signs of wound infection present

3 PLAN

Patient goals

1. The patient will regain physical mobility and ROM of all joints.
2. The patient will regain normal peripheral tissue perfusion.
3. The patient will regain skin integrity with a well-healed scar.
4. The patient will regain normal respiratory function.
5. The patient will become relatively pain free.
6. The patient will experience no dislocation of prosthesis, fixation device, or disruption of operative repair.
7. The patient will regain normal bowel and bladder elimination.
8. The patient will regain normal body temperature.

→ > >

4 IMPLEMENT

NURSING DIAGNOSIS	NURSING INTERVENTIONS	RATIONALE
Impaired physical mobility related to large incision, surgical implant, internal fixation or other device	Assess ROM of unaffected joints.	Data provide evidence of retention or loss of muscle strength.
	Assist patient to change positions in bed as permitted; may only be raised off back; may be turned to unoperative sides or may be turned side to side—varies with physician's order.	Changing positions helps relieve tired muscles and joints, increases circulation, and maintains strength.
	Teach isometric exercises such as quadriceps, triceps and gluteus setting; remind patient to do exercises q 4 h.	Isometric exercises provide muscle strength without changing position of joint. Muscle tension increases circulation to maintain strength and remove wastes.
	Instruct patient to do active ROM exercises to unaffected joints q 4 h.	Active exercises maintain functions of tissues inside and around joints.
	Secure consultation with physical therapy for resistive exercises or other isotonic exercises plus assistance for ambulation with ambulatory aid.	Professional guidance of experts provides optimal patient care for rehabilitation.
	Reiterate proper techniques for use of cane, crutches or walker within ordered weight-bearing restrictions. Monitor patient's use of ambulatory aid.	Repetition of instructions assures patient understanding. Monitoring provides for safe care or indicates need for additional teaching.
	Monitor patient's vital signs q 4 h.	Provides assurance of patient's condition and strength for ambulation
	Secure consultation with orthotist for fitting of splint or brace if needed.	Specialist provides latest techniques and facets for optimal care.
	Seek consultation with social services for home care equipment.	Social services assess need for home care equipment and for financial aid for continuity of care.
Altered peripheral tissue perfusion related to use of tourniquet in surgery, operative site, or preoperative condition	Assess neurovascular functions in all 8 parameters (see inside front cover); record findings and report abnormal findings to physician; do checks q 1-2 h as ordered; explain purpose of frequent checks	Trauma from herniated nucleus pulposus or from laminectomy or spinal fusion may give abnormal results such as numbness, tingling, radiating pain to hips or down legs, muscle weakness, and edema in back or incisional area. Understanding necessity of frequent checks should ease patient's concerns and anxiety.
	Observe operative site for signs of resolution of inflammation.	Initial inflammatory wound healing signs lessen in 2-3 days with decreased redness, edema, drainage, and wound tenderness.

NURSING DIAGNOSIS	NURSING INTERVENTIONS	RATIONALE
	Assist patient to log roll side to side if spinal fusion was done; two nurses are required to log roll the patient with one on each side the patient is turned "as a log" to the side; place pillows to back and between legs when on side to help patient maintain proper position; turn q 2-4 h.	Log rolling requires the patient to maintain the back straight without flexing back to maintain surgical correction.
	Assist patient to apply back brace, if ordered; assist to be up and to ambulate q 4 h.	Healing of bone grafts and operative site following spinal fusion requires 6-9 months or longer. Using a brace helps maintain surgical repair until healing has occurred.
	Encourage ROM exercises to unaffected joints q 4 h.	Exercises help maintain strength and help prevent stasis, which could lead to thrombophlebitis.
Impaired skin integrity related to drain in wound, incision, and sutures	Assess wound for size, location, drain and drainage, condition of dressing; assess for bleeding or type of drainage. Measure amount and character of drainage q 2 h × 4, q 4 h × 2, then q 8 h; recompress suction set-up.	Assessment provides indications for interventions. Wound drainage may initially be sanguineous for 4-6 h, then become serosanguineous, serous, and then clear. Drainage amount varies from 100 to 1000 ml, depending on type of surgery. Drainage or evacuation of drainage from wound is dependent upon negative suction and gravity drainage principles.
	Change dressing as ordered or as needed q 8-12 h; use aseptic technique for procedure; cleanse drainage from wound area. Replace dressings as necessary.	Removal of drainage from skin and wound areas prevents maceration of skin and lessens chance of infection. Aseptic technique prevents introduction of pathogens to area; covering wound with new dressings is usually done while drainage is still present.
	Observe drainage tubing for separation of cells and serum.	Separation of cells and serum (referred to as hematocrit sign) indicates stasis and cessation of flow; if early in postoperative period, separation may indicate blockage of drainage tubing; if separation is later (after 2 or more days), it means tubing can be removed from wound.
	Observe characteristics of drainage over time.	Drainage should become clear and minimal over 2-3 days; if it becomes yellow or green it may indicate presence of infection.

→ 〉 〉 〉

NURSING DIAGNOSIS	NURSING INTERVENTIONS	RATIONALE
	Observe wound for signs of healing, presence of hematoma or abscess, dehiscence, or evisceration; record and report untoward signs to physician: a hematoma or abscess will usually be opened and drained by the physician. Dehisced areas may be closed by resuturing, or application of steri-strips or butterfly dressings to reapproximate the wound edges; eviscerated tissues are usually replaced after the patient is returned to the surgical suite. Before replacement the eviscerated tissues must be kept moist with warm normal saline dressings.	Wounds go through inflammatory changes of redness, edema, tenderness and drainage in first 72 postoperative hours, then begin collagen growth phase for next 5-7 days. As wound closes, scar tissue forms, edges approximate, and drainage decreases and stops. A hematoma may develop near or in incisional area, with a soft, fluctuant area noted. An **abscess** is an area of fluctuant mass that is red, hot, and painful. **Dehiscence** is separation of a part of the wound edges and **evisceration** is separation of the wound edges with bulging out of internal tissues. The area of dehiscence must be kept moist to prevent drying out, cracking, and the development of infection. If a wound of a patient with internal fixation devices, total joint replacement, or an osteotomy becomes infected, it could develop into long-term infection, disability, and osteomyelitis.
	Turn or reposition patient q 2-4 h.	To prevent development of pressure areas.
	Observe all bony prominences for signs of pressure, tenderness or excoriation q 4 h.	Pressure areas may be reddened, white, or later, blue or discolored, depending on circulatory compromise or stasis.
	Massage around bony prominences q 4 h. **Do not** massage over reddened areas, only around them gently.	Massage increases circulation to an area. Reddening indicates injury to capillaries; massaging over them could increase damage.
	If a skin graft is present, observe the graft for color, temperature, edema, signs of adherence or loosening, and drainage; observe for presence of stent.	Grafts may be split or full thickness. They adhere by growth of new vessels into grafted area and adherence to subcutaneous tissues; graft may be slightly paler and cooler than surrounding tissues initially; may be slightly edematous; should not be easily movable, may be held in place by sutures or a stent, (packed dressing placed over graft and held in place with sutures criss-crossing over stent material).
	Roll skin graft area, if ordered, with applicators by gently rolling from center to all edges of graft. Be careful not to dislodge graft.	Helps prevent pooling of interstitial fluids and serum which could prevent graft adherence.
	If graft is split thickness, monitor donor site for inflammatory changes, signs of healing, and pain; remove and replace transparent dressing or medicated gauze q 8-12 h or prn.	Donor site will have serosanguineous drainage for 3-5 days; site will be reddened, edematous, and *very* painful because of exposed nerve endings in dermis. The donor site heals by regeneration of new dermal cells to close the area

NURSING DIAGNOSIS	NURSING INTERVENTIONS	RATIONALE
Impaired gas exchange RT anesthesia, bed rest, or operative site (shoulder or vertebral column)	Monitor patient's vital signs q 4 h; observe respiratory rates and nature of respirations, presence of dyspnea or shortness of breath.	Respiratory complications are reflected in temperature elevations and changes in rates and character of respirations—rates are increased and irregular, with dyspnea and some shortness of breath.
	Monitor breath sounds in all lobes q 4 h.	Decreased or absent breath sounds indicate infection in one or more lobes.
	Encourage deep breathing and coughing exercises q 2-4 h; observe color and amount of sputum, if cough is productive.	Deep breathing helps perfuse all areas of lung and aids oxygen–carbon dioxide exchange. If sputum is yellow or green, it indicates presence of infection.
	Encourage patient to curtail or stop smoking.	Smoking decreases aeration and perfusion in lungs.
	Encourage use of Respirex q 2 h or incentive spirometry q 4 h.	Use of respiratory aid increases lung perfusion.
	Assist patient to be up in chair or to ambulate as ordered.	Increases circulation, requires deep breathing, and aids perfusion.
	Observe effects of airplane splint or shoulder spica cast on patient's ability to deep breathe and cough thoroughly; notify physician if patient is unable to fully expand lungs.	Splint or cast may restrict ability to fully expand lungs; if unable to do so, periphery of lungs may not be well perfused, creating anoxia.
Pain (acute) related to surgical trauma and incision	Assess presence of pain, its duration, characteristics, amount, and site(s).	Pain is indicative of pressure, injury, anoxia, or other condition to nerve endings.
	Listen to patient's complaints of pain; discuss its severity, amount, and duration.	Discussing meaning of pain with patient increases understanding and tolerance.
	Assist patient to positions of more comfort q 2 to 4 h.	Changing positions helps relieve tired, sore, or painful tissues by relieving pressure on nerve endings.
	Teach patient relaxation techniques, visualization, or other pain-relieving techniques.	Relaxation techniques involve deep breathing exercises which enhance oxygenation and circulation, thereby relieving pain. Many types of pain are related to anoxia.
	Do all 8 neurovascular checks q 2-4 h as ordered; record findings.	Pain is sign of pressure on nerve endings; increasing pain is a sign of bleeding, increased venous pressure or other untoward sign, requiring additional care.
	Administer narcotic/analgesic medication q 3-4 h or encourage patient to use PCA medication more frequently; monitor for relief of pain.	Narcotics relieve pain through decreasing perception of pain. PCA pumps allow the patient to self-medicate to relieve pain. Therapeutic blood levels require regular administration of medications.

→ ❯ ❯

NURSING DIAGNOSIS	NURSING INTERVENTIONS	RATIONALE
	Measure compartment pressures if ordered; report pressures to physician.	Venous pressures in muscle compartments normally average 15-25 mm Hg. Venous pressures may increase from bleeding into traumatized tissues and from increased edema. Pressures ≥30 mm Hg are indicative of compartment syndrome, a severe complication which can result in death of muscles if the pressure is not relieved. A major indicator of compartment syndrome is *increased pain on passive movement.* Passive movement of distal joints increases stretch, thereby creating more anoxia and more pain.
	Monitor incisional area for signs of healing or of developing infection.	Pain is one indicator of healing—pain is lessened as healing progresses or inflammation lessens; infection increases pain from edema and abscess or pressure on nerve endings.
Potential for injury related to dislocation of prosthesis, or internal fixation devices or to disruption of operative repair.	Assess position of extremity or operative tissues in relation to body alignment; assess position of splint, brace, or dressings.	Postoperative position should be very similar to tissues of unoperative side, or as close to normal tissues as possible.
	Reiterate the need to maintain the desired position and the need for use of splint, brace, immobilizer, abduction pillow, traction or other equipment.	Auxiliary equipment may be required to help injured or weak tissues hold operative bones and tissues in desired postoperative position, if patient unable to maintain proper position.
	Teach patient/family member how to apply specific equipment.	Proper application provides safety and comfort. Self-application increases self-confidence and aids compliance.
	Monitor and adjust patient's position q 2-4 h.	Helps determine that proper positions will be maintained, and that adjustments will be made promptly if necessary.
	Teach patient how to assist with turning or transfer to chair and back to bed.	Understanding proper techniques helps patient participate actively and safely.
	Secure additional assistance, if necessary, while turning, lifting, positioning, or transferring patient.	The patient's condition, muscle strength, or operative repair may dictate need for additional nursing personnel for safe care for all involved.
	Investigate patient's statements of "feeling a pop," "can't move my arm or leg" or other complaints related to operative area; notify physician if unnatural position of limb, bulge, or mass noted.	Such statements could indicate loss of reduction, dislocation of prosthesis, wound dehiscence, or other untoward reaction in operative area.

NURSING DIAGNOSIS	NURSING INTERVENTIONS	RATIONALE
	Teach patient proper use of a cane, crutches or walker with ordered amount of limited weight bearing.	Proper use of ambulatory aid should prevent excessive or improper weight bearing or improper use of equipment.
	Provide the required equipment such as straight chairs, elevated toilet seats (toilet riser), crutch tips, shoulder and wrist supports or pads, elastic bandages or other required equipment as needed.	Use of proper equipment promotes safe care and helps prevent additional injury to the patient.
Constipation related to anesthesia and bed rest	Assess bowel sounds, distention, and last bowel movement.	Bowel sounds should be low-pitched and heard in all 4 quadrants; should be every 30 seconds related to peristalsis.
	Monitor and measure abdominal girth q 4 h; palpate amount of distention; percuss abdomen for hollow sounds related to distention or ileus.	Distention is noted by increasing abdominal girths; flatus in bowel sounds hollow on percussion.
	Ask patient if is expelling flatus and, if so, how frequently.	Passing flatus is indicative of return of bowel functions.
	Administer rectal suppository, if ordered; instruct patient to wait approximately 30 min to 1 hr to attempt bowel movement.	Rectal suppositories contain medications to draw fluid to the area to moisten and soften stool to make passage easier.
	When taking oral foods and fluids, administer laxative at bedtime.	Laxatives aid peristalsis and help bowel emptying.
	Encourage foods high in fiber and residue; force fluids to 3000 ml/day.	High fiber and residue create bulk in stool. Fluids help moisten stool for ease in passing stool.
	Examine stool for amount, color, and consistency.	Stool should be brown, soft, and formed in a moderate amount.
Altered patterns of urinary elimination related to bed rest, anesthesia, and surgical trauma	Assess intake and output q 4 h.	Postoperative urinary output may not occur for 8 or more hours after surgery due to trauma, decreased intake, or medications.
	Listen for complaints of feeling of fullness in bladder area; inability to void lying flat, or feeling of urgency to void.	Such complaints indicate need to void, and may require assistance (catheterization).
	If allowed up, assist patient to bathroom to void; make sure patient has brace on, if ordered.	Voiding is facilitated by privacy and "usual" bathroom area, and by upright position.
	If on bed rest, place patient on bedpan or place urinal; run water in sink; have patient put fingers in warm water. If patient is female, pour warm water over perineum.	Using suggested techniques aids voiding by relaxing bladder sphincters.

→ > >

NURSING DIAGNOSIS	NURSING INTERVENTIONS	RATIONALE
	If patient is unable to void, bladder palpation indicates fullness, and patient is uncomfortable, secure order for catheterization or for medication (bethanechol [Urecholine]) to relax bladder sphincter to aid voiding. Use strict aseptic technique with catheterization. Wait for medication to be effective—usually 30 minutes, if given.	Medications for pain relief may cause constriction of sphincters, especially morphine, Dilaudid and Meperidine. Catheterization may be required to prevent overdistention of the bladder. Bethanechol relaxes bladder sphincter to facilitate voiding.
	Increase fluid intake to 3000 ml daily, if tolerated.	Increased fluid intake aids renal perfusion and formation of urine.
Hyperthermia related to anesthesia or surgery	Assess vital signs q 1-4 h as ordered.	Body temperature rises about 1 to 2 degrees above normal for first 1 to 3 postoperative days; elevations above 100.6° F (38.1° C) require further investigation to determine cause.
	Monitor and listen to breath sounds in all lobes q 2-4 h.	Atelectasis is a complication after surgery if patient has inadequate pulmonary perfusion, or insufficient peripheral aeration and is noted by absence of breath sounds in one or more lobes; a common cause of elevated temperatures in first 24-48 h postoperative period.
	Monitor wound for signs of increasing or lessening inflammation; measure amount and character of drainage; change dressing q 4-8 h to observe wound characteristics and healing.	Wound infection can be the source of elevated temperatures. Infection can be noted by increased redness, edema, tenderness, and abscess formation or increased (purulent) drainage of wound.
	Listen for complaints of urinary frequency, burning, urgency when voiding; check color, odor, and amount of urinary output.	Urinary tract infection is characterized by frequency, urgency, burning, and decreased output; urine may be cloudy and have a noticeable odor.

5   EVALUATE

PATIENT OUTCOME	DATA INDICATING THAT OUTCOME IS REACHED
Patient regains physical mobility and ROM of all joints with assistance.	At discharge, was walking with crutches; could bend operative joints to nearly full ROM; remainder of joints had normal ROM; some muscle weakness remains in operative muscles.
Patient regains normal peripheral tissue perfusion.	All neurovascular checks are in normal ranges.

NURSING DIAGNOSIS	NURSING INTERVENTIONS	RATIONALE
Patient regains skin integrity with well-healed scar.	Incision edges well approximated with no sutures present; paper strips crossing incision; no signs of inflammation.	
Patient regains normal respiratory function.	Breath sounds clear and easily heard in all lobes; respiratory rate 16-20/min; no productive cough.	
Patient is relatively pain free.	Patient still takes nonnarcotic analgesics 2-3 times daily for soreness and discomfort in operative site; no other medications taken (except usual medications for concurrent chronic conditions).	
Patient experiences no dislocation of prosthesis or fixation devices or no disruption of operative repair.	X-rays show satisfactory placement of devices at time of discharge.	
Patient regains normal bowel and bladder elimination.	Bowel sounds active in all four quadrants; having daily bowel movement; intake and output equal; no urinary complaints.	
Patient regains normal temperature	Temperatures range between 98-98.6° F (36-37° C).	

PATIENT TEACHING

1. Teach patient about wound healing processes.
2. Teach patient proper positions and how to maintain them.
3. Teach patient proper exercise regimens.
4. Teach patient crutch walking and stair climbing (see
pages 188 to 189, 274)
5. Teach patient about foods having high fiber content.
6. Teach patient about neurovascular checks (see inside front cover).

Chemonucleolysis

Chemonucleolysis is the chemical reduction by an enzyme of a ruptured or herniating intervertebral disc.

The enzyme, chymopapain, is obtained from the papaya plant. It is injected intradiscally where it binds with and degrades the mucopolysaccharides in the disc. The mucopolysaccharides are primarily responsible for the hydration of the nucleus pulposus, and the intradiscal osmotic activity. With the degradation of the mucopolysaccharides, the disc no longer absorbs fluids and this loss of water content decreases intradiscal pressure, which relieves pressure on nerves, thereby lessening pain, and resolving radicular symptoms.

Chemonucleolysis is a controversial procedure because of adverse reactions and even deaths that have resulted from the procedure. It is still, however, being performed and is a viable option for patients with small ruptures of the nucleus pulposus.

CONTRAINDICATIONS AND CAUTIONS

Patients with prior lumbar surgery should not have chemonucleolysis.

A history of allergies, reactions to meat tenderizers or other allergens are contraindications.

Progressive neurologic deficit, evidence of spinal stenosis, spondylolisthesis, or spinal instability are other contraindications, as are degenerative changes or subluxation of the facet joints.

Pregnancy and prior injection with chymopapain are contraindications.

The patient should be aware that postinjection muscle spasms of the back are common.

Patients with large herniated discs or with sequestered nucleus (pieces of nucleus away from the rest of the nucleus) should not have chemonucleolysis.

Skin sites for insertion of needle must be free of open sores or lesions, which could cause transfer of pathogens into disc area.

PREPROCEDURAL NURSING CARE

1. Completion of all laboratory studies with results on chart and physician notified of results.
2. Assessment of allergy history must be thorough.
3. An intravenous infusion is initiated; and a heparin well is inserted.
4. No morphine, meperidine or urecholine should be given in the 24 hours preceding surgery.
5. Preoperative medications to be given may include cimetidine (Tagamet), 300 mg IV, diphenhydramine 100 mg IV and hydrocortisone 50-100 mg IV (may not be given to all patients).
6. A test dose of 0.2 ml of chymopapain may be given before the therapeutic dose.
7. Before chemonucleolysis, the patient may be in pelvic traction in Williams position in bed.

DIAGNOSTIC STUDIES AND FINDINGS

Diagnostic test	Findings
Erythrocyte sedimentation rate	Must be within normal limits (Normals: 0-9 mm/h males); ESR may be elevated in infection in the intervertebral disc, then chemonucleolysis would not be done
HLA-B27	Positive in ankylosing spondylitis; chemonucleolysis would not be done in presence of this condition.
Fasting blood sugar or glucose tolerance test	Done to rule out diabetes and diabetic neuropathy as a cause of sciatic symptoms
Skin test of chymopapain	Should show no wheal or allergic response
X-rays	
Discogram	Would show rupture of disc if present
Myelogram	Would show rupture of disc and pressure on nerve roots
CT	Will show herniation of nucleus pulposus
MRI	Excellent study to outline soft tissues to detect herniations of nucleus pulposus and to identify sequestered pieces

MEDICAL MANAGEMENT

DRUG THERAPY

Adrenergic agents: Epinephrine (Adrenalin), 1:1000, on hand.

Antihistamines (Histamine antagonists): Diphenhydramine (Benadryl), 50 mg on hand; cimetidine, 300 mg, on hand.

Narcotic analgesic agents (for postoperative use only): Morphine, 10-15 mg IM q 4 h PRN for severe pain or severe muscle spasms; meperidine, 75-100 mg IM q 3 h prn.

Non-narcotic analgesic agents: Aspirin, 600-1000 mg, PO q 4 h prn for enhanced pain relief.

Muscle relaxant/anti-anxiety agents: Diazepam (Valium), 2-5 mg IM q 4 h prn for muscle spasms. Intravenous 1000 ml 5% D/0.45 N/S at 75-100 ml/h for 8-12 h, then to "keep open" rate.

1 ASSESS

ASSESSMENT	OBSERVATIONS
Possible anaphylactic reactions	Pulse 96 (preop rates 84-90); BP 106/74 (preop 124/80; respirations 26 (preoperative 18); temperature 99° (preoperative 98.6° F (37° C); no rash or redness of skin noted; no wheezing or itching
Low (lumbar) back area for pain	Small dressing at insertion site of spinal needle; has slight edema of lumbosacral area; has muscle spasms intermittently in lumbosacral area that are very painful
Physical mobility	Still has "list" to one side; has sharp muscle spasms when turning or rising from bed; has sharp pain in lumbosacral area with radiation down leg
Bowel elimination	Bowel sounds present in four quadrants; abdomen moderately distended; no bowel movement since admission 20 h ago

2 DIAGNOSE

NURSING DIAGNOSIS	SUPPORTIVE ASSESSMENT FINDINGS
Potential for injury related to anaphylactic reactions	Had slight increases (84-96) in pulse rates after injection of chymopapain; BP readings lower each time than preoperatively; may have rash or wheezes
Pain related to muscle spasms or back pain postoperatively	Complains of intermittent, sharp muscle spasms at operative site; has sharp pain in lumbosacral area radiating down leg; asking for increased pain medication and for ice bag to back
Impaired physical mobility related to back pain and muscle spasms	States pain in back is same as preoperative pain with radiation down leg; has sharp spasms when turning or rising to upright position; walks with arm around shoulder of significant other; walks listing to side; walks hesitantly and slowly
Impaired gas exchange related to general anesthetic	Breathing is shallow, patient appears to "splint" when breathing
Altered bowel elimination related to ileus and decreased intake	Abdomen moderately distended and flatulent on percussion; no bowel movement to date; only IV intake since admission; eructating flatus and is nauseated

3 PLAN

Patient goals

1. The patient will experience no anaphylactic reaction to chymopapain.
2. The patient will have relief of back pain over time.
3. The patient will regain satisfactory physical mobility.
4. The patient will achieve satisfactory gas exchange.
5. The patient will regain usual bowel elimination.

→ > >

4 IMPLEMENT

NURSING DIAGNOSIS	NURSING INTERVENTIONS	RATIONALE
Potential for injury related to anaphylactic reactions	Assess for rash, hives, periorbital or perioral edema, flushed skin, anxiety, wheezing, and dyspnea q 1 h × 4, then q 2-4 h; check patient's skin over chest, back and legs for rash; if present, notify physician immediately.	Anaphylactic reactions can occur as long as 1-2 weeks postoperatively. Medications and medical care must be given immediately to overcome the allergic manifestations.
	Monitor vital signs q 1 h × 4, then q 2 h × 4, then q 4 h.	Blood pressure decreases, increases in pulse and respirations, and temperature changes may indicate shock or anaphylactic reaction.
	Remind patient of allergic manifestations before discharge and notify physician if they occur.	Safe care requires alerting patient to possible symptoms that would require medical attention.
Pain related to muscle spasms or back pain postoperatively	Assess for presence of back pain or muscle spasms q 1-2 h.	Chymopapain may precipitate muscle spasms in some patients.
	Maintain bed rest and assist patient to positions of comfort: bed flat or in Williams position; side-lying with pillows under knee; encourage to use bed controls to adjust to position of greater comfort; be sure trapeze is on bed.	Adjusting position rests tired or painful muscles. Positions may vary per patient. Self-participation in care increases confidence.
	Use heat or ice massage to low back area q 2-4 h prn; assess effects of each treatment; comply with patient's desire for heat or ice.	Heat is a vasodilator, and by bringing more blood to area helps remove wastes to lessen pain. Ice is a vasoconstrictor to lessen edema, thereby lessening pain.
	Administer narcotic, analgesic and muscle relaxant medications q 4 h prn.	Administering medications promptly and frequently over time helps maintain therapeutic blood levels.
	If permitted, immerse patient in whirlpool tub of warm water everyday.	Warm water relaxes tense muscles to lessen pain and spasms.
Impaired physical mobility related to back pain and muscle spasms	Assess ability and desire to reposition self.	May require additional interventions or assistance.
	Turn q 1-2 h; encourage ROM exercises to unaffected joints.	Exercises maintain muscle and joint strength.
	Reiterate techniques for transferring out of bed and ambulation; usually it is easier to rise from bed from side-lying position with knees flexed, with head of bed elevated to high Fowler's position. Patient places hands on nurse's shoulder to raise and pivot self to sitting position on edge of bed. Patient then stands with majority of weight on unaffected leg.	Transferring to upright position can be done comfortably, or, at least, with less increase in pain, when done using sound principles of transfer.

NURSING DIAGNOSIS	NURSING INTERVENTIONS	RATIONALE
	Allow to sit in chair only as desired; walking may be more comfortable for patient. Sitting in straddle position with arms on chair back may be desired. Use of a reclining chair reclined to 120 degrees with knees flexed higher than hips may be helpful.	Sitting puts greatest compressive forces on back and discs. Straddle position reduces weight on the buttocks and helps in keeping the back flat. Reclining chair helps "unload" the muscles and discs and puts the patient in a more comfortable flat-back position.
	Teach patient to "listen" to his/her back and legs and not to push beyond comfort to discomfort too quickly; instruct to take short, frequent walks rather than less frequent, longer walks.	Progress may be slow and steady as recovery proceeds.
	Teach patient to rest one foot on stool when standing at sink.	Resting foot on stool relieves muscle strain and pain to increase comfort.
Impaired gas exchange related to general anesthetic	Assess rate and depth of respiration Encourage deep breathing exercises q 2-4 h.	To determine recovery from anesthesia. Decreased air exchange may be related to discomfort.
	Note cough or production of sputum	Production of sputum indicates possible infection or irritation from anesthesia.
Altered bowel elimination related to ileus and decreased intake	Assess bowel sounds q 4 h; if no sounds heard, report to physician and record.	Bowel sounds should be heard in all four quadrants; sounds are related to peristaltic waves
	Gently percuss abdomen in all four quadrants; listen for hollow sounds.	Hollow sound is indicative of presence of flatus.
	Palpate abdomen and measure abdominal girth if distended q 4 h.	Measuring abdominal girth provides data of increased distention over time.
	Ask patient if is expelling flatus.	Expulsion of flatus indicates return of functions.
	Monitor food and fluid intake to determine tolerance; report prolonged anorexia, nausea, or vomiting.	Anorexia, nausea or vomiting are untoward signs indicating lack of bowel functions.
	Insert rectal suppository if patient unable to have bowel movement.	Suppositories draw more fluid into lumen of bowel and moisten stool mass to make passing stool easier.
	Check amount and consistency of stool.	Stool should be soft, firm, and of sufficient quantity in relation to intake.

5 EVALUATE

PATIENT OUTCOME	DATA INDICATING THAT OUTCOME IS REACHED
The patient has experienced no anaphylactic reaction.	Patient had no rash, wheezing, dyspnea, vital sign changes, or periorbital or perioral edema.
The patient is experiencing less pain over time.	Patient verbalizes relief of severe pain and muscle spasms; states still has some soreness in back and muscle weakness; states will be taking short walks frequently and will rest often when uncomfortable.
The patient is regaining physical mobility.	Patient verbalizes how to perform exercises prescribed; states will return to physician as appointment dictates; states will not return to employment until permitted; is able to move about without assistance.
The patient has satisfactory gas exchange.	Breath sounds clear in all lobes. Respirations deep and regular.
The patient has regained usual bowel elimination.	Bowel flatulence lessened; bowel sounds present in all four quadrants; has had soft, formed stool prior to discharge.

PATIENT TEACHING

1. Teach patient symptoms of anaphylactic reactions and to report them to physician.
2. Teach patient proper turning and transfer techniques.
3. Teach patient effects of heat and cold applications.
4. Teach patient proper standing positions.
5. Teach patient about resolution of inflammation of affected disc that occurs over time.
6. Teach patient to increase activities as condition permits.

Ilizarov Method for Treatment of Bone Defects

The **Ilizarov method** uses principles of tension-stress and controlled distraction to correct bone defects, deformity, limb-length discrepancies, and nonunion.

Dr. Gavriil Abramovich Ilizarov introduced a new external fixator and method for treating bone fractures in Russia in 1951. Since then he has continued to study biomechanics of bone structure, healing and regeneration and, in 1974, introduced a new technique for dealing with a variety of bone and soft tissue healing problems. The Ilizarov method involves using tension-stress and controlled distraction principles to care for patients with bone healing problems. Through use of a special external fixator, this technique can be used to correct or fill in bone defects, accomplish limb-lengthening through new surgical techniques, correct nonunion of fractures, and other conditions. The method provides hope and healing for many patients with difficult management conditions as well as a method to increase heights for many short-statured persons.

The principle of tension-stress allows for gradual controlled distraction of bone ends that stimulates bone production and supports new growth of surrounding tissues. The new tissues grow along the same lines as the distraction force vector.[89] The Ilizarov method also is based on the concept that the size and shape of bone are influenced by the load applied to the bone and by its blood supply.[89]

Essential to success of treatment by the Ilizarov method for treating bone conditions is use of the Ilizarov external fixator, which is applied before surgery. The surgical procedure involves a special osteotomy-corticotomy technique that transects only the bone cortex while preserving its blood supply and bone marrow, endosteum, and periosteum. Corticotomy is cutting the cortex of the bone, commonly done at the proximal or distal metaphyses where the bone is cancellous and nutrient arteries can be preserved. Capillary blood flow in an extremity in an Ilizarov fixator during a period of distraction can be increased 160% to 300%, and during the period of bone maturation and regeneration, a 30-40% higher than normal blood flow was maintained when the apparatus was removed.[89] With such increased blood supply, an increase in the load on a bone then leads to an increase in bone size.

Corticotomy transects the bone cortex while preserving the medullary canal. The cut bone ends are distracted at the rate of 1 mm per day, as this rate had been determined through research to promote maximal bone growth without creating ischemia or delayed maturation. Through specially designed auto-distractor areas on the fixator, the bone may be distracted at scheduled times during the day, so long as the total distractions do not exceed 1 mm per day. Distractions begin 7-10 days after the corticotomy to take advantage of the new bone cell growth (osteogenesis) stimulated by the corticotomy, again through research determined to be 7-10 days postcorticotomy, although this period is shorter in pediatric patients.[89]

The Ilizarov apparatus not only allows limb lengthening but also permits concurrent treatment of osteomyelitis, nonunion, or deformity. Additionally, weight bearing and range of motion of adjacent joints are continued throughout the course of treatment.

The Ilizarov fixator consists of a system of rings and semirings, connected with 1 mm pitch threaded rods or special telescoping rods. One full turn of a nut at the end of the rod changes the distance between the rings by 1 mm.[89] Angulations in bones can be changed up to

15 degrees through special washer couples between the ring and rod. Stability is added to the fixator with additional rods to both sides of the ring. A wire with a stopper (the "olive" wire), unique to the Ilizarov fixator, allows force to be applied directly to a bone fragment to correct deformity, aid in fracture reduction, prevent undesirable displacement of bone during limb lengthening as well as increase the stability and rigidity of the fixator.[77] The fixator permits three-dimensional corrections, including rotation, angulation, manipulating of length, and translation.

Advantages of the Ilizarov method over other techniques include that it is less invasive, allows immediate weight bearing, has few failures and complications, operates on the healthy bone rather than the pathologic bone, and treats not only the bone defect and nonunion, but also any preexisting infection, deformity, or limb-length discrepancy.

PREPROCEDURAL NURSING CARE

1. Observe for type of injury, condition, infection, or other reason for use of Ilizarov method, e.g., limb lengthening; observe scars, drainage, and soft tissue.
2. Observe alertness and awareness of patient; note any infection or history of past illnesses or other conditions.
3. Observe temperature, pulse, respirations, and blood pressure; observe height and weight curves and percentiles according to norms.
4. Assess neurovascular status—observe color, temperature, edema, pain, movement, sensation, and capillary refill.
5. Observe gait and weight bearing and use of cane, crutches, or walker.
6. Assess ROM; observe for limitations or hesitance to use joint.
7. Observe interactions between patient and family/significant others.
8. Observe for complaints of or evidence of pain; observe for medication use or other pain-control measures.
9. Observe for ability to understand discussions, answer questions, alertness, and appropriateness of behavior to situation.

1 ASSESS

ASSESSMENT	OBSERVATIONS
Physical mobility	Observe ability to move self, or willingness to help move self and touch fixator to reposition; observe ROM of all unaffected joints and joints distal to operative site
Postoperative pain amounts, types and sites	Pain be acute, sharp, and initially unrelenting, but relieved by medications; specific types and amounts of pain may be related to past pain history, drug abuse or fear related to unfamiliar apparatus or outcome of treatment
Peripheral tissue perfusion	Observe all neurovascular data: color, temperature, capillary refill, edema, pain, movement, sensation as compared with unoperative limb; observe all entrance and exit sites for rods or wires for edema, drainage, and color
Skin integrity	Observe all skin areas for signs of pressure, color changes, or soreness; observe entire fixator for pressure areas on skin
Ability to do self-care	Initially, may be hesitant to do own care; if upper extremity has fixator, assess ability to do bathing, feeding self, and grooming; will be hesitant to do required turning of nuts to create the distraction needed for bone growth
Skin integrity around fixator and operative site	Operative incision(s) for corticotomy is (are) small, approximately 1-2 cm, covered with sterile dressings; there are multiple rods and rings that can cause pressure on multiple skin areas; drainage from rod sites will initially be serosanguineous, then clear and minimal after 3-5 days; edema around rod sites is initially slight to moderate, becoming slight in 3-5 days

2 DIAGNOSE

NURSING DIAGNOSIS	SUPPORTIVE ASSESSMENT FINDINGS
Impaired physical mobility related to corticotomy and Il-izarov apparatus	Initially, patient hesitant to move due to pain and presence of fixator; should be able to move all unaffected joints, and in day or so postoperatively should be able to move fixator by grasping rings with hands; may have first physical therapy on 1st postoperative day.
Pain related to surgical procedure	Pain may be sharp, constant and unrelenting on day of surgery but should respond to medications; some pain may be related to fear or presence of fixator.
Altered peripheral tissue perfusion related to surgical procedure and Il-izarov apparatus	Color of operative limb will be paler than contralateral limb; it will be cooler and more edematous; pain as stated above; movement of operative limb will be passive, but ROM in other joints normal; capillary refill in 2 to 3 seconds; sensory deficit may be slight numbness in operative areas or in distal tissues

NURSING DIAGNOSIS	SUPPORTIVE ASSESSMENT FINDINGS
Impaired skin integrity related to surgery and Ilizarov treatments	Will have small, 1-2 cm incision(s) for corticotomy covered with dressings; drainage from incision should be serosanguineous; Ilizarov apparatus will have multiple rods entering and exiting skin areas, which may have slight to moderate edema, slight redness, and slight serosanguineous drainage
Self-care deficit related to surgery and Ilizarov apparatus	Deficit varies with upper or lower limb; if upper, will need assistance with bathing, grooming, preparing foot for eating, and dressing self; if lower, care deficits less except for dressing self and transfer activities; hesitant to do required turns of nuts to create distraction needed for bone growth.

3 PLAN

Patient goals

1. The patient will achieve physical mobility and bone healing or regeneration following treatment with Ilizarov technique.
2. The patient will achieve pain-free mobility after Ilizarov treatments.
3. The patient will regain satisfactory peripheral tissue perfusion after treatments.
4. The patient will regain normal skin integrity after healing.
5. The patient will actively participate in self-care during Ilizarov treatments for length of time required.

4 IMPLEMENT

NURSING DIAGNOSIS	NURSING INTERVENTIONS	RATIONALE
Impaired physical mobility related to corticotomy and Ilizarov apparatus	Assess ability to ambulate with crutches preoperatively.	Data are useful for teaching and for postoperative care.
	Explain that patient will be up and stand several times on first postoperative day.	Ambulation will proceed as patient is able. Weight bearing enhances bone formation and growth.
	Explain use of wheel chair postoperatively, along with use of crutches for short areas of ambulation, as to bathroom.	Use of wheel chair increases distances patient can travel from room without tiring. Crutches facilitate ambulation for short distances initially and will be used during latter stages of rehabilitation.
	Secure physical therapy consultation for postoperative exercises.	Specialists provide optimal care.
	Assist as needed with ROM exercises q 4 h.	Active exercises maintain muscle strength and mass.
	Teach family or significant others how to assist patient to rise from bed and to ambulate.	Teaching family or significant others increases their comfort and independence and encourages patient independence also.
	Encourage intake of fluids and foods from all food groups; assist with completing menu planning as needed and food selections.	Intake of high quality foods and fluids helps maintain muscle strength and body weight for long convalescent period of up to 6 months.

→ › ›

NURSING DIAGNOSIS	NURSING INTERVENTIONS	RATIONALE
	Teach crutchwalking techniques if use of crutches is new to patient (see pages 188-189, 274).	Use of proper crutchwalking technique facilitates recovery and provides for safe care and helps prevent possible trauma or additional injury.
Pain related to surgical procedure	Assess for presence, amount, severity, type, and duration of pain; ask patient to describe and quantify pain on scale of 1-10 (10 most severe).	Care can be individualized if patient data are current and are used by health team members.
	Apply ice bags to site of corticotomy.	Ice decreases edema and lessens muscle spasms to lessen pain and decrease inflammation.
	Adjust patient's position q 2-3 h; elevate limb if ordered.	Changing patient's position eases tired muscles and increases circulation to remove wastes to lessen pain and soreness.
	Encourage patient to self-medicate via PCA pump or administer medication as ordered q 3-4 h.	Self-medicating methods increase the patient's sense of control and independence related to pain management. Avoid use of aspirin and other antiinflammatory medications as they are counterproductive in this treatment.
	Check sites of pain to determine its cause; ask patient if pain is increasing or is different from previous pain episodes.	Pain is an indication of pressure on nerve endings; it may also be an indicator of a developing complication.
	Encourage patient to participate in diversionary activities such as card games, board games or musical activities; encourage telling jokes or listening to funny movies or tapes.	Diverting one's attention lessens focusing on amount of discomfort or pain present. Laughter releases endorphins which relieve pain naturally. Laughter also diverts attention to lessen focus on pain.
	Encourage visits from family, friends and others as patient's condition permits.	Visits increase patient's self-esteem and also divert attention for periods of time.
Altered peripheral tissue perfusion related to surgical procedure and Ilizarov apparatus.	Assess neurovascular status as ordered q 2 h.	Surgical procedure sets processes of inflammation into action, noted by redness, edema, temperature increases, pain and altered functions.
	Check capillary refill q 1-2 h.	Capillary refill should occur in 2-4 seconds. Refill of 4-6 seconds is sluggish and should be reported if it persists. Corticotomy plus application of Ilizarov apparatus with programmed adjustments is used on the principle that tension-stress increases the blood supply to the operative site from 160%-300%[89] to enhance healing of affected tissues. Color should be pink.

NURSING DIAGNOSIS	NURSING INTERVENTIONS	RATIONALE
	Listen to patient's complaints of numbness or tingling if present; note presence of and amount of edema, and whether increasing or decreasing.	Numbness or tingling indicate pressure on sensory nerves and may be caused by edema. Edema may be secondary to the inflammatory process but should decrease soon after the surgical procedure is done (approximately in 3-5 days).
	Monitor systemic temperatures and feel skin in operative sites.	Systemic temperature elevations should only persist for 1-3 days, then continue downward toward normal. Skin surfaces should feel warm in operative area related to increased blood supply.
	Encourage or assist patient to turn and adjust positions frequently.	Moving, turning and changing position increase peripheral perfusion and lessen pressure on dependent tissues.
	Encourage deep breathing exercises and use of incentive spirometer q 2 h.	Deep breathing increases oxygen intake and pulmonary perfusion, as well as increasing peripheral perfusion and exchange of carbon dioxide and other wastes in tissues.
Impaired skin integrity related to surgery and Ilizarov treatments	Assess surgical area for signs of inflammation, infection, and wound healing.	Initially the wound area is edematous, reddened and hot due to surgical incision. Inflammatory changes lessen in 3-5 days, edema will lessen, incisional area will be less hot and serosanguineous drainage will markedly decrease or stop in 5-7 days.
	Do wound (incisional) care as ordered.	Initial dressings may remain in place 1-3 days or be changed as needed. Wound may be left undressed after drainage ceases and skin edges are adhered.
	Inspect pin sites once per shift to note increased redness, edema or drainage; if present, report changes to physician.	Signs of infection include marked redness, edema, purulent drainage and pain.
	Inspect Ilizarov apparatus for integrity and tightness of wires and nuts once per shift.	All health team members should understand how apparatus functions and its make-up to note untoward changes in its normal configuration.
	Place pillows under apparatus or limb as desired by patient.	Pillows lessen direct pressure on tissues to lessen tenderness or pain.
	Administer ordered antibiotics q 4-6 h.	Antibiotics are administered to prevent infection.
	Offer back massage in AM and PM.	Massage stimulates circulation to ease sore or tense muscles and enhances patient's circulation throughout body.

→ 〉 〉

NURSING DIAGNOSIS	NURSING INTERVENTIONS	RATIONALE
Self-care deficit related to surgery and Ilizarov apparatus	Assess self-care abilities.	Data are needed for individualized care.
	Assist patient with hygienic care as needed.	Patient may be able to perform own care if lower extremity is involved and upper limbs are healthy.
	Teach patient how to turn nuts to accomplish the distraction technique; significant others are also taught procedures; have patient and significant others practice using wrenches and turning nuts.	Distraction is done by turning the proper nuts ¼ turn q 6 h day and night so total is 1 mm/24 h. Nuts are marked for proper direction to be turned and how far.
	Discuss ways to modify clothing to cover apparatus such as use of pressure sensitive straps or snaps, larger-sized clothing, leisure (sweatpants) clothing or others.	Clothing should be modified for ease in donning or removing and to lessen chances of catching on apparatus.

5 EVALUATE

PATIENT OUTCOME	DATA INDICATING THAT OUTCOME IS REACHED
Patient is achieving physical mobility and bone healing (union) and regeneration following treatments.	X-rays show bone union is occurring over time; angiograms show increased blood flow; no infection is present; bone mass is increased
Patient is achieving comfort and pain-free mobility.	Patient no longer taking narcotic medications and only occasionally takes acetaminophen for soreness; presently using crutches until bone mass is sufficiently strong (may be in Ilizarov apparatus 4-6 months, depending on purpose of procedure). States walks easily without pain.
Patient is regaining satisfactory peripheral tissue perfusion.	Neurovascular checks are all within normal limits; skin is warm and pink.
Patient is regaining normal skin integrity as healing progresses.	Areas of skin around Ilizarov fixator are clear of drainage and are warm and nonedematous; areas are growing hair again; has no tender or hot areas around fixator pins.
Patient actively participates in self-care.	Patient does own distraction turns after discharge to home; patient makes own observations of skin condition and Ilizarov apparatus and checks observations with family members; keeps scheduled appointments; ambulates with crutches frequently and as needed.

PATIENT TEACHING

1. Teach patient about operative procedure and explain meaning of terms.
2. Teach patient and significant others about the Ilizarov apparatus and how it will be used to repair the injured tissues.
3. Teach patient and significant others self-care techniques required by the operation and the apparatus.
4. Teach patient about narcotics for pain and use of PCA pump.
5. Teach patient about effects of antiinflammatory medications as hindering goals of operation.
6. Teach patient about crutch walking techniques.
7. Teach patient about food groups for nutritional intake.

Rehabilitation

Rehabilitation is the process of restoring function, regaining function, or regaining mobility after or because of an orthopaedic disease, condition or trauma. Rehabilitation consists of the definitive measures directed toward lessening the sequelae of a permanent disability, if or when present.

Rehabilitation services are needed because of the number of persons who suffer severe or disabling injuries each year. It has been estimated that 10,000 or more persons are paralyzed yearly, with 5,000 of them having quadriplegia. Approximately 1 in 10 severely disabled persons uses rehabilitation services. There are presently 15 to 20 rehabilitation regional centers in the United States for severely injured patients.

The process of rehabilitation should begin as soon as the severely injured person is admitted to a hospital for emergency care. The rehabilitation team may be available at the initial admitting hospital or the patient may be transferred to a nearby regional rehabilitation center after his/her condition has been stabilized and the extent of the permanent disabilities has been determined.

The rehabilitation team is composed of many health care personnel with the patient as the center and most important member of the team. The team is under the guidance and leadership of one or more rehabilitation or physical medicine physicians. At one time or another additional members of the rehabilitation team may be nurses, physical and occupational therapists, social workers, dietitian, psychiatrist, psychologist, orthotists, prosthetists, recreational therapists, vocational or educational counselors, speech therapists, pharmacists, and possibly anesthesiologists for pain management. Some

responsibilities of each of these team members are listed in Table 13-1. The patient and family members also have significant responsibilities for the quantity and quality of the ultimate recovery of the patient.

Initial evaluation of rehabilitation potential is made as early as feasible after the injuries and while the emergency care to stabilize the patient's condition is proceeding. Goals for the patient's rehabilitation are determined *with* the patient and family members and the health team members, as the medical and surgical treatments are undertaken with the rehabilitation goals in consideration. The patient's specific anatomic and functional deficits must be determined so the patient and team can focus on the patient's potential for return of function. Plans outline the specific treatments with a general time frame for the treatments needed to accomplish the treatment goals and contraindications for any individual treatment are determined. Treatment plans are reviewed periodically to determine their pertinence toward achievement of the goals with evidence of long-term continuity of care incorporated into the rehabilitation efforts.

One of the primary goals of rehabilitation is to bring the patient from the horizontal to vertical position as soon as possible. Being in an upright position gives a great psychologic boost to the patient, to say nothing of the physical benefits to the patient's body. Benefits of being upright early can be noted in less cardiovascular deconditioning and improved food and fluid intake to aid gastrointestinal functioning, lessen nitrogen/calorie imbalances, improve muscle strength and joint movements, and hopefully deter development of pulmonary or peripheral vascular complications. The more severe

Table 13-1

REHABILITATION TEAM AND FUNCTIONS OF MEMBERS

Member	Functions
Physical medicine physician	Leader of rehab team; develops medical care plan with patient and other health team members; coordinates care with other team members; provides on-going evaluation of patient's progress toward goals of care; provides medical/surgical care as needed by patient.
Nurses	Provide bedside patient care; develop nursing care plan with and for the patient and family; coordinate care of and with allied health personnel; provide on-going evaluation of nursing care plan to identify possible problems and recommend changes in care, if needed.
Physical therapists	Provide therapy through various modalities to help patient regain muscle and joint functions; may assist with exercise regimen, ambulation, heat or cold therapies, massage, and others as deemed part of the patient's care plan; teach self-care related to specific treatments, wrappings, use of exercise equipment, and others; provide input to other rehab team members regarding patient's progress toward goals (see Figure 13-13).
Occupational therapists	Teach patient self-care techniques, special exercises or activities to relearn previous skills or to adapt remaining muscles to necessary skills; evaluate home situation and make recommendations for needed adjustments, if any; provide input to other rehab team members regarding patient's progress toward goals.
Psychiatrist/psychologist	Assess patient's reactions to present condition; help patient adapt or adjust to loss of functions, if needed; does psychometric testing to determine patient's need for counseling or other therapy, if any.
Orthotist/prosthetist	Measure and fit patient for specific orthosis, splint, or prosthesis needed; adjust orthotic devices as needed; provide input to rehab team members regarding application of orthosis or prosthesis as patient progresses toward goals (see Figure 13-14).
Dietitian	Makes nutritional assessment to determine nutritional needs to maintain protein/calorie balances; monitors daily intake for adequacy and necessary changes; provides input to rehab team regarding patient's progress.
Social worker	Makes financial assessments related to medical insurance, finances, and concerns for long-term care; seeks health care facilities for extended care; provides input to rehab team regarding financial and long-term care arrangements.
Pharmacist	Provides input to rehab team members related to medication regimen for pain and infection control; evaluates patient's responses to medications and recommends changes to rehab team, if needed.
Speech therapist	Assists patient to regain or improve communication skills, if needed; provides input to rehab team members regarding special training or equipment needed by patient.
Vocational counselor	Assists patient to adjust to disabilities related to work or employment possibilities if adjustments needed; helps patient make transition from rehab center to home and/or employment setting with regard to disabilities.

the patient's injuries and the more body organ systems affected, the greater the potential for complications such as sepsis or shock to occur. Multiple organ failure, with its high mortality, is directly related to the number of organ systems involved.

NURSING CONSIDERATIONS

Emergency assessments and care have been discussed previously related to trauma and will not be repeated here. However, a summary of rehabilitation considerations is appropriate here. During the rehabilitation period each of the following factors must be considered by the rehabilitation team members.

Patient factors: age, sex, types and severity of injuries, education, family roles and responsibilities, financial situation, including insurance coverage, psychologic state, and personal motivation.

Physical factors: Integumentary tissues: *open areas,* wounds, incisions, *pressure areas,* bony prominences, presence of rashes, subcutaneous fat or padding around bony prominences, turning and positioning programs or schedules, presence of traction, external fixators, skin color and temperature.

Cardiovascular tissues: vital signs, changes in blood pressure, pulse or respirations, *presence of hemorrhage or shock,* capillary refill, presence or absence of periph-

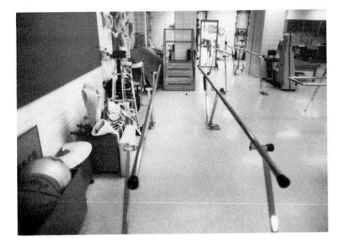

FIGURE 13-13
Physical therapy room for rehabilitation through a variety of strengthening techniques. (Courtesy The Ohio State University, Columbus, Ohio.)

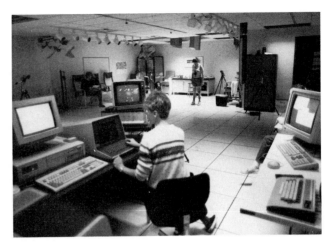

FIGURE 13-14
Gait analysis laboratory for research, analysis, and modification as needed of gaits of injured persons or persons with amputations. (Courtesy The Ohio State University, Columbus, Ohio.)

eral pulses, arterial peripheral vascular disease, venous problems such as varicose veins or stasis ulcers, edema.

Pulmonary tissues: history of smoking, cough, *shortness of breath*, presence, change in or absence of breath sounds, pneumothorax, hemothorax, fractured ribs, production of sputum, dyspnea, use of accessory muscles to breathe, presence of mechanical ventilator or endotracheal tube, presence of or history of asthma, bronchitis or emphysema, fat or pulmonary embolism, *respiratory distress syndrome.*

Gastrointestinal tissues: presence of anorexia, nausea, or vomiting, *hematemesis*, diarrhea, constipation, fecal impaction, presence of, change in or *decrease in bowel sounds*, appetite, food intake, ability to feed self, abdominal distention, bloating, eructation of gas, gastric burning or pain, history of hiatal hernia or gastrointestinal ulcer, abdominal pain or tenseness, melena, fluid intake, likes and dislikes of foods, hemorrhoids, ostomy.

Genitourinary tissues: urinary output, hematuria, urinary sugar and acetone, history of urinary tract diseases or calculi, *presence of indwelling catheter*, urgency, frequency or burning, incontinence, prostatic enlargement, past prostatic surgery, vaginal bleeding, menstrual history, gynecologic surgery, bladder sphincter control, pregnancy, sexually transmitted disease, sexual dysfunction from trauma.

Musculoskeletal: injury to specific tissues (tendons, cartilage, bones, muscles, joints, intervertebral discs, *vertebrae*, synovium, ligaments), open fractures, multiple fractures, loss of part or all limb from trauma, presence of traction equipment, external or internal fixation devices, fractures of hip or cervical vertebrae, *pelvic fracture*, paralysis, muscle spasms, sensory changes or loss

of sensation, muscle wasting or atrophy, ROM of joints, contractures, malunion, ability to use ambulatory aid or transfer to wheel chair or bed.

Endocrine tissues: presence of hypothyroidism or hyperthyroidism, diabetes, hypoglycemia, hyperglycemia, insulin therapy, adrenal hypofunction or hyperfunction, stress reaction, amenorrhea, lowered sperm count, temperature elevations.

Nervous tissues: change in motor or sensory functions, pain, *paralysis*, hemiplegia, paraplegia, quadriplegia, loss of bowel or bladder control, radicular pain, referred pain, "trigger" point, inability to feel a specific tissue or part.

Psychologic factors: mood, grief, disinterest, hostility, anger, frustration, withdrawal, history of mood disorders, suicidal ideation, sadness, crying periods, regression, dependence, previous drug or alcohol dependence, history of absence from school or job.

Treatments offer relief from pain and accompanying muscle spasms that frequently result from low back injury. Medical interventions can prevent long-term disability and chronic pain. However, there are still a disturbing number of low back pain patients whose pain source is not specifically known and for whom treatment is often hit or miss. Some of these patients eventually become "chronic pain patients."

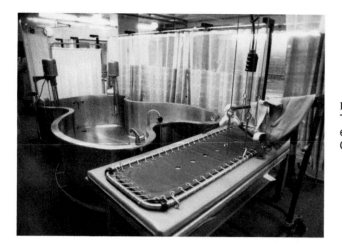

FIGURE 13-15
The Hubbard tank is used for exercise hydrotherapy without the effects of gravity. (Courtesy The Ohio State University, Columbus, Ohio.)

THERAPEUTIC USES OF HEAT OR COLD

Principles for use	Types of applications
Heat	
Produces vasodilation, increases circulation, decreases muscle spasms, relaxes tight muscles, increases cell metabolism, increases velocity of nerve conduction, reduces pain, increases inflammatory response,	Hot packs, infrared applications, diathermy, ultrasound, hydrotherapy (Figure 13-15)
Cold	
Vasoconstriction, decreases circulation, reduces muscle spasms, decreases edema, decreases pain, lowers pain threshold, slows velocity of nerve conduction, lowers inflammatory response, lowers muscle contractility,	Ice pack, gel packs, ice massage, vapocoolant spray, slush pack

VARIOUS THERAPIES USED DURING TREATMENT OR REHABILITATION

Exercise programs	Physical therapy	Medications
Active ROM	Heat or cold	Analgesics
Passive ROM	Rest, including bed rest	Narcotic analgesics
Flexion/extension	Elevation	Muscle relaxants
Strengthening	Traction	Nonsteroidal antiinflammatories
Isometric	Biofeedback	Steroids
Isotonic	Transcutaneous electrical	Antibiotics
Hyperextension (for some	nerve stimulation (TENS)	Immunosuppressives
conditions)	Massage	
Endurance	Orthotic devices	
Resistive	Relaxation techniques	
Coordination		

CHAPTER 14

Patient Teaching Guides

Patient education about musculoskeletal diseases, diagnostic tests, treatments, or special checks is a vital part of nursing. Nurses teach patients and families in many settings as patients undergo diagnostic or therapeutic care. Frequently more than one explanation or teaching session is required because of the patient's condition, the setting, or time constraints. Patient Teaching Guides help facilitate teaching and learning and provide a means to individualize the patient's instruction by comparing information in the teaching guide with the patient's specific condition.

Written teaching guides provide (1) ready sources for teaching in clinics, physicians' offices, outpatient ambulatory care, and in-hospital settings; (2) information for later review and directions for self-care at home; and (3) a measure of assurance to patients and family members for compliance and security regarding observations, the patient's response to self-care or treatments, or untoward signs to report to the physician.

More than one guide may be needed for a particular patient; for example, a person in a cast may need to be taught not only about cast and skin care but also about circulation checks, crutch walking, and bone and joint conditions. All guides should be available and should be used to help the patient gain a thorough understanding of his or her condition.

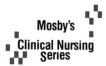
Strains and Sprains

The terms *strain* and *sprain* are used for some musculoskeletal injuries. Although these injuries differ in severity and tissues affected, they are often treated in similar ways.

A **strain** involves overstretching or overuse of a muscle, ligament, or tendon. You may feel pain, weakness, or numbness in the injured area. The area might be swollen, and you may find it difficult to use it, move it, or bear weight on it.

A **sprain** involves the tearing of a muscle, ligament, or tendon around a joint. You may have swelling, pain, and bruising, and you may be unable to use, move, or bear weight on the injured joint. A sprain is more serious than a strain and demands more intense treatment.

Treatment for strains and sprains

Remember the term RICE and what it stands for, and you will know how to treat a strain or sprain.

R = *Rest.* Let the injured area rest. The severity of the injury will determine how long you will need to rest the limb.

I = *Ice.* Applying ice packs to the injured area can keep swelling and bruising down. You will need to apply ice for 48 to 72 hours or longer, depending on how severe your injury is.

C = *Compression.* Elastic bandages are most commonly used to wrap the injured area, although sometimes a circular cast is used for severe sprains. The bandage should be wrapped firmly around the injury, but not so tightly that blood flow is restricted.

E = *Elevation.* The injured part must be elevated to at least heart level to help reduce swelling. (The foot should be higher than the knee and the hand higher than the elbow). Don't elevate too high, however, because you could reduce blood flow. You can use a sling to elevate your arm if that is the injured area.

Some serious sprains may require a cast, a splint, or a brace, some of which are inflated with air.

Circulation checks

If you or your doctor wraps the injured area in a bandage or cast, there are circulation checks that you must do to make sure the bandage or cast is not too tight. A too-tight bandage or cast can cut off the blood supply to the injured area and to the hands, fingers, feet, or toes; it can also press on muscles and nerves and damage them.

There are eight parts to a thorough circulation check. You need to do all eight.

1. **Color**—The injured part is usually paler than the surrounding tissues. If the area is very red, purple, or blue, you should call your doctor, although bruised areas are usually bluish.
2. **Temperature**—The injured part is usually cooler than the surrounding tissues. Call your doctor if it feels warm or hot.
3. **Swelling**—The injured part will be more swollen, but the skin around it should not be tight. Call your doctor if there is swelling or skin tightness.
4. **Pain**—You will have some dull, aching pain in the injured area. Call your doctor if you feel a sudden increase in the type or severity of pain.
5. **Change of function**—You should be able to bend or flex the fingers or toes on an injured limb. Call your doctor if you can't bend them, even though it might hurt a little when you do so.
6. **Sensory perception**—Call your doctor if you are in a cast and the toes or fingers of your injured limb are numb or tingling or feel as if they are asleep. If you are wearing a bandage, loosen it.
7. **Capillary refill**—Push down on a fingernail or toenail of the injured limb. The pink color of the nail should return in 2 to 4 seconds. If the color takes longer than 4 seconds to return and you are wearing a cast, call your doctor. If you are wearing a bandage, loosen it.
8. **Compare**—Compare the injured side (arm, leg) to the other side (arm, leg). Do you notice any difference? Comparing is a good way to notice changes in color, temperature, and swelling.

These eight checks can also be done right after you suffer an injury. Follow the instructions given above.

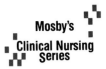
Arthritis

What is arthritis?

Arthritis is a disease of the joints. The word *arthritis* means joint inflammation. There are more than 100 kinds of arthritis that affect more than 36 million people in the United States. Arthritis causes serious disability in many people. Osteoarthritis and rheumatoid arthritis are the two major kinds of arthritis. Osteoarthritis, or degenerative joint disease, is a noninflammatory arthritis that affects 16 million people in the United States. Rheumatoid arthritis is an inflammatory arthritis that affects 7 million people in the United States; when it occurs in children, it is called juvenile rheumatoid arthritis, or Still's disease.

What is a joint?

To understand how arthritis affects your joints, you must know how your joints are made up. The joint is the point of contact of two or more bones. The bone ends of the joint are covered with cartilage, which provides a smooth surface for movement. The synovium is a membrane that surrounds the joint and secretes a fluid that lubricates the cartilage and the joint. The whole joint is enclosed in the tough, protective joint capsule. Ligaments connect the bones and keep the joints stable.

What is osteoarthritis?

Osteoarthritis usually affects people who are over 35 years of age. Sometimes it can begin at an earlier age because of joint injury or overuse. Men and women are affected equally before the age of 55, but there is a higher incidence of osteoarthritis in women over 55. Ninety percent of people over 60 show some signs of osteoarthritis. When the cause of osteoarthritis is unknown, it is called primary osteoarthritis. When the cause is known, such as obesity, injury, and repeated use of the joint (such as the shoulder and elbow joints of baseball pitchers), it is called secondary osteoarthritis.

Osteoarthritis destroys the joint cartilage of the major weight-bearing joints—the hips, knees, and spinal column. The disease usually affects only one or two joints. With osteoarthritis, the cartilage of the joints gradually wears away with weight bearing and movement in the joint.

As the disease progresses, so much of the cartilage is destroyed that the bone ends begin to rub against each other. Bony spurs develop around the joint, and pain and inflammation result.

Osteoarthritis is not only the most common type of arthritis, it is also the most easily managed. Osteoarthritis is diagnosed based on the patient's medical history, a physical examination to determine which joints are affected, blood tests, and x-rays. A sample of synovial fluid from the affected joint may also be taken. The main symptom of osteoarthritis is restricted motion in the joint, along with a deep, aching pain during movement and at night, and joint deformity.

What is rheumatoid arthritis?

Rheumatoid arthritis is a chronic disease, meaning that those who have it must live with it the rest of their lives. Rheumatoid arthritis affects children between 8 and 15 years of age and adults between 25 and 55 years of age. It rarely occurs in those over 55. It is two to three times more common in women than in men, and it has a tendency to run in families. Seventy percent of the people affected are over 30 years of age.

The cause of rheumatoid arthritis is unknown. A possible explanation is that it is an autoimmune (or self-immune) disorder, which means that the body is attacking itself, especially the lining of the joints. An infectious agent also could be a cause. Rheumatoid arthritis affects the smaller joints of the hands, wrists, feet, and ankles before it affects joints such as the hips, knees, and elbows. The disease is symmetric and bilateral, meaning that it affects the same joints on both sides of the body.

Rheumatoid arthritis affects the synovium, which becomes inflamed (red, swollen, painful, and warm) as if reacting to an infection. The synovium secretes more fluid, making the joint more swollen. Later, the cartilage also becomes involved and eventually becomes rough and pitted. Ligaments and tendons also become inflamed, scarred, and shortened by the disease, contributing to the deformities often noticed in the hands and wrists of people with rheumatoid arthritis.

The main symptoms of rheumatoid arthritis are pain and loss of function in the joints. Other symptoms include morning stiffness in one or more joints, warmth in the joints, swelling in at least one or two joints, a tingling or prickling sensation in the hands or feet, tiredness, weight loss, and a feeling of ill health. As the disease progresses, nodules form under the skin, cysts (water-filled masses) develop in the synovium and bone, and the joints and surrounding bone and tissue become deformed. Rheumatoid arthritis is diagnosed based on the symptoms, a physical examination, x-rays, blood tests, and other laboratory tests.

How are osteoarthritis and rheumatoid arthritis treated?

Many treatments for osteoarthritis and rheumatoid arthritis are similar. The goals of the treatments are to relieve pain, minimize joint destruction, maintain the range of motion in the joint, and increase the strength of the joint.

1. Drugs such as salicylates (aspirin) and nonsteroidal antiinflammatory drugs (NSAIDs) are used to relieve pain and reduce inflammation. Steroids, which are injected directly into the joint, may also be used. Steroids may also be given orally to patients with rheumatoid arthritis, but not to those with osteoarthritis.
2. Good nutrition and careful weight control are important, especially for patients who are overweight.
3. Hot and cold treatments and ultrasound treatments are used to relieve pain and improve joint flexibility.
4. Exercises are prescribed to strengthen the muscles and tissues supporting the joint and to maintain as much joint motion as possible.
5. The use of crutches, canes, or walkers may be prescribed to protect the joints from stress. Splints are also used to maintain proper joint positions.
6. Learning less stressful ways to accomplish daily activities and home management are part of the treatment process.

The most common surgical treatment for osteoarthritis is total joint replacement. Hip joints are the most commonly and successfully replaced joints, but the elbow, shoulder, knee, and ankle joints can also be replaced. With rheumatoid arthritis, the first surgical treatment is removal of the synovium; total joint replacement is a later alternative.

Comparison chart

	Osteoarthritis	Rheumatoid arthritis
Causes	Obesity	Autoimmune disorder?
	Injury	
	Joint overuse	Infectious agent?
	Heredity/gene defect	
	Sometimes unknown	
Persons affected	90% of those over 60 yr	Children 8-15 yr
		Adults 25-55 yr
	More women than men over 55 yr	More women than men
Joints	Hips, knees, shoulders, spinal column	Hands, wrists, feet, ankles
Treatment	Aspirin, ibuprofen and other NSAIDs, steroids (only into joint)	Aspirin, ibuprofen and other NSAIDs, steroids (oral and into joint), gold compounds, immune suppressants
	Weight control, good nutrition	Weight control, good nutrition
	Hot and cold treatments	Hot and cold treatments
	Exercise	Exercise
	Crutches, canes, walkers	Crutches, canes, walkers, splints
	Joint replacement	Rest
		Removal of synovium
		Joint replacement (later)

What is Osteoporosis?

Osteoporosis is the most common metabolic bone disease. It results from the loss of calcium in the bones, causing the bones to become brittle and susceptible to breaking. Osteoporosis, which means "porous bone," is also called the "silent disease," because it is usually not diagnosed until the person suffers a fracture, or broken bone. Osteoporosis affects 15 million to 20 million people in the United States. Women are affected eight times more often than men.

Osteoporosis primarily affects the vertebrae and the hips, wrists, and rib bones. Fractures can occur without any outside force being placed on the bones, especially in the spinal column. Hip bones are most often broken. Women suffer hip fractures two to three times more often than men. The vertebrae may compress and cause a stooped appearance or outward curvature of the back. The result is loss of height and back pain.

How do bones function?

Bone is a living tissue that is being formed and shaped continuously. Bones go through a process of formation (building up the bone) and resorption (breaking down the bone for other uses) throughout your life. Bones store calcium for other body functions, and the body takes the calcium out by resorption. Bone mass, or the amount of bone in your body, increases as you grow through childhood, adolescence, and into adulthood. Bone mass is at its greatest when you are about 35 years of age. Up to that time the process of formation occurs faster than the process of resorption. However, as you age, resorption naturally occurs faster than formation, resulting in a gradual decrease in bone mass. Bones become brittle and susceptible to fractures. Women suffer the greatest loss of bone mass within the first 5 years after menopause (the ceasing of menstruation). The decrease in bone mass is slower in men.

Why are women affected more often?

One out of four women, and half the women over 65 years of age, have osteoporosis to some extent. Most are white women who have gone through menopause. Generally, blacks have greater bone mass than whites, and men have greater bone mass than women. Petite women with small bones and thin bodies have very small bone masses. Thus women are at greater risk of developing osteoporosis if they have a Caucasian or Oriental background or are petite.

Osteoporosis is also caused by low estrogen levels that occur in women after menopause. Although the role of estrogen is not clear, it is linked to the processes of bone formation and resorption. Estrogen is thought to reduce bone resorption, to reduce calcium loss through the kidneys, and to increase calcium absorption in the digestive tract. Estrogen protects women who have had an inadequate intake of calcium in their growing years. However, when estrogen levels drop after menopause, bone resorption in women increases greatly.

What are the risk factors?

Two major factors for osteoporosis are lack of exercise and inadequate intake of calcium, vitamin D, and protein. Osteoporosis caused by calcium and vitamin D deficiencies affects men and women 70 to 85 years of age. Other risk factors contributing to the disease are these:

1. A family history of osteoporosis
2. Smoking and consuming too much alcohol and caffeine, which interfere with the absorption of calcium
3. Prolonged use of drugs or medications such as steroids, magnesium-based antacids such as Maalox, and heparin
4. Diseases and hormonal disorders such as rheumatoid arthritis, liver disease, certain cancers, and an overactive thyroid
5. Poor calcium absorption in the intestines

Although osteoporosis primarily affects middle-aged or older people, it can occur in young adults. Injuries that result in paralysis or long periods of immobility can lead to osteoporosis.

How is osteoporosis diagnosed?

Osteoporosis is diagnosed by several methods. A physical examination can reveal bone thinning. X-rays can show bone loss of 25% to 40% or more, but they are only helpful in later detection. A more specialized x-ray technique (computed tomography) can detect bone loss as slight as 2%, which is useful in measuring a patient's response to therapy. Absorptiometry, another specialized x-ray technique, can detect bone loss of as little as 2% in the wrist and hand.

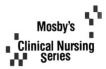

Mosby's
Clinical Nursing
Series

Treatment of Osteoporosis

The goals of treatment are to prevent further bone loss, to increase bone formation, and to prevent fractures. Treatment is designed to your needs, based on your age, the extent of bone loss, and whether you have fractured bones. In some patients bone loss has been reduced or stopped with an increased intake of calcium and vitamin D. But your doctor should oversee your vitamin D intake, because too much is harmful. For women, treatments of estrogen or estrogen combined with progestin have been effective in reducing and preventing further bone loss. Again, your doctor should monitor the treatment so that you avoid harmful side effects. Some studies indicate that the compound sodium fluoride, given with calcium and vitamin D, stimulates bone formation. All of these treatments must be monitored by your doctor. Regular treatments include a proper diet, estrogen replacement therapy for women, medication for back pain, and moderate exercise.

The calcium-rich diet

A diet rich in calcium can help slow or prevent the loss of bone. Dietary calcium from foods is absorbed better than calcium from supplements. Many calcium-rich foods are also high in protein, vitamin D, phosphorus, and fiber. Some calcium-rich foods include the following:
1. Milk and milk products, such as yogurt, ice cream, and cheese
2. Fish, such as sardines (with bones) and salmon
3. Dark green vegetables, such as broccoli and collard greens
4. White vegetables such as bok choy and cauliflower
(A rule of thumb: If the vegetable grows above the ground, it is high in calcium.)
For comparison, 8 ounces of milk contain 300 mg of calcium. Children need 400 to 700 mg of calcium per day. The requirement increases to 1,300 mg per day for adolescents and then drops to 1,000 mg per day for adults. After menopause, women need 1,500 mg per day. About 400 international units (IU) of vitamin D, which aids in the absorption of calcium, are needed daily. Vitamin D–fortified milk and multi-

ple vitamins are good sources of vitamin D. See your doctor for a diet plan for you. Keep alcohol intake moderate, and avoid smoking, beverages with caffeine, and eating too much protein, as these may increase bone loss.

Exercise

Exercise is vital for keeping bones strong. Exercises such as walking and swimming that put moderate stress or weight on your bones can help slow or prevent osteoporosis. Exercise increases the rate of bone formation, strengthens muscles, increases bone density (mass), improves circulation, and enhances the absorption of nutrients such as calcium. Just do it!

Home safety measures

Home safety is also an important preventive measure for people with osteoporosis. Here are some guides for you:
1. Use only large area rugs that won't slide or move or rugs with nonskid under surfaces.
2. Avoid waxing floors, because that makes them slick.
3. Provide adequate lighting in every room to prevent falls.
4. Use nonskid strips in the shower or bathtub.
5. Install handrails on the stairs and in the bathtub.
6. Avoid long cords that could cause you to trip or fall.
You should be careful doing any activity. Falling, getting up from a chair, bending deeply, or straining to open a window can cause severe strain or can cause bones to break. Call your doctor if you have pain, swelling, or stiffness after a fall or an unusually strenuous activity.

Your doctor may also suggest using devices such as a sock applier, shoe horn, and long-handled sponge (for bathing) to aid you in daily activities. Wearing rubber-heeled shoes may be suggested to protect your back from stress during walking. The doctor may suggest that you use a cane or walker to relieve stress on your back and joints, to help you maintain your balance, and to reduce the risk of falling.

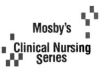
Scoliosis

Scoliosis is a condition in which the spine curves abnormally to the left or right side. People with scoliosis can't straighten their backs and may appear to lean to one side. In some severe cases, the spinal curve can become so pronounced that the spine takes on the shape of the letter S or an elongated C.

What causes scoliosis and who is affected?

Children and adults can be affected by scoliosis. Most cases of scoliosis in children have no known cause, but the condition does seem to run in families. Curvature of the spine in children may be present at birth or may occur because of muscular dystrophy and cerebral palsy. Poor posture does not cause scoliosis.

Both boys and girls can have scoliosis, although girls are seven times more likely to suffer from severe curvatures. The condition sometimes worsens as the child enters the teenage years. However, most cases of scoliosis in children are mild, and the degree of spinal curving is minimal. A few cases of childhood scoliosis can worsen in adulthood.

Diagnosis and treatment

Scoliosis must be treated as early as possible so that the spinal curves do not become severe. Parents, school nurses, pediatricians and physicians should watch for the early signs:

- One shoulder higher than the other
- One hip higher than the other
- One shoulder blade more prominent than the other
- Greater space between the arm and body on one side when the child's arms hang loosely at her sides
- Rib prominence and sideway curvature of the spine when the child bends forward

The earlier the diagnosis of scoliosis is made, the sooner orthopedic treatment can begin and the more effective that treatment will be. Each case of scoliosis is different, so what works for one patient may not work as well for another.

Exercise is an important part of treatment for scoliosis. Sit-up pelvic tilts, hyperextension of the spine, and special breathing exercises are a few of the exercises the orthopedist may prescribe.

A **brace** is the most common treatment for mild and moderate curvature. The brace's function is not to correct the curve—it is to prevent the curve from getting worse. Occasionally a child will show some improvement in the curve and body alignment after wearing a brace.

There are two types of braces. The **Milwaukee brace** is a high-profile brace, which means that it extends up into the hairline. It is a commonly used brace and is prescribed when the upper thoracic vertebrae are involved as well as the lumbar vertebrae. The **Boston brace** is a low-profile brace and doesn't extend as far up the back and neck. It is prescribed when the curves are lower or less severe.

A brace must be worn 23 hours a day. It may be taken off for 1 hour a day to exercise or swim.

Sometimes the brace will not prevent the curve from worsening. Other treatments then must be considered. **Electrical muscle stimulation** occasionally has been effective for certain types of curves. This treatment is done at night and can take the place of or supplement use of the brace. However, muscle stimulation is ineffective for most patients.

If the scoliotic curves become progressively worse, surgery may be necessary. Surgery can help straighten the curves and help prevent complications when scoliosis becomes severe.

Skin and brace care

Because a brace must be worn 23 hours a day, it is very important to take care of it and the skin under and around the brace. It is vital to keep the skin clean. A shower or bath should be taken daily. A small amount of powder or cornstarch can be sprinkled on the skin where the brace rests. A T-shirt is worn under the brace to help prevent chafing.

Check for reddened or tender areas daily or have a family member check areas of your back that are hard to see. If the brace rubs in any spot, have the doctor check the fit of the brace. It may need to be adjusted. The brace should not rub or chafe. It is important that red or tender areas not become open sores.

The brace should be kept clean. Wash plastic or metal parts with soap and water; keep all padded areas dry to prevent bunching up of the padding or skin irritation.

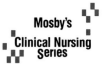
Low Back Pain

Your lower back hurts. Does it help to know that you are not alone? Eighty percent of the population suffers from low back pain. Both young people and older people are affected, although the chances you will have low back pain increase as you age.

The history of back pain

Your lower back is made up of five vertebrae and accompanying disks, nerve roots, muscles, and ligaments. A healthy back has all its vertebrae aligned and is supported by strong hip, back, and abdominal muscles. Low back pain begins when something goes awry among all these bones, disks, ligaments, and muscles. However, this area contains so many nerve endings that the cause of low back pain may be hard to discern. To help diagnose why you have low back pain, your doctor will ask you some questions:

- How and when did your pain begin?
- Were you injured?
- Did the pain begin after you performed a strenuous activity?
- Where is the pain? Is it only in your back or does it also go down your hip and leg?
- Is the pain constant or only occasional?
- Do coughing and sneezing make it worse?
- What kind of work do you do?

Your doctor will examine your back, check your muscle tone and posture, and may do abdominal, rectal, and pelvic examinations. X-rays may be taken. When a disk problem is suspected, a myelogram may be needed. The doctor will inject a special solution into the spinal canal, which allows the disk to show up on x-rays. Other x-rays, such as a computed tomography (CT) scan or a magnetic resonance imaging (MRI) examination, may be done before the myelogram. A CT scan or MRI study may show the disk problem so that a myelogram is not needed.

Diagnosis

From the test or x-ray information, your doctor should be able to make a diagnosis. Following are some possible causes of low back pain:
1. Poor posture, lack of exercise, and obesity: These are some of the most common causes of back pain and the most easily corrected.

Poor posture, weak abdominal and back muscles, and extra weight (especially on the abdomen) put a strain on your back. This strain can make your back susceptible to injury.
2. Osteoarthritis: A result of the aging process, osteoarthritis produces bony spurs on the vertebrae and narrows the disks, which can cause pain from pressure on nerve pathways.
3. Injury: Usually injury to the back means a strain or sprain. Lifting, bending, standing, or sitting improperly can stretch or tear the back's muscles and ligaments.
4. Ruptured disks: Sometimes a back injury can result in a ruptured (or slipped) disk. The disk shifts and presses on nerve endings, producing great pain. Sometimes the spinal nerves can be pinched, and you may feel pain that radiates down your hip and leg. See a doctor if you have this kind of pain, because muscle weakness and nerve damage can result if the disk continues to pinch the nerve.
5. Other causes of back pain: Osteoporosis, which occurs mainly in postmenopausal women and involves small fractures of the vertebrae; Reiter's syndrome, which affects adult men and can produce arthritis that affects the back; spondylolisthesis, which occurs when one vertebra moves forward onto another; infection, which can mimic a ruptured disk and may require examination of the spinal fluid; and spinal tumors, which may be discovered through MRI studies.

Preventing back pain

Good posture when sitting or standing is very important for a healthy back. When sitting, make sure both feet are flat on the floor and that your knees are level with your hips. Sit with your back firmly against the back of the chair. A rolled-up towel or small pillow between your lower back and the chair back can support your lower back. When standing, stand with one foot up on a stool if possible and change positions often. Stand as straight as possible. When walking, keep your head high, tuck in your chin slightly, keep your abdominal muscles tight, and tilt your pelvis to maintain a natural low back curve.

The following **rest positions** can help relieve back tension by straightening the spine:

1. Stand upright and place your hands in the small of your back; bend backward slowly and hold this position for 30 to 60 seconds.
2. Sit on a chair. Lean forward and lower your head to your knees. Hold for 2 to 5 minutes.
3. Lie with your back flat on the floor and place your legs on a chair. For best results hold this position for 15 minutes.

Lifting should be done with the knees, not the back. Bend your knees when you lift something. Don't lift heavy things any higher than your chest. Get someone to help you.

Sleeping takes up one third of your life. It is important that you sleep on a firm mattress. Sleep on your side with your knees bent or on your back with a pillow under your knees. Sleeping on your stomach can cause back strain.

Exercise is important for maintaining the back's natural curve and for strengthening the back and abdominal muscles. These muscles will support your back and help protect it from injury and strain. The following exercises are meant for people who have a healthy back or who have recovered fully from a back injury. (If you are recovering from a back problem, do **only** the exercises prescribed by your doctor.)

Knee-to-chest lift: 1. Lie on your back on the floor with knees bent and feet flat on the floor. 2. Draw both knees up to your chest. 3. Place both hands around your knees and pull them firmly against your chest. 4. Lower your legs and return to the starting position. 5. Repeat 5 to 10 times.

Single leg lift: 1. Lie flat on your back on the floor, left knee bent, left foot flat on the floor. 2. Slowly raise your right leg as high as you comfortably can. 3. Hold for five counts. 4. Slowly return the leg to the floor. 5. Bend your right knee and put your right foot flat on the floor; raise your left leg and hold for five counts. 6. Repeat 5 to 10 times for each leg.

Pelvic tilt: 1. Lie flat on your back on the floor, knees bent, feet flat on the floor. 2. Firmly tighten your buttock muscles. 3. Hold for five counts. 4. Relax buttocks. 5. Repeat 5 to 10 times. Be sure to keep your lower back flat against the floor.

Half sit-ups: 1. Lie flat on the floor on your back, knees bent, feet flat on the floor, hands on chest. 2. Slowly raise your head and neck to the top of your chest. 3. Reach both hands forward and place them on your knees. 4. Hold for five counts. 5. Slowly return to starting position. 6. Repeat 5 to 10 times.

Elbow props: 1. Lie face down with your arms beside your body and your head turned to one side. Stay in this position for 3 to 5 minutes, making sure that you relax completely. 2. Remain face down and prop yourself on your elbows. Hold this position for 2 to 3 minutes. 3. Return to starting position and relax for 1 minute. 4. Repeat 5 to 10 times.

Remember:
- Don't exercise if you are having pain.
- Start slowly and gradually increase the number of repetitions for each exercise.
- Exercise every day, once in the morning and once at night. Exercising only occasionally can actually do your back harm.

Treatments for low back pain

The treatment prescribed for your back will depend on the diagnosis of your back pain. Recovery may be slow and frustrating, but follow your doctor's instructions completely and be patient.

Bed rest may be the first thing that is prescribed. Bed rest is extremely important, because your back needs time to heal, particularly if it has been injured.

Medication, hot or cold compresses, and **back support** may also be prescribed.

Transcutaneous electrical nerve stimulation *(TENS) units* can provide relief for severe back pain.

Hospitalization may be required to ensure bed rest. Sometimes patients are put in *traction* to alleviate pressure on the spinal nerves.

Surgery is occasionally needed for problems that do not respond to treatment.

Injections into the intervertebral disks can be given in some cases as an alternative to surgery for ruptured disks. **Physical therapy** may be recommended to begin rehabilitating your back. **Exercise programs** can begin once your back is on the mend.

Changes in life-style are sometimes necessary so you don't reinjure your back. If your work requires heavy lifting, your doctor may recommend that you request a less strenuous job.

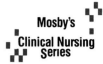

Mosby's
**Clinical Nursing
Series**

Ruptured Disks

Ruptured disks, sometimes called herniated disks, can cause severe back pain and disability. Ruptured disks are serious and demand medical treatment.

Disks and how they rupture

Most ruptured disks (95%) occur in the lower back. A disk is a soft, cushioning pad of cartilage that lies between each vertebra in the spine. These disks give the back the flexibility it needs to move and bend and at the same time absorb the shock of these movements. Each cartilage disk has a jellylike center to help the disk absorb shock.

Poor posture, injury, and the aging process can cause disks to wear out. The jellylike center of the disk may begin to bulge through the cartilage. A sudden movement or extreme stress on the lower back (such as picking up a child) can cause the disk to rupture (herniate) through its protective cartilage. The ruptured disk can pinch or irritate spinal nerves. Sudden, sharp, often disabling pain results. The pain may radiate down from the lower back into the buttocks and down the thigh and leg. This type of pain is called sciatica, because the sciatic nerve is being pinched. You must seek medical treatment for this type of pain, because nerve damage can result if the condition is left untreated.

Treatment

Because you must give your back a chance to heal completely, bed rest is extremely impor-tant. Your doctor may also prescribe a muscle relaxant and/or a pain-killing medication such as aspirin or a nonsteroidal antiinflammatory drug such as ibuprofen. You may need to wear a back brace or a cervical collar if a cervical disk rup-tures. Hot or cold packs can help relieve pain and inflammation. Once your back pain has sub-sided, physical therapy can begin to help strengthen your back muscles and regain mobil-ity.

If you still have pain, numbness, or disability after these conservative treatments, your doctor may recommend other tests and probably sur-gery. You may have a CT scan, a myelogram, or an MRI study (magnetic resonance imaging) to help diagnose the condition of your disks. If sur-gery is needed, it is best to have it done soon af-ter the disk ruptures to help prevent permanent nerve damage and to get you on your feet again. There are many forms of surgery that can be performed, and your doctor will discuss the op-tions with you.

Some patients with ruptured disks may be treated with chymopapain in a process called **chemonucleolysis.** Chymopapain is an enzyme extracted from the papaya plant; it can dissolve the part of the disk that is pressing on the spinal nerve and causing pain. However, chemonucle-olysis is a controversial procedure that can cause some potentially serious complications. Your doctor will explain the risks and the benefits of chemonucleolysis with you before you have the procedure done.

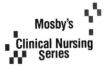

Mosby's
Clinical Nursing
Series

Preventing Future Back problems

Once your back has healed, you'll need to know how to help prevent reinjury.

Good posture when sitting or standing is very important for a healthy back. When sitting, make sure both feet are flat on the floor and that your knees are level with your hips. Sit with your back firmly against the back of the chair. A rolled-up towel or small pillow between your lower back and the chair back can support your lower back. When standing, stand with one foot up on a stool if possible and change positions often. Try to stand as straight as possible. When walking, keep your head high, tuck in your chin slightly, tighten your abdominal muscles, and tilt your pelvis to try to maintain a natural low back curve.

Rest positions such as the following can help relieve back tension by straightening the spine:

1. Stand upright and place your hands in the small of your back; bend backward slowly and hold this position for 30 to 60 seconds.
2. Sit on a chair or stool. Lean forward and lower your head to your knees. Hold for 2 to 5 minutes.
3. Lie with your back flat on the floor and place your legs on a chair. For best results hold this position for 15 minutes.

Lifting should be done with the knees, not the back. Bend your knees when you pick something up. Don't try to lift heavy things any higher than your chest. Get someone to help you if the load is too heavy.

Sleeping takes up one third of your life. It is important that you do this sleeping on a firm mattress. Sleep on your side with your knees bent or on your back with a pillow under your knees. Sleeping on your stomach can cause back strain.

Exercise is very important for maintaining the back's natural curve and for strengthening the back and abdominal muscles. These muscles will support your back and help protect it from injury and strain. The following exercises are meant for people who already have a healthy back or who have recovered fully from a back injury. (If you are recovering from a back problem, you must do only those exercises prescribed by your doctor.)

Knee-to-chest lift: 1. Lie on your back on the floor with knees bent and feet flat on the floor. 2. Draw both knees up to your chest. 3. Place both hands around your knees and pull them firmly against your chest. 4. Lower your legs and return to the starting position. 5. Repeat 5 to 10 times.

Single leg lift: 1. Lie flat on your back on the floor, left knee bent, left foot flat on the floor. 2. Slowly raise your right leg as high as you comfortably can. 3. Hold for five counts. 4. Slowly return the leg to the floor. 5. Bend your right knee and put your right foot flat on the floor; raise your left leg and hold for five counts. 6. Repeat 5 to 10 times for each leg.

Pelvic tilt: 1. Lie flat on your back on the floor, knees bent, feet flat on the floor. 2. Firmly tighten your buttock muscles. 3. Hold for five counts. 4. Relax buttocks. 5. Repeat 5 to 10 times. Be sure to keep your lower back flat against the floor.

Half sit-ups: 1. Lie flat on the floor on your back, knees bent, feet flat on the floor, hands on chest. 2. Slowly raise your head and neck to the top of your chest. 3. Reach both hands forward and place them on your knees. 4. Hold for five counts. 5. Slowly return to starting position. 6. Repeat 5 to 10 times.

Elbow props: 1. Lie face down with your arms beside your body and your head turned to one side. Stay in this position for 3 to 5 minutes, making sure that you relax completely. 2. Remain face down and prop yourself on your elbows. Hold this position for 2 to 3 minutes. 3. Return to starting position and relax for 1 minute. 4. Repeat 5 to 10 times.

Remember:
- Don't exercise if you are having pain.
- Start slowly and gradually increase the number of repetitions for each exercise.
- Exercise every day. Exercising only occasionally can actually do your back harm. It is much better for your back if you exercise it once in the morning and once at night.

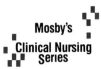
Transcutaneous Electrical Nerve Stimulation (TENS)

You have been given a transcutaneous electrical nerve stimulation unit, commonly called a TENS unit, to help control your pain. There are a few things you should know about your unit, such as how it works, how to use it, and how to care for it and your skin.

What is TENS and how does it work?

Let's say that your lower back is causing you severe, constant pain. Pain messages travel along the nerves from your injured back to your brain. Your brain receives the message and reacts. The result is that you feel pain. A TENS unit can stop these pain messages before they reach your brain, thereby stopping the pain.

A TENS unit is a pocket-sized, battery-operated device that provides mild, continuous electrical current through the skin by use of two to four electrodes. The electrodes are taped onto the skin, and lead wires connect the electrodes to the device. It is this mild electrical current that blocks or modifies the pain messages and replaces them with a buzzing, tingling sensation. It is also thought that TENS may stimulate the body's production of endorphin, a natural pain reliever.

Pain relief can vary from patient to patient. You may need to use your TENS unit only occasionally, or you may need it constantly. Often people find that they need to use it less and less as time goes by.

How to use your TENS unit

Your TENS unit is very easy to use if you follow a few basic procedures:

1. Apply a thin coat of gel over the entire electrode.
2. Make sure each electrode is placed securely on the skin. Electrodes should be placed close to the site of pain.
3. Tape the electrodes firmly to your skin.
4. Slowly turn the intensity (output) knob until you feel a slight tingling or buzzing on your skin. You may find that you have to increase the intensity if you are still feeling pain or decrease the intensity if the tingling sensation becomes uncomfortable.

How to care for your TENS unit

1. Turn the TENS unit off before removing it.
2. After removing the electrodes from your skin, wipe them with an alcohol and water mixture.
3. Do not use the TENS unit if you will be getting wet or will be perspiring heavily. If the unit does get wet, it must be allowed to dry thoroughly before you use it again.
4. The electrodes should be replaced if the adhesive surface separates from the backing or if they no longer stay firmly on your skin.
5. After a while the battery pack will need to be recharged or the batteries replaced. If your skin does not tingle when the intensity is increased, this usually means the batteries are weakening.

Skin care

1. After you remove the electrodes, cleanse the skin well.
2. Apply a lotion to the electrode placement sites after each TENS treatment.
3. Watch for any redness on your skin where the electrodes were placed. If you see redness or rash, use hypoallergenic tape to secure the electrodes. If the redness or rash persists, try putting the electrode at different sites.

Casts

So now you or a member of your family is wearing a cast. The cast is only one of several devices used to promote the healing of broken bones. Doctors also use traction and pins, or a combination of these three, to help heal broken bones. The cast has the advantage of being less expensive, requiring little care on your part, and allowing you to move around. The cast also encloses and immobilizes the broken bone and injured soft tissues to prevent movement that could cause further injury and to keep the bone in place for proper healing.

Your cast may be made of plaster or of a synthetic material such as fiberglass. Although the plaster cast is heavy, the doctor can mold a plaster cast more easily for a close fit over severe injuries. The synthetic cast is lightweight and easier to move around, making it good for elderly patients. Your cast has a name. If it covers your forearm or lower leg, it is a **short arm** or **short leg** cast. A **long leg** cast covers the whole leg, and a **hanging** cast covers the whole arm and forearm. The **body** cast encircles the chest and abdomen, whereas the **Minerva** cast covers the chest, neck, and head with openings for the ears, face, and arms. The cast that covers the hips and one or both legs is the **hip spica** or **spica** cast.

Things to watch for

Your cast will be warm at first because of the setting process. However, warm areas on the cast later on may indicate infection, and you should notify your doctor at once.

You should watch for increased pain or soreness under the cast, particularly around bony prominences such as the wrist or ankle, that is not relieved by repositioning the body. Check the skin color and temperature periodically. When the tip of a finger or the big toe that protrudes from the cast is squeezed until it is white, the pink color should return within 2 to 4 seconds. If skin color does not return within 4 to 6 seconds or if the skin is red, blue, white, or discolored, notify your doctor. If fingers or toes are cool, cover them. If they do not warm up in 20 minutes, call your doctor. Call your doctor immediately if any of these other symptoms occur:

- An increase in swelling
- A tingling or burning sensation
- An inability to move muscles around the cast
- A foul odor around the edges of the cast
- Any drainage, which may show through the cast
- Any cracks or breaks in the cast

Home Cast Care

The first 24 hours

Your cast needs at least 24 hours to dry if it is plaster. Avoid handling it as much as possible. When you do have to move the cast, such as when you change your body position, use only the palms of your hands and support the cast under your joints. You want to avoid putting indentations in the cast that will put pressure on the skin inside. You may use a fan placed 18 to 24 inches from the cast to aid its drying in the first 24 hours. You should be sure to expose the whole cast for drying, and do not cover it with linen for the first 24 hours.

Keep the cast and extremity above the level of the heart for at least 48 hours by propping your cast up on firm pillows. Put ice directly over the fractured area for 24 hours, but be sure to enclose the ice in a plastic bag to keep the cast dry. Move the parts of your body above and below the cast regularly to aid circulation and relieve stiffness. Massaging the joints and extremities around the cast will also improve circulation.

How to care for your cast

If you have a plaster cast, do not get the cast wet because it will lose its strength. To keep the cast clean and dry, you should cover it with plastic when bathing, using the toilet (if it is a spica cast), or going out in rain or snow. You may use a damp cloth and scouring powder to clean soiled spots on the cast. Be sure to brush away plaster crumbs or other objects from the edges of the cast, but do not remove any padding.

If you have a synthetic cast and you do not have any wounds under the cast, your doctor may allow you to bathe and swim with it. You should use only a small amount of mild soap around your cast and should rinse under your cast thoroughly. If you swim in a pool or a lake, be sure to rinse both the inside and outside of the cast to flush out any dirt and chemicals. Dry your cast and stockinette thoroughly each time they get wet to avoid excess moisture on your skin. Use a towel to blot moisture off the cast, then dry it with a hair dryer set on low. When your cast does not feel cold and damp, it is dry.

Skin care is very important during the time a cast is worn. Do not insert objects under the cast, because you could scrape the skin or add pressure and cause an infection or sore under the cast. You should use powders and lotions only outside the cast so that the skin stays clean and soft. Powder inside a cast can cake and cause sore areas.

Do not walk on a leg cast for the first 48 hours. If you are allowed to walk on it, be sure to walk on the walking heel. If your arm is in a cast, be sure to use your sling for support and comfort.

Once your cast has been taken off, you should not try to scrub away the flaky skin and old skin cells all at once. Soften and condition your skin with dampened cloth and Woolite, which contains enzymes that loosen the dead cells so they will wash off easily without injuring the remaining skin cells. Gently wash the skin with water and Woolite, let the Woolite stay on the skin for 5 to 10 minutes, then rinse it off thoroughly. Pat your skin dry—do not rub it, because you could cause a sore to develop. After the skin is dry, apply a moisturizing lotion. Repeat the cleaning and lotion the next day, after which your skin should be nearly normal again.

The part that was in the cast may be sore and weak for several days or longer. You may need to limit use of the part for a period of time (1 to 4 weeks) until the muscles have become stronger. You may also need to take a mild pain medication such as aspirin or acetaminophen for a day or so to relieve the soreness of reuse.

Also, you may have some swelling of the part after the cast is removed. Elevating the part for 1 to 3 days should help relieve the swelling.

Remember, it takes time for the muscles and joints that had been injured and were in the cast to regain their strength, flexibility, and full functions. Try to build up to full use over 1 to 4 weeks, so these tissues have time to adjust to being used again. Easy does it.

Traction

Traction involves the use of a pulling force either directly or indirectly to bones. Traction can be used to prevent or reduce muscle spasms, keep a joint or other part of the body from moving, or restore a fractured bone to its normal position. There are two main types of traction—skin and skeletal.

Skin traction

Skin traction is applied to the skin surfaces, usually by a pelvic belt, head halter, traction boot, or moleskin straps covered with elastic wraps. It is attached to ropes and weights appropriate to the age and condition of the patient. Skin traction uses lower amounts of weight because skin cannot tolerate the pull of large amounts of weight over long periods. Thus skin traction is sometimes used intermittently or for short periods while skeletal traction, once applied, is always continuous and is used for longer periods and with heavier weights.

Skin traction is used to treat muscle injuries, bone fractures, ruptured or herniated discs, muscle contractures, and arthritic conditions. It can be applied to an arm, the head, a leg or the pelvis. Some types of skin traction, such as the head halter and Buck extension, can be used at home. Considerations for use of skin traction at home include:

1. Look over all areas of the skin where the traction is to be applied. The traction will pull on the skin and could cause additional injury to the already compromised skin. It should not be applied over open sores, rashes, bruises, marked swelling, or raised moles or warts.
2. Do not shave the skin under the areas where the traction is to be applied. Shaving could cause small cuts that could become inflamed under the traction.
3. Make sure the skin is clean and dry to prevent chafing or maceration caused by excess water on the skin.
4. Be sure you have an explanation of the traction equipment and how it is to be applied. Have the instructions in writing so there is no chance of forgetting a vital piece of information. Also, have the phone number of the physician ordering the traction and the supplier of the equipment to clarify any concerns you

may have after the traction is in use.
5. Find out if the weights can be removed at times—especially at night. The doctor may give an order that the patient can be in 2 hours, then out 2 hours, and off at night. Being in traction at night often prevents the patient from relaxing muscles to allow rest and sleep.
6. Usually the patient will receive relief of muscle spasms and pain from the effects of the traction. If the spasms or pain increase, however, be sure to notify the doctor. Adjustments in the amount of weights, positions, or time in traction may be needed for benefits to be achieved. At times, the use of traction may need to be stopped if there are adverse reactions.
7. Usually, you will be shown how to count the arterial pulses in the extremities or area in traction, how to feel for temperature, color, and swelling. You will also be shown how to wrap the elastic bandages (if used) properly to prevent overtightness leading to more swelling, numbness or tingling, or throbbing under the bandages. Elastic bandages should be removed and reapplied more loosely if these symptoms occur after the traction has been applied.
8. If possible, an orthopedic technician, a nurse, or a physical therapist should check the traction while in use at home. Arrangements can be made with your doctor.

Skeletal traction

When the injury is severe and demands longer periods of immobilization, skeletal traction is needed. Skeletal traction is applied directly to the bone by nails or pins inserted into the bone. Because your bones can tolerate more pressure than your skin, up to 30 pounds of pull may be applied by means of weights, ropes, and pulleys.

Skeletal traction must be done in a hospital. Your doctor and nurse will tell you on what you are allowed to do while in traction. Many times you can help with your own personal care. The one important thing to remember is not to disturb the traction apparatus or remove any weights. Skeletal traction must remain in continuous use until the doctor says it can be removed, usually when bone healing has occurred or when surgical repairs are done so healing can continue at home and out of traction.

Crutch Walking

Your doctor has prescribed crutches for you, and you need to know how to use them correctly.

Walking with crutches if you can bear some weight on both legs: Move one foot and leg and the crutch in the *opposite* hand forward at the same time; then move the other crutch and opposite foot and leg forward. Continue to move one crutch and the opposite foot and leg forward with each step.

Walking with crutches if no weight is to be borne on one leg (e.g., a foot and leg are in a cast but are not to bear any weight): Put all your weight on your unaffected foot and leg. Move both crutches and the foot and leg in the cast forward about 8 to 10 inches. Shift your weight to your wrists and hands and step forward with the unaffected leg. Rest, if needed, then continue to walk in the same way. Always move the crutches and the foot in the cast forward at the same time.

Remember: When you have a cast on your leg, always keep the casted foot in front of the other foot when you use crutches; this helps prevent you from stubbing your toes, catching the cast, or aggravating the injury by putting more weight on the foot than allowed.

Sitting down in a chair: Walk up close to the chair. Turn, then back up until you feel the chair touching the back of your knees. Hold the handgrips of both crutches with one hand, and with the other hand reach for the arm (or seat) of the chair. Lower yourself into the chair by bearing your weight on the handgrips of the crutches and the chair handle. Slide your affected leg forward as you sit.

Getting up from a chair: Place both crutches on one side. Put one hand on top of both handgrips and put the other hand on the chair arm (or seat if the chair has no arm). Push up from the chair until you are standing. Place a crutch under each arm. Make sure the chair is strong enough that it won't tip when you push up with the hand on the chair.

Going up stairs with one crutch in each hand: Walk up close to the bottom steps. Put all your weight on your handgrips, and step up to the next step with your unaffected leg and foot. Then bring your body, affected leg, and crutches up to the same step. Be sure your crutches are centered on the step, so you feel secure and don't feel as if you're falling backward.

Going down stairs with one crutch in each hand: Walk up near the edge of the top step. Bend your hips and place both crutches and the affected leg on the next lower step. Put your weight on the crutches, and bring the unaffected leg down to the same step. Continue down the stairs in the same way.

Going up stairs if there is a bannister: Walk up close to the stairs. Place both crutches under the arm opposite the bannister, and grasp both handgrips. Grasp the bannister with your free hand. Put all your weight on your hands, and lift the unaffected foot and leg up to the next step. Bring the crutches, your body, and the affected leg up to the same step. Continue up the stairs in the same way.

Going down stairs if there is a bannister: Put both crutches in one hand, holding them together at the handgrips and under the arm. Put the other hand on the bannister. Move the affected leg and the crutches down to the next step, but do not put any weight on the affected leg if it is to bear no weight. Put all weight on your hands and wrists on the crutches and the bannister, and step down with the unaffected leg. Continue down the stairs in same way.

Precautions

If you stop to rest while using crutches, rest without leaning your shoulders on the shoulder pads over the tops of the crutches. If you lean too long or put too much pressure in the axillary (armpit) area, you can injure the nerves and cut off the circulation down your arms. Instead, put your weight on your wrists, handgrips, and unaffected leg, and hold your crutches nearer your chest. You will know you've put too much pressure on the nerves in your axillary area if you develop numbness and tingling down the arm to the thumb. Such numbness and tingling should go away quickly if you stop leaning your shoulders on the crutch tops. If the numbness does not go away, notify your doctor.

Avoid walking on slick floors and throw rugs, since your crutch may slip. Keep the crutch tips clean, because dirt and dust can build up and make them slippery. Be sure to replace worn crutch tips.

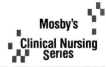

Total Hip Replacement

A painful hip can take all the joy out of life. But thanks to modern medicine, you don't have to live with the pain. A total hip replacement can relieve the pain and stiffness and give you a smoothly functioning hip again.

The hip

The hip is a simple ball-and-socket joint, located where the thigh bone joins the pelvis. A healthy hip moves painlessly, because smooth cartilage allows the ball (the head of the thigh bone) to glide easily in its socket. However, when osteoarthritis attacks the hip, the cartilage wears away and the bones start rubbing together. Bony spurs can form inside and around the hip joint, making walking and getting up from a chair extremely painful. Osteoarthritis is the most common cause of hip problems, although rheumatoid arthritis, injury, and loss of blood supply to the hip can also damage the joint.

Hip prostheses

Hip prostheses resemble the parts of a normal hip. The prostheses are a cup (usually made of plastic), which replaces your worn hip socket; a ball (made of metal), which replaces the worn head of your thigh bone; and the stem, which is connected to the ball and which may or may not be cemented into the thigh bone (uncemented components fit tightly into bone, which grows into and around them).

Should you have hip replacement surgery?

In order to decide whether you are a candidate for hip replacement, your orthopedic surgeon will need to do several things:
1. Assess the condition of your hip. How much pain you are feeling and how much mobility you have are two important considerations in determining whether you need the prostheses.
2. Take your medical history. You will be asked about prior injuries, medication you are taking, and any other joint problems you may have.
3. Take x-rays of your hips for comparisons.
4. Possibly take some fluid from your hip (called joint aspiration) to determine if infection is present.
5. Do blood tests to check for other irregularities.
6. Do an electrocardiogram to check heart functions.

If you are a candidate for hip replacement surgery, the doctor will then discuss the benefits and risks of surgery with you. The benefits of course, are that you will have a painless, mobile hip and you will be able to return to most of the activities you enjoy. The risks include possible infection, pneumonia, and blood clots. These complications are unlikely, but you need to know about them.

The surgical procedure

First you will be given a general or spinal anesthetic. Then your surgeon will make an incision and prepare your hipbone for implantation of the prostheses. The parts of the prostheses (ball and stem and socket) are implanted separately and then brought together. The incision is closed after a small tube is inserted to help drain fluids from the hip joint area.

Complications

Sometimes complications such as blood clots, infection, and joint dislocation develop after surgery. Notify your nurse and surgeon if you experience any of the following symptoms:
- Pain, soreness, swelling, or redness in the calf muscles of either leg
- Increased pain in the operative area
- Redness, swelling, or puslike drainage from the area around the incision.
- Fever
- Cough that produces yellow or green phlegm or shortness of breath

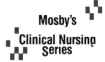

Recovery After Total Hip Replacement

It is important that you keep your hip in the proper position for a period of time after surgery. You will be positioned to keep your hip from bending, and an abduction pillow will keep your legs apart and prevent them from turning inward.

Physical therapy will begin as soon as possible to help strengthen the muscles around your hip and to help you regain your hip's mobility. Walking begins soon after, first with a walker, then crutches, then a cane. Your balance may seem unsteady at first but will improve as you progress with your walking.

As soon as your initial recovery is satisfactory, you will be discharged from the hospital and sent home. Here are some things to remember as you continue to recover at home:

Your new hip has limited range of motion, up to 90 degrees. The prostheses can slip out of position unless you follow a few precautions.

- Avoid crossing your legs or ankles while standing, sitting, or lying.
- Sit with your feet 6 inches apart.
- When sitting, keep your knees below your hips (sit on a pillow, if possible, to keep hips higher).
- Avoid bending over at the waist. Use a **long-handled shoehorn** and sock aid to help you put on and take off shoes and socks. A **reacher** can help you grab objects that are too high or too low for you to reach.

You should avoid putting excess weight on your new hip. Use crutches, then a cane until your hip heals.

Your balance may be shaky for awhile.
- Use handrails on stairs.
- Wear low-heeled shoes.
- Be sure your floors are free of things that could trip you—throw rugs, phone or electrical cords, and small objects. Avoid wet or waxed floors.
- If riding in a car, stop every hour or so to get out and walk around for several minutes to increase circulation to your legs. Your doctor will tell you when you can drive (approximately 3 months after surgery).

Exercises

These exercises may be started while you are in the hospital. They will speed recovery and help you to walk sooner. Repeat each exercise 5 to 10 times, twice a day. Your doctor will prescribe these exercises for you.

1. Lie flat on your back, and lift the affected leg straight off the bed about 12 inches. Hold for 5 seconds, then relax.
2. Sit with your feet on the floor, and lift the knee of the affected leg straight off chair about 4 inches. Hold for 5 seconds, then relax.
3. Lie on your unaffected side with a pillow between your knees. Try to lift the affected leg straight off the pillow. Hold for 5 seconds, then relax.

The following exercises should be done while you stand and hold onto something stable. Repeat 5 to 10 times; do twice daily or as ordered by your doctor.

1. Bend your affected leg, and bring it up toward your chest. Do not exceed a 90-degree angle. Straighten the leg again.
2. Point your hips, knees, and feet straight in front. Slowly move your affected leg out to the side and then back again to the other leg.
3. Bend your knee, and move your leg backward. Do not arch your back. Return the leg to the starting position.

Continue with these exercises when you return home. Make walking a part of your daily routine. Start walking for 10 minutes three times a day, and work up to 30 minutes once a day.

Your new hip does not have quite the range of your original hip, but you eventually should be able to do most of the things you did when your hip was healthy.

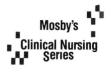

Total Knee Replacement

The knee is one of the hardest working joints in the human body. However, when the knee becomes stiff and painful, you may find even a simple thing, such as walking, an unbearable experience. Now, thanks to breakthroughs in surgical materials and techniques, you may be able to have your knee replaced. You won't be able to do some things with your new knee, such as play strenuous sports, but you can look forward to returning to most of your daily activities—pain free.

The anatomy of the knee

The knee is a complex, weight-bearing joint that rolls, rotates, and glides whenever you walk or climb stairs. The major bones of the knee are the femur (upper leg bone), the tibia (larger lower leg bone), the fibula (smaller lower leg bone), and the patella (kneecap). Muscles and ligaments keep the knee in place and give it strength and flexibility. Cartilage covers the ends of the bones of the knee and provides smooth surfaces for easy movement. When the cartilage wears away because of injuries or osteoarthritis, the bones begin to rub together and bone spurs may develop. Movement becomes difficult and painful. Rheumatoid arthritis and poor leg alignment can also cause knee damage and pain.

Knee prostheses

The replacement parts for the knee (prostheses) are similar to your own knee. The **femoral component** covers the end of your femur, the **tibial** and **fibular components** cover the top of your tibia and fibula, and the **patellar component** covers the underside of your kneecap. One or all parts of your knee may need to be replaced, depending on the condition of your knee joint. Your knee problem will be carefully diagnosed and evaluated by your orthopedic surgeon before a decision is made on knee replacement surgery; the surgeon also will decide on the best prosthesic design and whether **cement** will be used to hold the prostheses in place. (As with hip replacements, uncemented prostheses fit tightly into the bones, which grow into and around the components.)

Should you have knee replacement surgery?

In order to decide whether you are a candidate for knee replacement, your orthopedic surgeon will need to do several things:
1. Assess the condition of your knee. How much pain you are feeling and how much mobility you have are two important considerations in determining whether you need prosthesic replacement.
2. Take your medical history. You will be asked about prior injuries, medication you are taking, and any other joint problems you may have.
3. Take x-rays of both knees, even though only one may be replaced. Both are x-rayed for comparisons.
4. Possibly take some fluid from your knee (called joint aspiration) to determine if infection is present.
5. Do blood tests to check for other irregularities.

Your surgeon should also tell you about the possible complications of surgery, which are pneumonia, infection, blood clots, loosening of the prostheses, and nerve loss. These complications are unlikely, but you need to know about them before you decide to have surgery.

The surgical procedure

First you will be given a general or spinal anesthetic. Then your surgeon will make an incision and prepare your knee for implantation of the prostheses by reshaping and resurfacing the bones of your knee joint. Surgery should take 2 to 3 hours, depending on the condition of your knee. When the surgery is finished, the incision will be closed and a small tube will be placed in the incision to help drain fluid from the operative area.

Recovery After Total Knee Replacement

You will spend the first few days after surgery resting and recovering. Gentle circulation exercises will begin, and your knee may be exercised by a continuous passive motion machine (CPM).

Physical therapy will soon begin to help your knee regain its strength and mobility. You will begin walking, first with a walker, then with crutches, and then with a cane. Once you have recovered fully from surgery and you can bend your knee and walk well with a walker or crutches, you can go home.

Recovery at home

There are a few signs you need to watch for after you are home. Call your surgeon if you experience any of the following:
- Increased knee pain
- Swelling in your leg or knee
- Any unusual pain in your knee, or increased pain in your knee
- Any fluid leakage from your incision
- Shortness of breath or chest pain
- Any other symptom you don't understand
- Pain or swelling of the calf muscle in either lower leg

Following are some strengthening and range-of-motion exercises you can do at home. These exercises will help strengthen your leg muscles and help your knee regain its mobility and flexibility. They will be prescribed by your doctor.

1. Lie on your back in bed with a towel under your ankle. Push your affected knee down into the mattress. Hold for 5 seconds. Relax. Repeat 6 times.
2. Lie on your back in bed with a towel under your ankle. Push your heel down into the mattress. Hold for 5 seconds. Relax. Repeat 6 times.
3. Lie on your back in bed. Slide the heel of your affected leg back toward your buttocks while you bend your knee. Hold for 5 seconds. Repeat 6 times.
4. Lie on your back. As you tighten your thigh muscles, lift your affected leg about 12 inches. Hold for 5 to 10 seconds. Slowly lower your leg. Repeat with other leg. Do 6 times each leg.
5. Sit in a chair. Slowly raise your foot, then bring it back under you as far as possible. Repeat with other leg. Do 6 times each leg.

If you follow your surgeon's guidelines and do your exercises and physical therapy faithfully, your new knee should provide you with years of comfortable mobility.

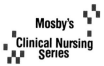

Mosby's
Clinical Nursing
Series

Total Shoulder Replacement

The shoulder is the most flexible joint in the body. However, this flexibility makes the shoulder prone to wear and injury. Sometimes the shoulder becomes so painful and stiff that replacement surgery becomes necessary.

The shoulder's anatomy

The shoulder is a ball-and-socket joint, much like the hip. The ball-like head of the humerus (upper arm bone) fits into a socket called the **glenoid fossa,** which is formed by the **scapula** (shoulder blade) and the **clavicle** (collarbone). Tendons, muscles, and ligaments hold these three bones in position. The shoulder allows the arm to move around in a full circle, back and forth, and up and down. A healthy shoulder moves easily and painlessly, but a shoulder that has been damaged by injuries, osteoarthritis, or rheumatoid arthritis moves much less freely and often painfully. Sometimes so much damage is done that a total shoulder replacement becomes necessary.

Should you have shoulder replacement surgery?

To decide whether you are a candidate for shoulder replacement, your orthopedic surgeon will need to do several things:
1. Assess the damage done to your shoulder, such as how much pain you are in and how much mobility you have left—two important considerations to determine whether you need a replacement.
2. Take your medical history by asking about prior injuries, medications you may be taking, and any other joint problems you may be experiencing.
3. Take x-rays of your shoulder.
4. Possibly take some fluid from your shoulder (joint aspiration) to determine if infection is present.
5. Take blood tests to check for other irregularities.

If you are a candidate for shoulder replacement surgery, the doctor will then discuss the benefits and risks of surgery with you. The benefits are, of course, a pain-free, mobile shoulder and a return to most of the activities you enjoy. The risks include dislocation, possible infection, pneumonia, and blood clots. These complications are unlikely, but you need to know about them.

The surgery

You will be given a general anesthetic. Your orthopedic surgeon will make an incision and prepare your shoulder for implantation of the prostheses. One part of the prosthesis is metal and one part is plastic. The metal part is placed into the shaft of the humerus, and the plastic part is placed into the glenoid area of the shoulder. The prostheses are usually then cemented into place. A small tube is inserted to help drain fluids out of the area, and the incision is closed.

Complications

Sometimes complications such as blood clots, infection, and joint dislocation arise after surgery. Notify your nurse and orthopedic surgeon if you experience any of the following symptoms:
- Pain, soreness, swelling, or redness in the calf of one of your legs
- Increased pain in the shoulder area
- Redness, swelling, or puslike drainage from the incision
- Fever
- Decreased ability to move the shoulder and arm

Recovery

Recovery from shoulder replacement surgery takes approximately 3 to 6 months for full movement to return. Your doctor will prescribe specific exercises for you to do to regain your joint mobility.

CHAPTER 15

Musculoskeletal Drugs

ANTIINFLAMMATORY MEDICATIONS

SALICYLATES

The salicylates have antipyretic, analgesic, antiinflammatory, and antirheumatic effects. Aspirin and other salicylates are metabolized to salicylic acid. Diflunisal, although not a true salicylate, is similar in structure and effects. The drugs' antiinflammatory and analgesic actions are related to inhibition of prostaglandin synthesis. Aspirin, but not other salicylates, irreversibly inhibits platelet aggregation after even a single dose. This effect lasts for the life span of platelets (7 to 10 days). Single doses of aspirin may prolong bleeding time.

Indications: Relief of mild to moderate pain and as an antipyretic and antiinflammatory drug in a variety of disorders, including rheumatoid arthritis, osteoarthritis, and other conditions causing musculoskeletal pain.

Usual dosage: See Table 15-1. Aspirin and other salicylates are available in a variety of forms and in combination with many other drugs. All forms are administered orally. Sodium salicylate may also be administered by injection but is rarely used therapeutically by this route.

Precautions/contraindications: Use with caution in patients with liver disease, vitamin K deficiency, hypoprothrombinemia, peptic ulcer disease, or gastric irritation; also in patients taking anticoagulants. Patients with allergies, asthma, and nasal polyps are at increased risk for a hypersensitivity reaction characterized by rhinitis, urticaria, and asthma. Contraindicated in patients with gastrointestinal bleeding, hemophiliacs, or patients with known hypersensitivity to salicylates. Cross-sensitivity may exist between salicylates, nonsteroidal antiinflammatory drugs, or tartrazine dye. Use during pregnancy may adversely affect the fetus, and use near term may increase antipartum or postpartum hemorrhage.

Side effects/adverse reactions: Allergic and anaphylactic reactions may occur. Nausea, heartburn, and other gastrointestinal (GI) disturbances are most commonly reported. Repeated large doses of salicylates may lead to chronic salicylate intoxication, or "salicylism," which includes dizziness, tinnitus, (ringing in ears), altered hearing, GI disturbances, central nervous system (CNS) depression, mental confusion, sweating, thirst, and hyperventilation. Tinnitus and hearing loss are the most common signs of chronic intoxication. (See the box on page 281, "Salicylate Toxicity.")

Pharmacokinetics: Salicylates are readily absorbed through the GI tract. Serum levels depend on gastric pH, the presence of food, gastric emptying time, the presence of buffering agents or antacids, and drug preparation. Enteric forms have less reliable absorption. The drugs are converted to salicylic acid during absorption and are eliminated primarily through the kidneys. Excretion depends on urinary pH and increases with increased urinary pH.

Interactions: Salicylates are highly protein bound and may displace or be displaced by other protein-bound drugs. The risk of bleeding increases when salicylates are administered with oral anticoagulants. Salicylates are antagonistic to uricosuric medications. When salicylates are administered with corticosteroids, salicylate levels may decrease. Use of alcohol while using salicylates, particularly aspirin, increases the risk of gastric irritation and ulceration.

Nursing considerations: Monitor patients taking high doses for signs of toxicity; instruct the patient about symptoms to report to the physician. Discontinue use if dizziness, ringing in ears, or hearing changes occur. Aspirin or products containing aspirin are generally discontinued 1-2 wk before surgery. Administer with caution in asthmatic patients, and assess for bronchospasm after administration. Children or teenagers should not take salicylates for flu symptoms or chickenpox without first consulting their physician because of a strong association between the use of salicylates (especially aspirin) during a viral illness and the develop-

Table 15-1

SALICYLATES

Generic name	Trade name	Average dose	Maximum daily dosage
Aspirin (acetylsalicylic acid, ASA)	Many trade names	325-650 mg q 4 hr* 3.6-5.4 g/day in divided doses† 5-8 g/day‡	5-8 g
Magnesium salicylate	Doan's, Magan, Mobidin	650 mg 3 times/day	4,800 mg
Choline salicylate	Arthropan	870 mg q 3-4 hr	6,960 mg
Salsalate	Disalcid Mono-Gesic Salflex Salsitab	3,000 mg/day in divided doses	
Diflunisal	Dolobid	Initial dose 1 g, followed by 500 mg q 8-12 hr	1,500 mg

Salicylate combination	Trilisate Three strengths available:
	  500 mg salicylate: 293 mg choline salicylate
	                              362 mg magnesium salicylate
	  750 mg salicylate: 440 mg choline salicylate
	                              544 mg magnesium salicylate
	  1,000 mg salicylate: 587 mg choline salicylate
	                                725 mg magnesium salicylate		

*Dosage for minor aches and pains.
†Dosage for arthritis and rheumatic conditions.
‡Dosage for acute rheumatic fever.

ment of Reye's syndrome. An analgesic, such as acetaminophen, should be used in this situation. Evaluate the pain effectiveness of antirheumatic therapy by assessing joint mobility and relief. Monitor for signs of increased bleeding tendencies or GI bleeding, including black, tarry stools, bleeding gums, or bruising.

SALICYLATE TOXICITY

Gastric ulceration or gastric irritation
Gastrointestinal bleeding that can be significant
Tinnitus (ringing in ears)
Dyspepsia or heartburn
Acid-base imbalances
Prolongation of clotting
Hypoglycemia
Asthmalike reaction
Convulsions and respiratory failure may occur in severe intoxication.

NONSTEROIDAL ANTIINFLAMMATORY DRUGS

The nonsteroidal antiinflammatory drugs (NSAIDs) are a group of drugs that all, to varying degrees, have antipyretic, antiinflammatory, and analgesic effects. Although their exact mechanism of action is not understood, these drugs appear to exert most of their effects by inhibiting the synthesis of prostaglandin. Peripheral vasodilatation may contribute to the antipyretic effect. These drugs provide symptomatic relief but do not alter the course of the underlying problem. There is little information to serve as a guide in selecting the most appropriate drug for each patient; rather, the choice often depends on personal preference, convenience, cost, and clinical experience.

Indications: Primarily for antiinflammatory action in the treatment of musculoskeletal disorders (rheumatoid arthritis and osteoarthritis) and to relieve mild to moderate pain. Ibuprofen is available over the counter in doses up to 200 mg/tablet. All other NSAIDs are available by prescription.

Table 15-2

NONSTEROIDAL ANTIINFLAMMATORY DRUGS (NSAIDS)

Generic name	Trade name	Dosage*	Maximum daily dose
Propionic acid			
Fenoprofen	Nalfon	300-600 mg, 3-4 times daily	3,200 mg
Flurbiprofen	Ansaid	50-100 mg, 2-4 times daily	300 mg
Ibuprofen	Advil, Nuprin, Motrin, and others	200-800 mg, 3-4 times daily	3,200 mg
Ketoprofen	Orudis	25-75 mg, 3-4 times daily	300 mg
Naproxen	Naprosyn	250-500 mg, 2-4 times daily	1,250 mg
Naproxen sodium	Anaprox	275-550 mg, 2-4 times daily	1,375 mg
Indole			
Indomethacin	Indocin Indo-Lemmon Indometh	25-75 mg, 3-4 times daily	200 mg
Sulindac	Clinoril	150-200 mg, twice daily	400 mg
Tolmentin	Tolectin	200-400 mg, 3-4 times daily	2,000 mg
Fenamate			
Meclofenamate	Meclomen, Meclodium	50-100 mg, 3-4 times daily	400 mg
Mefenamic acid	Ponstel	250 mg, 4 times daily	1,000 mg
Oxicam			
Piroxicam	Feldene	20 mg, daily	20 mg
Phenylacetic acid			
Diclofenac	Voltaren	25-75 mg, 2-4 times daily	200 mg

*All doses are oral.

Usual dosage: See Table 15-2.

Precautions/contraindications: Contraindicated in patients with known sensitivity to salicylates or other NSAIDs because of the potential for cross-sensitivity. Fenoprofen and mefenamic acid should not be administered to patients with significant renal impairment.

Side effects/adverse reactions: Minor upper GI symptoms are common when using NSAIDs. Long-term use may lead to more serious GI toxicity, including ulceration, perforation, and bleeding. Renal toxicity may occur.

Pharmacokinetics: NSAIDs are rapidly and almost completely absorbed after oral administration and are highly protein bound. Metabolism occurs in the liver, with renal excretion of metabolites.

Interactions: Bleeding time may be prolonged when oral anticoagulants are administered with NSAIDs. The antihypertensive effects of beta-blocking drugs may be reduced by NSAIDs. Indomethacin may blunt or block the antihypertensive effects of captopril, on angiotensin-converting enzyme inhibitor.

Nursing considerations: Patients who do not respond well to one NSAID may have a better or different response to another. Administration with narcotic analgesics may cause an additive analgesic effect. NSAIDs may be administered with food to decrease GI irritation.

Prozalone Derivatives

Phenylbutazone and oxyphenbutazone, a metabolite of phenylbutazone, have potent analgesic and antiinflammatory effects. These two drugs have actions similar to other NSAIDs but with a very high incidence of adverse effects. Because of the potential for serious adverse effects, use of these drugs is generally limited to short-term therapy of acute symptoms that do not respond to more conservative therapy such as nonsteroidal antiinflammatory drugs. If a therapeutic effect has not been noticed after 1 wk of therapy, the drug should be discontinued. The lowest possible effective dose should be used.

Indications: Relief of pain and inflammation related to inflammatory and degenerative musculoskeletal conditions. Recommended for use only after other NSAIDs have been tried without satisfactory effects. Usual dosage: Phenylbutazone (Azolid, Butazolidin) and oxyphenbutazone: 300-600 mg/day in 3-4 divided doses administered orally, with meals to prevent GI upset. Maintenance doses may be as low as 100 mg/day.

Precautions/contraindications: Adverse reactions are more common in patients over 40 years of age. Drug treatment should be limited to 1 wk in patients over age 60. Administer with caution to patients with preexisting renal disease that may be aggravated by drug treatment. Contraindicated in patients under 14 years of age or in those with known hypersensitivity to phenylbutazone or who have a bronchospastic reaction to aspirin and NSAIDs.

Side effects/adverse reactions: Phenylbutazone can cause aplastic anemia and agranulocytosis. Long-term administration of phenylbutazone has been associated with renal toxicity. Liver function tests may be elevated in some patients.

Pharmacokinetics: GI absorption is rapid and nearly complete. The drugs are highly protein bound and are metabolized in the liver. The major metabolite of phenylbutazone is oxyphenbutazone.

Interactions: The effects of antiinflammatory drugs, oral anticoagulants, oral hypoglycemics, sulfonamides, and phenytoin may be increased by phenylbutazone.

Nursing considerations: A complete physical examination, medical history, and laboratory studies (blood count and urinalysis) should be completed before starting therapy and periodically during treatment. Instruct the patient in the proper dosage, and not to exceed the prescribed dose. Tell her to discontinue the drug immediately and call her physician if any of the following symptoms occur: blurred vision; sore throat; mouth lesions; symptoms of anemia; unusual or excessive bruising or bleeding; epigastric pain; black, tarry stools; skin rashes; edema; or sudden weight gain. Patients should be warned that the drug may impair mental alertness and physical coordination. Taking the drug with food or milk may reduce GI upset.

Corticosteroids

Although their precise mechanism of action is not known, corticosteroids have been used for years to treat inflammation. Naturally occurring glucocorticoids, such as cortisol and cortisone, have effects also associated with mineralocorticoids (sodium retention, potassium excretion, hypertension). The development of synthetic glucocorticoids has produced agents with enhanced antiinflammatory effects and reduced mineralocorticoid effects. Qualitative differences among the synthetic antiinflammatory steroids is minimal; differences involve the potency of the antiinflammatory effects and their duration of action.

Indications: *Systemic therapy:* Adjunct short-term therapy in rheumatic disorders, bursitis, tenosynovitis, gouty arthritis, osteoarthritis, epicondylitis, maintenance therapy in selected cases of rheumatoid arthritis. *Intraarticular or soft tissue administration:* Synovitis, acute gouty arthritis, tenosynovitis, posttraumatic osteoarthritis.

Usual dosage: The use, dosage, and administration of corticosteroids vary widely. Table 15-3 lists some of the glucocorticoids used in treating musculoskeletal disorders.

Precautions/contraindications: Use with caution in patients with peptic ulcer, heart disease or hypertension with congestive heart failure (CHF), infection, psychosis, diabetes, osteoporosis, glaucoma, or herpes infection.

Side effects/adverse reactions: Side effects are uncommon with short-term therapy (less than 1 wk) but increase with the duration of therapy. Undesirable effects that may occur during prolonged systemic use at high doses include truncal obesity and cushingoid features, hyperglycemia, sodium retention with edema, hypertension, weight gain, muscle wasting, acne, hypokalemia, peptic ulcers, osteoporosis, increased intraocular pressure (glaucoma), cataract development, psychosis, and exacerbation of infections. Adrenal function is suppressed when these drugs are administered over a long period.

Pharmacokinetics: Onset of action: Slow. Plasma half-life: prednisone, 60 min; methylprednisolone, 78-188 min. **Route of elimination:** Metabolized in the liver with renal excretion.

Interactions: Requirement of insulin or hypoglycemic agents may increase. Phenytoin, phenobarbital, rifampin, and possibly ephedrine may increase metabolism of corticosteroids and reduce the effectiveness of a given dose. Oral contraceptives may inhibit corticosteroid metabolism.

Nursing considerations: Children treated for prolonged periods should have periodic eye examinations to detect the development of cataracts. Monitor all patients for development of adverse effects. Patients on long-term therapy must have the drug dose tapered slowly to avoid adrenal insufficiency (Addison's syndrome). Assess all patients for signs of adrenal insufficiency during withdrawal of systemic therapy. During periods of stress, patients recently withdrawn from systemic steroids should have treatment resumed. Caution patients against overusing joints in which symptomatic relief has been obtained through the use of steroids, because the inflammatory response may still be present.

Table 15-3

GLUCOCORTICOIDS USED IN MUSCULOSKELETAL DISORDERS

Generic name	Trade name	Dosage	Administration
Cortisone	Cortone acetate	25-300 mg/day	PO
		20-300 mg/day	IM
Hydrocortisone	Cortef	20-240 mg/day	PO
		⅓-½ oral dose q 12 hr	IM
Hydrocortisone cypionate	Cortef	20-240 mg/day	PO
Hydrocortisone sodium phosphate	Hydrocortone Phosphate	7.5-120 mg/day	IV, IM, or SC
Hydrocortisone sodium succinate	A-hydroCort, Solu-Cortef	100-500 mg/day	IV, IM
Hydrocortisone acetate	Biosone	5-75 mg	Intraarticular, intralesional, or soft tissue injection
Prednisone	Deltasone, Liquid Pred, Metiocorten, Orasone, Pansol-S, Prednicen-M, Sterapred	5-60 mg/day	PO
Prednisolone acetate	Articulose, Key-Pred, Niscort, Predaject, Predcor	4-60 mg	Intraarticular, intralesional, and soft tissue injection
Prednisolone tebutate	Nor-Pred, Predalone, Predcor TBA	4-20 mg	Intraarticular, intralesional, and soft tissue injection
Prednisolone sodium phosphate	Hydeltrasol, Key-Pred-SR, Pediapred, Predicort	4-30 mg	Intraarticular, intralesional, and soft tissue injection
Triamcinolone	Aristocort, Atolone, Kenacort	8-16 mg/day	PO
Triamcinolone diacetate	Aristocort, Amcort, Cenocort Forte, Tac-D and others	5-40 mg	Intraarticular, intralesional, and soft tissue injection
Triamcinolone acetonide	Cenocort A-40, Kenoject, Kenalog, Tac-40, and others	2.5-40 mg	Intraarticular, intralesional, and soft tissue injection
Triamcinolone hexacetonide	Aristospan	2-20 mg	Intraarticular, intralesional, and soft tissue injection
Methylprednisolone	Medrol, Mepolone	4-48 mg/day	PO
Methylprednisolone sodium succinate	A-methaPred, Solu-Medrol	10-40 mg	IV, IM
Methylprednisolone acetate	Depo-Medrol, depMedalone-40, Depoject, Duralone, Medralone, and others	40-120 mg/wk	IM
		40-80 mg	Intraarticular and soft tissue injection
Dexamethasone acetate	Dalalone L A, Decaject-LA, Dexoacen LA-8, and others	4-16 mg	Intraarticular and soft tissue injection
Dexamethasone sodium phosphate	Ak Dex Alba Dex, Dalalone, Sezone, Solurex, and others	0.8-4 mg	Intraarticular injection
Betamethasone sodium phosphate (3 mg/ml) and Betamethasone acetate (3 mg/ml)	Celestone Soluspan	0.25-2 ml	Intraarticular, intralesional, and soft tissue injection

MUSCLE-RELAXANT MEDICATIONS

CENTRAL-ACTING MUSCLE RELAXANTS

As an adjunct to rest, physical therapy, and other measures, muscle relaxants are used in the treatment of many painful musculoskeletal disorders. These drugs generally are central-acting medications; that is, they do not directly relax tense skeletal muscles. The exact mechanism of action is not known for many of these drugs, but their effect may be due in part to their sedative properties or CNS depression. Painful muscle spasm associated with acute conditions usually requires only short-term therapy. Some muscle relaxants are used on a long-term basis in the treatment of muscle spasticity associated with upper motor neuron disorders

Table 15-4

CENTRAL-ACTING SKELETAL MUSCLE RELAXANT MEDICATIONS

Generic name	Trade name	Dosage*
Used as an adjunct to other measures to relieve acute painful musculoskeletal conditions		
Carisoprodol	Rela, Sodol, Soma, Soprodol	350 mg 3-4 times/day
Chlorphenesin carbamate	Maolate	400-800 mg 4 times/day
Chlorzoxazone	Paraflex, Parafon Forte	250-500 mg 3-4 times/day
Cyclobenzaprine	Flexeril	10 mg 3-4 times/day
Diazepam	Q-pam, Valium, Zetran	2-10 mg 3-4 times/day
		2-5 mg q 3-4 hr (IV or IM)
Metaxalone	Skelaxin	800 mg 3-4 times/day
Methocarbamol	Delaxin, Marbaxin, Robaxin	0.5-1.5 g 4 times/day
		1-2 g (IV or IM)
Orphenadrine citrate	Banflex, K-Flex, Marflex, My-olin, Norflex, O-Flex	100 mg 2 times/day
		60 q 12 hr (IV or IM)
Used in the treatment of muscle spasticity associated with upper motor neuron disorders		
Baclofen	Lioresal	40-80 mg/day
Diazepam	Q-pam, Valium	2-10 mg 3-4 times/day
		2-5 mg q 3-4 hr (IV or IM)

*All doses are oral unless otherwise noted.

in conditions such as stroke, spinal cord injury, cerebral palsy, and multiple sclerosis.

Indications: See Table 15-4.

Usual dosage: See Table 15-4.

Precautions/contraindications: Carisoprodol is contraindicated in patients with porphyria. Administer chlorphenesin carbamate or metaxalone with caution to patients with impaired liver function. Methocarbamol should not be administered to patients with known or suspected renal impairment.

Side effects/adverse reactions: Many of the muscle relaxants may impair mental function and cause drowsiness, dizziness, mental confusion, or other mild CNS symptoms. Allergic, idiosyncratic, and hypersensitivity reactions have been reported. Abrupt withdrawal from baclofen may cause hallucinations and seizures.

Pharmacokinetics: Varies.

Interactions: Use of alcohol or CNS depressants with a central-acting muscle relaxant may result in additive CNS depression. Mild GI disturbance may also be caused by many of these muscle relaxants. Cyclobenzaprine closely resembles the tricyclic antidepressants, which may cause hypertensive crisis, convulsions, and death when administered with a monoamine oxidase (MAO) inhibitor. Cyclobenzaprine may cause a similar response if administered to a patient receiving an MAO inhibitor.

Nursing considerations: Instruct the patient to use caution when performing hazardous tasks and to avoid alcohol and CNS-depressant medications. Caution patients receiving baclofen that they must not stop taking the drug abruptly.

DIRECT-ACTING MUSCLE RELAXANTS

Dantrolene (Dantrium) differs from central-acting drugs in that it produces relaxation by acting on a site within muscle fibers.

Indications: Control of spasticity in cases of upper motor neuron dysfunction.

Usual dosage: Initially 25 mg/day PO, increased to 100 mg 2-4 times/day.

Precautions/contraindications: Do not administer to patients with liver disease.

Side effects/adverse reactions: Idiosyncratic or hypersensitivity reactions leading to potentially fatal liver disorders may occur. Dantrolene may cause photosensitivity and CNS effects similar to the central-acting muscle relaxants; the CNS sedative effects are usually transient. Gastrointestinal disturbances, including diarrhea, constipation, and GI bleeding, have occurred.

Pharmacokinetics: Approximately 70% of the oral dose is absorbed. The drug is metabolized in the liver.

Interactions: CNS drugs may have an additive effect.

Nursing considerations: Liver function studies should be performed at the start of therapy and monitored at intervals during therapy. Caution the patient to avoid CNS-depressant drugs and to watch for signs of hepatotoxicity (skin rash, pruritus, bruising, tarry stools, and yellow discoloration of the skin, eyes, or urine)

ANTIGOUT MEDICATIONS

The use of drugs in the treatment of gout is aimed at relieving the acute attacks and preventing recurrences. Drugs used in the acute attacks include NSAIDs and the more specific agent, colchicine. Additional drug therapy is aimed at reducing hyperuricemia.

The specific actions of colchicine are not well understood; however, the drug reduces the inflammatory response to acute gout attacks. The drug is not an analgesic. Administration should begin at the first signs of a gout attack. Delaying administration even a few hours reduces the drug's effectiveness.

Indications: Relief of pain associated with acute gout attacks.

Usual dosage: *Oral:* Initial dose of 0.5-1.2 mg, followed by 0.5-1.2 mg q 1-2 hr until pain is relieved or side effects (nausea, vomiting, or diarrhea) occur. *Intravenous:* 1-2 mg initially, followed by 0.5 mg q 6 hr to a total dose of 4 mg.

Precautions/contraindications: Colchicine should not be administered to patients with serious renal, GI, or cardiac disorders. The drug should not be administered by subcutaneous or IM routes, because it causes severe local tissue irritation. Long-term use increases the risk of neutropenia, anemia, alopecia, and azoospermia.

Side effects/adverse reactions: The most common adverse effects are GI disturbances after oral administration. Local irritation or thrombophlebitis may occur following injection. Bone marrow suppression may occur following long-term therapy.

Pharmacokinetics: Absorption is good after oral administration; excretion is through the kidneys and in bile.

Interactions: Colchicine has been shown to reversibly induce malabsorption of vitamin B_{12}.

Nursing considerations: The drug should be stored in dark, tight containers. The IV drug may be diluted with normal saline but not 5% dextrose and should be administered over 2-5 min. Because of the potential for toxicity, some have suggested that the IV dose not be repeated for several weeks. The patient should be instructed to take the drug as soon as possible when an acute gout attack occurs to receive maximum benefit from the drug.

URICOSURIC DRUGS

One method of treating gout is to increase the kidneys' excretion of uric acid. Uric acid is filtered through the glomeruli, secreted in the proximal tubule, and actively reabsorbed. Uricosurics affect both transport systems (secretion and reabsorption) to increase excretion of uric acid. Useful uricosuric drugs include probenecid and sulfinpyrazone. As the concentration of uric acid excreted increases, it is possible to exceed the solubility level; at this point uric acid will precipitate out in the urinary tract. Alkalinization of the urine increases the solubility of uric acid, and increasing urine volume helps prevent precipitation.

Probenecid

Probenecid (Benemid, Probanlan) increases renal excretion of uric acid; this reduces serum levels, which in turn retards uric acid deposition and increases resorption of uric acid deposits.

Indications: Treatment of increased serum urate levels associated with gout; adjunct therapy with penicillins and cephalosporins to increase and prolong serum antibiotic levels.

Usual dosage: Gout: 0.25 g 2 times/day for 1 wk, then 0.5 g 2 times/day; with antibiotics: 2 g/day.

Precautions/contraindications: Therapy should not begin during an acute gout attack; it is contraindicated in patients with known hypersensitivity, blood dyscrasias, or uric acid kidney stones.

Side effects/adverse reactions: Therapy may exacerbate gout; increased excretion of uric acid may lead to formation of urate stones, especially during initial therapy. The drug may cause GI upset.

Pharmacokinetics: Probenecid is well absorbed in the GI tract, highly protein bound, with renal excretion of metabolites; increased dosage may be needed in patients with reduced renal function.

Interactions: Probenecid decreases renal excretion of most penicillin and cephalosporin antibiotics. The decreased renal excretion may lead to serum levels two to four times normal. The drug is sometimes administered with penicillins to increase the effectiveness. Salicylates and pyrazinamide decrease the effectiveness of the drug. Probenecid reduces excretion of aminosalicylic acid, clofibrate, dyphylline, dapsone, indomethacin, methotrexate, naproxen, pantothenic acid, rifampin, sulfonamides, and sulfonylureas, leading to increased serum levels unless dosages of these drugs are reduced.

Nursing considerations: Increased urine output and alkalinization of the urine reduces the risk of uric acid stone formation. Instruct the patient to drink at least 2.5 L/day. GI upset may be minimized by taking the drug with food. If taking the drug precipitates an acute gout attack, the drug may be continued and an additional anti-gout medication, such as colchicine administered. Advise the patient to avoid aspirin or other salicylates that will reduce the drug's effectiveness.

Sulfinpyrazone

Sulfinpyrazone (Anturane, Aprazone) is a uricosuric that also has antithrombotic effects and inhibits the effects of platelets. The drug suppresses development of tophi and may reduce existing uric acid deposits.

Indications: Treatment of increased serum urate level associated with gout.

Usual dosage: Initially 200-400 mg/day in 2 doses; dosage may be increased to 800 mg/day.

Precautions/contraindications: Do not administer to patients with active peptic ulcer or GI inflammation.

Side effects/adverse reactions: May cause GI disturbances, blood dyscrasias, rash; bronchospasm has occurred in patients with aspirin-induced asthma.

Pharmacokinetics: Sulfinpyrazone is well absorbed in the GI tract and highly protein bound. About half of the absorbed dose is excreted unchanged in the urine.

Interactions: Salicylates decrease the effectiveness of the drug. The effects of some sulfonamides may be potentiated. The effects of tolbutamide and warfarin may be increased, because sulfinpyrazone inhibits hepatic metabolism of these drugs.

Nursing considerations: Same as those for probenecid.

Allopurinol

Allopurinol (Lopurin, Zurinol, Zyloprim) acts differently from the uricosuric agents. It decreases both serum and urinary uric acid by inhibiting the formation of uric acid; the uricosuric agents work by increasing uric acid excretion. Allopurinol has no analgesic or antiinflammatory effect and is not helpful in the management of acute gout attacks; however, it is quite effective for long-term therapy in reducing uric acid with little toxicity. Long-term use may be associated with slow reabsorption of tophi.

Indications: Treatment of gouty arthritis; management of patients with malignancies who are undergoing oncologic treatment that results in hyperuricemia; management of patients with recurrent calcium oxalate calculi.

Usual dosage: Gout: 100-800 mg/day; daily dosages over 300 mg are taken in divided doses.

Precautions/contraindications: Acute attacks of gout may occur during initial treatment. Discontinue drug immediately if rash or other sign of hypersensitivity occurs.

Side effects/adverse reactions: Skin rashes are the most common adverse reactions and may progress to more severe and even fatal hypersensitivity reactions. Drowsiness may occur occasionally.

Pharmacokinetics: About 90% of the orally administered drug is absorbed. Allopurinol is excreted primarily through the kidneys. Oxipurinol is an active metabolite with a long half-life.

Interactions: Administration with thiazide diuretics may increase the potential for toxicity. Allopurinol may increase the half-life of oral anticoagulants, but it has not been shown to increase their effects. Administration with cytotoxic drugs may increase bone marrow suppression. Uricosuric drugs enhance excretion of allopurinol. Unlike the uricosuric agents, salicylates do *not* antagonize the effects of allopurinol.

Nursing considerations: If GI disturbances are a problem, the drug should be taken after meals. Instruct the patient to drink enough liquids to maintain a urine output of more than 2 L/day. Warn the patient that the drug may cause drowsiness and to use caution when driving or performing hazardous tasks. The patient should be instructed to notify his physician immediately if he develops a skin rash. Because acute gout attacks often increase in frequency during the first 6-12 mo of therapy, colchicine is usually administered concurrently during the first 3-6 mo.

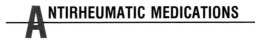

ANTIRHEUMATIC MEDICATIONS

ANTIMALARIAL DRUGS

Chloroquine (Aralen) and hydroxychloroquine (Plaquenil) are 4-aminoquinolone compounds that are most commonly used in the treatment of malaria. They are used to treat rheumatoid arthritis in patients whose symptoms cannot be adequately controlled by salicylates or NSAIDs. The mechanism of action and the drugs' effect on rheumatoid arthritis are not well understood.

Indications: Treatment of acute or chronic rheumatoid arthritis; treatment of chronic discoid and systemic lupus erythematosus; suppression and relief of *Plasmodium* species malaria; treatment of extraintestinal amebiasis.

Usual dosage: For rheumatoid arthritis: Chloroquine, 150-300 mg/day; hydroxychloroquine, 200-600 mg/day.

Precautions/contraindications: Irreversible retinopathy has occurred with long-term or high-dose therapy. In patients with psoriasis or porphyria, these drugs may precipitate a severe attack. Use with caution in patients with hepatic disease or alcoholism. Avoid concurrent use with other drugs that may cause skin sensitization and dermatitis, such as phenylbutazone and gold compounds.

Side effects/adverse reactions: GI disturbances, hypotension, headache, blood abnormalities. Hemolysis may occur in individuals with glucose 6-phosphate dehydrogenase (G6PD) deficiency. Dermatologic effects such as pruritus, pigmentary changes, eruptions, and other dermatoses and bleaching of hair may occur.

Pharmacokinetics: The drugs are absorbed readily from the GI tract and persist in the body for a prolonged period. Excretion is through the kidneys and is enhanced with urinary acidification.

Interactions: Kaolin or magnesium trisilicate may decrease absorption of 4-aminoquinolone compounds.

Nursing considerations: Monitor complete blood counts (CBCs) during prolonged therapy. Administer with food to minimize GI disturbances. Side effects and adverse reactions are most common with acute high-dose treatment. A response may not occur for several weeks or months; discontinue if no response is seen in 4-6 mo. Salicylates, NSAIDs, and glucocorticoids may be administered concurrently with these drugs.

GOLD COMPOUNDS

Gold arrests the progression of the bone and articular destruction in rheumatoid arthritis but does not have analgesic properties. The mechanism of action is unknown; however, long-term therapy leads to a gradual reduction in symptoms. Prolonged therapy is needed for gold compounds to achieve their effect. Improvement may be seen after 6-8 wk or may take as long as 6 mo. Three gold preparations are available: auranofin (Ridaura) is administered PO and contains about 29% gold; aurothioglucose (Solganal) and gold sodium thiomalate (Myochrysine) are administered IM and contain roughly 50% gold.

Indications: Actively progressing rheumatoid arthritis that does not respond to less toxic antiinflammatory agents and conservative treatment.

Usual dosage: *Auranofin:* 6 mg/day PO; if response is inadequate after 6 mo, the dose may be increased to 9 mg/day. *Aurothioglucose:* Weekly injections, IM, 10 mg first week, 25 mg second and third weeks, then 50 mg/week until a total of 0.8-1 g has been administered; maintenance dose is 50 mg q 3-4 wk. *Gold sodium thiomalate:* Weekly injections, IM, 10 mg first week, 25 mg second week, 25-50 mg third and subsequent weeks until a total of 1 g has been administered; maintenance dose is 25 mg-50 mg q 2 wk, and interval may be increased to q 3-4 wk if clinical cues are stable.

Precautions/contraindications: Contraindicated in patients with previous toxicity, pregnancy, serious renal or liver dysfunction, and blood dyscrasias.

Side effects/adverse reactions: GI disturbances are the most common side effects with orally administered gold therapy. Commonly seen adverse reactions include dermatitis, pruritus, stomatitis, pharyngitis, a metallic taste, and GI disturbances. Arthralgias may occur for 1-2 days after the first few injections. A blue-gray skin discoloration (chrysiasis) may develop, especially in areas exposed to strong light. Gold-induced nephritis or blood dyscrasias are more serious effects.

Pharmacokinetics: Gold is widely distributed in body tissues, and after prolonged therapy the concentration in synovial fluid of inflamed joints will be several times the concentration in other tissues. It can take as long as a year for all the gold to be removed from the body after prolonged therapy. Excretion is through feces and the kidneys.

Interactions: Do not administer antimalarials with gold. Gold is not administered with penicillamine, because the later will remove most of the gold. Salicylates, NSAIDs, and corticosteroids may be administered with gold therapy.

Nursing considerations: Rule out pregnancy and perform urinalysis, blood and platelet counts, and liver function tests before beginning therapy and periodically during therapy. Injections should be administered only IM, preferably intragluteally. Instruct the patient to remain recumbent for 10 min after injection, and observe for at least 15 min after administration. Instruct the patient to avoid strong light and to report any skin or mucous membrane lesions.

PENICILLAMINE

A metabolite of penicillin, penicillamine (Cuprimine, Depen) is similar to gold in its antiinflammatory effect on rheumatoid arthritis. Like gold, penicillamine has a latency period of several months before therapeutic effects are observed, and its mechanism of action is not clearly understood. Because of the high incidence of adverse reactions, this drug is reserved for patients who have not responded to conservative therapy or gold therapy.

Indications: Actively progressing rheumatoid arthritis that does not respond to less toxic antiinflammatory agents and conservative treatment.

Usual dosage: Initial therapy is 125-250 mg/day, increased at 1- to 3-month intervals until a therapeutic response, toxicity, or a daily dose of 1-1.5 g is obtained. Maintenance doses are individualized at the level needed for effect (500 mg-1.5 g/day).

Precautions/contraindications: Contraindicated in pregnant patients or in those with renal insufficiency. Penicillin allergy is *not* a contraindication to penicillamine therapy.

Side effects/adverse reactions: About 40% of patients receiving penicillamine will have significant adverse effects that require discontinuation of the drug. Cutaneous and mucous membrane reactions are the most common side effects. GI disturbances and loss of taste may occur. Leukopenia or thrombocytopenia may occur and may lead to aplastic anemia in some patients. Renal dysfunction, autoimmune reactions, alopecia, mammary hyperplasia, and psychologic changes have been reported. Drug fever may occur, usually associated with skin eruptions.

> ## GOLD TOXICITY
>
> As many as one third of all patients undergoing gold therapy experience some form of toxicity. Signs of serious gold toxicity include a fall in hemoglobin, platelets, or white blood cells; protein in the urine; persistent diarrhea; pruritus, rash, or stomatitis. Any of the above symptoms should be considered a toxic reaction to gold until proven otherwise.
>
> Toxic reactions may occur during gold therapy or after it is stopped. The incidence of toxic reactions does not appear to be related to the serum gold level but does increase with higher total doses.
>
> Monitoring of patients during gold therapy should include urinalysis, blood and platelet counts (usually every other week), and liver function tests.
>
> Gold administration should be discontinued immediately if a toxic reaction is noted. Minor reactions may resolve spontaneously. More serious reactions may be treated with systemic corticosteroids for symptomatic relief. Severe reactions may require administration of a chelating agent in addition to corticosteroids. Therapy for toxic reactions may be continued for several months.

Pharmacokinetics: Approximately half of the oral dose is absorbed. Absorption is increased if the drug is taken 1½ hr after meals. The drug is excreted in the urine and feces.

Interactions: Gold therapy, phenylbutazone, and antimalarial or cytotoxic drugs should not be administered with penicillamine. Penicillamine has the potential to interfere with the absorption of may drugs. Salicylates, NSAIDs and corticosteroids may be used in conjunction with Penicillamine.

Nursing considerations: Penicillamine should be taken 90 min after meals and at least 1 hr apart from any other drug. Instruct the patient about the signs of toxic reactions and that he should notify the physician if they occur. CBCs (including platelets) and urinalysis should be performed bimonthly for the first several months and at least monthly during therapy.

IMMUNOSUPPRESSIVE AGENTS

Immunosuppressive agents have proved useful in treating some patients with severe rheumatoid arthritis. Because of the high potential for serious adverse effects, these drugs are used only in severe cases after more conventional treatments have failed to provide satisfactory effects. Azathioprine (Imuran) is an immunosuppressive agent that has been approved for use in treating rheumatoid arthritis. Symptoms may not improve until the patient has had 6-12 wk of therapy.

Indications: Only for the treatment of adult patients with severe, active, erosive rheumatoid arthritis that does not respond to conventional management.

Usual dosage: 50-100 mg/day; beginning at 6-12 wk and thereafter, the dose may be increased every 4 wk if the initial response is inadequate and toxicity does not develop. The maximum dose is 2.5 mg/kg/day, with the lowest effective dose used for maintenance.

Precautions/contraindications: Not for use in pregnant patients or in those with hypersensitivity to the drug. Patients with poor renal function may need reduced doses.

Side effects/adverse reactions: Severe bone marrow depression may occur, usually late in the course of therapy, and may be dose related. Azathioprine increases the patient's risk of neoplasm. Serious infections are a common risk in patients with immune suppression.

Pharmacokinetics: Absorption is good from the GI tract. The drug is metabolized in the liver, and metabolic products are excreted primarily through the kidneys.

Interactions: The metabolism of azathioprine is decreased by allopurinol.

Nursing considerations: Monitoring of blood counts is essential during therapy, and the patient should be instructed to report any unusual bleeding or bruising. Signs and symptoms of infection should be reported to the physician.

CYTOTOXIC DRUGS

Cytotoxic drugs, which are used primarily in the treatment of neoplastic diseases, have had only limited success in the treatment of rheumatoid arthritis. Because of their many serious adverse effects, these drugs are limited to severe cases that do not show a satisfactory response to conventional treatment. Cytotoxic drugs are used as part of a comprehensive treatment program, including other drug and nondrug therapies. There is no evidence that cytotoxic drugs stop rheumatoid arthritis permanently or reverse its progression; rather, these drugs slow the progression of the disease. Improvement generally is greatest during the first 6 mo. of therapy and decreases during prolonged treatment.

Table 15-5

HISTAMINE H₂ ANTAGONISTS

Generic name	Trade name	Dosage	Administration
Cimetidine	Tagamet	200-400 mg q 6-8 hr	Oral, IM, IV
Famotidine	Pepcid	20-40 mg q 12 hr or at bedtime	Oral
		20 mg q 12 hr	IV
Nizatidine	Axid	150 mg twice daily or 300 mg at bedtime	Oral
Ranitidine	Zantac	150 mg twice daily or 150-300 mg at bedtime	Oral
		50 mg q 6-8 hr	IM, IV

Methotrexate (Rheumatrex, Folex)

Indications: Severe, active, and progressive rheumatoid arthritis that does not respond to conventional treatment.

Usual dosage: Optimum dosage is based on individual response; usual dose ranges from 5 to 15 mg once weekly, administered PO or parenterally.

Precautions/contraindications: Use with extreme caution in any patient, particularly with systemic illnesses or organ dysfunction.

Side effects/adverse reactions: Because of the low therapeutic index and high toxicity, the drug rarely produces a therapeutic effect without some evidence of toxicity. The drug's greatest toxic effects are seen in bone marrow and the GI tract. GI lesions are often the first signs of toxicity and may be reversible. Bone marrow suppression is a more severe toxicity that is commonly seen. Methotrexate therapy has been associated with significant hepatic and pulmonary effects, in addition to some alteration in almost all body systems.

Pharmacokinetics: Methotrexate is widely distributed in body tissues, with high concentrations found in the liver and kidneys long after the drug has been discontinued. The drug is excreted through the kidneys with little metabolism.

Interactions: NSAIDs should be avoided in patients taking high doses of methotrexate, since a sometimes fatal toxicity has been reported when the two drugs are administered in high doses together.

Nursing considerations: Live virus vaccination should not be administered to patients receiving methotrexate. Patients should be instructed very carefully in their drug regimen in order to avoid a potentially fatal overdose. Monitor these patients closely for signs of adverse reactions and instruct the patient in self-monitoring and reporting of adverse effects to the physician. The therapeutic response of methotrexate is usually seen within 3-6 wk.

Cyclophosphamide

Another cytotoxic drug that has had some success in treating severe, active, and progressive rheumatoid ar-

thritis is cyclophosphamide (Cytoxan). Like methotrexate, it is a highly toxic drug that is used in patients who fail to respond to other, less toxic treatments.

ANTIULCER MEDICATIONS

Patients receiving high doses of salicylates or NSAIDs for musculoskeletal disorders are prone to developing GI irritation, erosions, or ulcers. Many of these patients are also treated with anti-ulcer agents to prevent gastric damage. A class of medications commonly used are the histamine H₂ antagonists (or H₂ blockers). These drugs block histamine receptors in the stomach, thereby greatly reducing gastric acid production for most patients. Histamine H₂ antagonists are widely prescribed for numerous GI conditions when a reduction in gastric acid volume is desirable. They have proven to be effective and to have a low incidence of adverse effects.

Indications: Treatment of gastric ulcers and prevention of NSAID and salicylate damage.

Usual dosage: See Table 15-5.

Precautions/contraindications: Use with caution in patients with renal or liver dysfunction.

Side effects/adverse reactions: Cimetidine has a weak antiandrogenic effect. Nizatidine and ranitidine have been reported to elevate liver enzymes.

Pharmacokinetics: Histamine H₂ antagonists are partly metabolized and excreted through the kidneys.

Interactions: Cimetidine reduces hepatic metabolism of many drugs, including warfarin-type anticoagulants, phenytoin, diazepam, and propranolol and others, leading to the possibility of increased drug levels or toxicity. Other histamine H₂ antagonists do not exhibit this effect. Taking these drugs with antacids may interfere with drug absorption.

Nursing considerations: Monitor patients receiving cimetidine for increased effects of drugs metabolized in the liver. Stagger dosing of antacids and histamine H₂ antagonists.

GASTRIC ACID SECRETION INHIBITOR MEDICATION

Misoprostol (cytotec) is a recently developed medication given to prevent gastric ulceration associated with arthritis pain medication, such as aspirin, and with NSAIDs.

Indications: Misoprostol is indicated for patients with a high risk of developing gastric ulceration, and for patients taking daily doses of aspirin-containing or NSAIDs.

Usual dosage: Adult dose is 200 μg 4 times/day with food.

Precautions/contraindications: Misoprostol should not be given to women with childbearing potential or who are pregnant because it may cause a miscarriage. It should also not be taken by persons with an allergy to prostaglandins.

Side effects/adverse reactions: Misoprostol can cause neausea, headache, vomiting, flatulence, menstrual cramping, menstrual irregularity, and skin rash. Adverse reactions include diarrhea, which may be dose-related and self-limiting with dose reduction, and miscarriage.

Pharmacokinetics: Misoprostol inhibits basal and nocturnal gastric acid secretion and acid secretion in response to a variety of stimuli. It also can increase mucus production and bicarbonate production in the stomach. It is rapidly absorbed, with a half-life of 20 to 40 minutes. It is excreted in the urine.

Interactions: Misoprostol may decrease effects of aspirin in about 20% of patients. It does not affect actions of diazepam if it is administered 2 h apart from diazepam.

Nursing considerations: Instruct the patient to notify her physician on the first day of a missed menstrual period so the medication can be discontinued in the event she is pregnant.

Appendix

SPECIAL ASSESSMENT TECHNIQUES FOR MUSCULOSKELETAL TISSUES

Examination or Test (Sign)	Site and Technique	Normal Findings	Abnormal Findings
Adams	**Vertebral column:** Person bends forward at waist with arms dangling forward.	Spinal column remains centered without lateral curvature or asymmetric prominences.	Person may have asymmetric prominences of one side of chest or lumbar region related to juvenile scoliosis.
Adson	**Upper extremities and radial pulse:** Locate and palpate radial pulse while abducting, extending and externally rotating patients's arm; ask patient to take a deep breath and turn head to arm being tested.	Pulse should remain strong.	Marked decrease or absence of radial pulse could indicate presence of extra cervical rib, tightened neck muscle, or thoracic outlet syndrome.
Allen maneuver	**Elbow and shoulder;** Examiner flexes patient's elbow while shoulder is extended horizontally and laterally rotated. Patient turns head to opposite shoulder. Examiner palpates radial pulse.	Pulse may diminish but remain palpable.	Pulse becomes absent when head is rotated away, indicative of thoracic outlet syndrome.
Allis (Galeazzi test)	**Knees of child ages 3-18 months:** Child lies supine with knees flexed and hips flexed to 90 degrees.	Knees should be of same height.	One knee higher than the other is indicative of congenital dislocation of the hip or shortened femur.
Apley	**Thigh, leg, and knee:** Person lies prone with knee flexed to 90 degrees. Examiner uses own knee to hold down patient's knee, then examiner rotates tibia medially and laterally, combined first with distraction, then with compression.	Patient should experience no pain or discomfort.	If pain is greater with rotation and distraction than with compression, patient may have a ligament injury; if compression produces more pain meniscus may be injured or torn.
Babinski	**Sole of foot:** Examiner strokes plantar surface along outside of patient's foot, using a pointed object.	Toes may curl down toward sole. Normally baby up to 2-3 weeks of age will have positive test, as shown in right-hand column.	If test is positive (abnormal), big toe will extend and toes will splay (spread or abduct) as one indication of an upper motor neuron lesion.
Ballottement (patella or patellar tap)	**Knee: Extended:** Examiner lightly taps patella.	Patella moves only slightly.	Patella moves easily, indicative of fluid in knee capsule.

Examination or Test (Sign)	Site and Technique	Normal Findings	Abnormal Findings
Barlow	**Hips of infant:** Examiner performs Ortolani's test (see below) and then uses the thumb to apply pressure backward and outward on the inner thigh (used in infants up to 6 months of age).	Head of femur should remain in acetabulum.	"Unstable" hip is indicated if head of femur slips out over posterior lip of acetabulum and then reduces again when thumb pressure is removed.
Brudzinski (**Hyndman**)	**Leg and neck:** Person lies supine. Examiner raises patient's leg with hip medially rotated and knee extended (leg straight), then flexes hip until patient complains of tightness or pain; then lowers leg until there is no pain, patient then flexes neck to put chin to chest.	No increase or indication of pain with neck flexion thus no radicular or spinal nerve problems.	Increased pain with neck flexion indicates stretching of dura mater of spinal cord; pain that does not increase with neck flexion may indicate tight hamstring muscles or lumbosacral joint problems.
Brush, stroke or wipe	**Knee:** Examiner strokes upward on medial side of patella 2-3 times with palm and fingers of one hand while stroking downward on lateral side of patella.	Small wave or bulge of fluid may be noted because joint normally holds 5-7 ml of synovial fluid.	Bulge or wave of fluid noted in medial distal border of patella.
Bunnel-Littler	**Metacarpophalangeal joint of hand:** Examiner attempts to flex proximal interphalangeal joint while metacarpophalangeal joint held slightly extended (patient is passive during examination).	Proximal interphalangeal joint can be flexed.	Proximal interphalangeal joint cannot be flexed, indicative of contracture of joint capsule or tight intrinsic muscle.
Cage	X-ray view of head of femur.	No osteoporosis of head of femur.	Translucent, osteoporotic area on lateral side of epiphysis of head of femur.
Camel	**Lateral side of knee and patella:** Examiner views knee and patella area from the side.	Generally only one "hump" (patella) is noted.	An abnormally high patella (one "hump") permits the examiner to note prominence of infrapatellar fat pad (second "hump").
Chvostek	**Facial nerve of cheek:** Lightly tap facial nerve over cheek in front of ear (site of entry of nerve to face).	No twitch of face or cheek.	Twitch or contraction of cheek and lip caused by hypocalcemia
Clarke	**Patella:** Examiner presses down slightly proximal to upper pole or base of the patella with web of hand, while patient lies supine with the knee relaxed. Patient is asked to contract quadriceps while examiner presses down.	Normally, patient should be able to complete and maintain contraction without pain.	Pain with pressure and inability to maintain contraction may indicate chondromalacia of the patella.
Cozen	**Elbow:** Examiner stabilizes elbow with thumb resting on lateral epicondyle. Patient is asked to make fist, pronate forearm, radially deviate and extend wrist while examiner resists motion.	No pain should be felt against resistance in lateral epicondyle of humerus.	Sudden, severe pain in the area of the lateral epicondyle is felt with persistence. This is one test for tennis elbow.

Continued.

Examination or Test (Sign)	Site and Technique	Normal Findings	Abnormal Findings
Cram	**Leg and knee:** Examiner does straight leg raise to produce pain; then knee is slightly flexed to reduce pain; thigh remains raised; examiner applies pressure on popliteal area to reproduce pain.	Straight leg raising usually does not produce pain.	Pain is associated with radicular pain from inflamed or ischemic sciatic nerve, from pressure on sciatic nerve.
Cullen	**Umbilicus:** Examiner inspects umbilical area of abdomen.	Skin area is pinkish or same as other skin areas of patient's body.	Bluish discoloration around umbilicus may indicate intraabdominal bleeding.
Drawer	**Knee: Flexed to 90 degrees:** Examiner sits on patient's foot for stability; then places hands around upper tibia and draws leg forward.	Can move tibia forward up to 6 mm.	More than 6 mm forward movement with anterior cruciate ligament tears, or medial collateral ligament tears.
Faber	**Leg, knee, and hip:** With patient supine, examiner places patient's foot of test leg on top of opposite knee, then slowly lowers leg in abduction to table by pressing on knee.	Leg will fall to table and rest parallel to other leg.	Test leg remains above opposite leg, indicating spasm of iliopsoas muscle or some pathologic process of sacroiliac joint. This test is also known as Patrick test.
Finkelstein	**Wrist:** Ask patient to make fist with thumb inside; examiner grasps fist and deviates fist toward ulnar side while holding forearm stable.	Only slight pain may be noted over abductor pollicis longus and extensor pollicis brevis tendons.	Moderate to severe pain over abductor and extensor tendons of thumb may indicate tenosynovitis, also called deQuervain's or Hoffman's disease.
Froment	**Thumb and index finger** Patient holds piece of paper between thumb and index finger while examiner tries to pull it away.	Terminal phalanx of thumb will remain extended.	Flexion of the terminal phalanx of the thumb is abnormal and indicative of ulnar nerve paralysis and paralysis of the adductor pollicis muscle.
Gaenslen	**Hip and leg:** Patient lies on side with lower leg flexed to chest and upper leg hyperextended at hip; examiner stabilizes pelvis while extending upper leg (test leg). **or:** With patient supine and one leg flexed at knee to chest, patient extends other leg off edge of table; patient draws both legs up to chest, then slowly lowers test leg down into extension.	Usually no pain is noted.	Pain may be noted in sacroiliac joints which may be due to sacroiliac pathology, hip conditions, or L4 nerve root lesion.
Golfer's elbow	**Medial epicondyle of elbow:** Examiner palpates medial epicondylar area while forearm is supinated and elbow and wrist are extended.	No pain should be noted or felt.	Pain is felt over medial epicondyle.
Homan	**Ankle and foot:** Examiner passively dorsiflexes patient's foot toward tibia.	No pain in calf muscles should be felt, nor tenderness in calf stated.	Pain in calf muscles, along with tenderness on palpation, may indicate deep vein thrombosis.

Examination or Test (Sign)	Site and Technique	Normal Findings	Abnormal Findings
Hughston	**Knee:** With patient lying supine with 80-90 degree knee flexion and hip flexed to 45 degrees, examiner rotates patient's foot medially slight amount, then sits on foot to stabilize it; examiner pushes tibia posteriorly at knee.	Each knee should move or rotate minimally or in similar smounts in relation to each other.	If tibia of one leg moves or rotates excessively in comparison with other leg, it may be due to injury to one or another of following structures; posterior cruciate or posterior oblique ligaments, medial collateral ligament, posteromedial capsule, anterior cruciate ligament, or semimembranous capsule.
Kernig	**Head and neck:** Patient lies supine and flexes head on chest with own hands placed at back of head.	No complaints of pain.	May have pain along spinal column into legs, indicative of dural irritation.
Lachman	**Leg and knee:** Patient lies supine; examiner holds patient's knee between full extension and 30 degrees flexion; femur is stabilized with one of examiner's hand while moving proximal aspect ot the tibia forward with other hand.	Tibia should remain firm as it is moved forward.	As tibia is moved forward, there may be soft, mushy feeling indicative of anterior or posterior cruciate ligament injury.
Laguere	**Hip and leg:** With patient lying supine, examiner flexes, abducts, and laterally rotates hip, applying overpressure at end of range of motion; examiner stabilizes pelvis on opposite side by holding down anterior iliac crest area.	Should have no pain or discomfort in hip or sacroiliac joint.	Pain in sacroiliac joint on same side as tested hip joint may indicate hip pathologic process.
Macintosh	**Leg and knee:** With patient lying supine and hip flexed to 20 degress, examiner holds patient's foot with one hand while other hand flexes knee 5 degrees by placing heel of hand behind fibula over lateral gastrocnemius muscle with tibia medially rotated. Examiner then applies a valgus stress to knee. If leg is then flexed 30-40 degrees, tibia will reduce or jog backward, producing a feeling of "giving way."	Should not have feeling of instability.	Feeling of instability or "giving way" may indicate injury to cruciate or lateral collateral ligaments, or the posterolateral capsule.
McMurray	**Knee and leg:** With patient supine, legs extended, examiner cups heel in hand and flexes leg fully and places other hand on knee joint with fingers on medial jointline and thumb on lateral joint line; leg is rotated internally and externally, then is gently extended as the examiner palpates medial joint line.	No clicks or sounds should be felt or heard.	Click in knee joint may indicate tear of medial meniscus.

Continued.

Examination or Test (Sign)	Site and Technique	Normal Findings	Abnormal Findings
Milgram	**Leg:** With patient lying supine, examiner asks patient to raise straight legs about 2 inches off table.	Usually can hold both legs up for about 30 seconds.	If elevation cannot be maintained, it may indicate pressure on spinal cord from herniated disc.
Naffsiger	**Neck:** With patient lying supine, examiner compresses jugular veins about 10 seconds (face will flush); asks patients to cough.	No pain or discomfort is noted.	Pain or discomfort may indicate pressure on spinal cord from herniated disc.
Ortolani	**Hips and thighs of infant:** With infant lying supine, examiner abducts and externally rotates flexed thigh.	No sounds or clicks are noted.	Click may be heard or felt as femoral head slides over acetabular rim, indicative of congenital hip dislocation or dysplasia.
Phalen	**Wrists:** Examiner has patient flex wrists tightly against each other at right angles and hold position for 1 min.	No discomfort or tingling is noted.	Numbness or tingling of thumb or fingers may indicate carpal tunnel syndrome.
Quick	**Hips, knees, and ankles:** With patient standing, examiner has patient squat down as far as possible and bounce two to three times, then stand up. NOTE: Persons with arthritis, pregnant women, and elderly persons should not do this test.	Should have no difficulty squatting or bouncing.	Pain or inability to squat and bounce may indicate pathologic process in ankles, knees, or hips.
Schober	Posterior pelvis: Examiner marks point midway between "dimples of pelvis" at the level of 2 vertebra, then marks points 0.5 cm and 1.0 cm above that level and measures distances between these points; patient is asked to flex forward and distances are remeasured.	Some change in distances indicate normal flexion in vertebrae.	No differences with flexion between marks may indicate lack of mobility in vertebral column.
Speed	**Arm and shoulder:** With patient's forearm supinated and elbow completely extended, examiner resists patient's efforts at shoulder forward flexion.	No tenderness should be noted over bicipital groove.	Tenderness in bicipital groove may indicate bicipital tendinitis.
Supraspinatus	**Shoulder and arm:** Examiner applies downward pressure to arms while patient holds arms abducted to 90 degrees in neutral (no) rotation; then patient rotates and angles arm so thumb faces toward floor.	Arm and shoulder should be able to resist pressure without pain or weakness	Pain or weakness may indicate tear of rotator supraspinatus muscle or tendon.
Thomas	**Leg and knee:** With patient lying supine, ask patient to flex sound leg to chest.	Opposite leg should remain flat.	Flexion contracture may be indicated if opposite leg moves up off table.

Examination or Test (Sign)	Site and Technique	Normal Findings	Abnormal Findings
Thompson	**Achilles tendon:** With patient lying prone or kneeling on chair with feet over edge of table or chair, examiner squeezes calf muscles.	Patient's foot will plantar flex when muscle is squeezed.	Lack of or inability to plantar flex foot is usually indicative of a ruptured Achilles tendon. Note: At times, even with rupture patient can plantarflex by action of long extensor leg muscles.
Tinel	**Volar surfaces of wrist and elbow:** Examiner taps area between olecranon and medial condyle (for ulnar nerve) or taps volar surface at center of wrist (for median nerve).	No tingling should be noted with tapping of ulnar or median nerves.	Tingling along ulnar nerve pathway may indicate neuroma or ulnar tunnel syndrome, tingling of fingers along median nerve pathway indicates carpal tunnel syndrome.
Trendelenberg	**Posterior iliac crests:** With patient standing, examiner has patient raise one leg and flex knee; examiner observes level of iliac crests; then has patient stand on leg and raise other leg and again observes iliac crests.	Iliac crest and pelvis opposite weight-bearing leg should rise to maintain balance.	Iliac crest and pelvis opposite weight-bearing leg drops lower if gluteus medius muscles are weak or injured, or if there is hip pathologic process.
Weber	**Hand:** With patient's hand immobile on firm surface, examiner uses paper clip to apply pressure on two adjacent points simultaneously to determine smallest distance at which patient can distinguish two stimuli. Patient must not be able to see area being tested.	Should be able to detect two points very close together referred to as threshold for discrimination.	Inability to detect two points close together may indicate insufficient nerve/muscle regeneration.
Wilson	**Knee:** With patient sitting with knee flexed over table; patient extends knee with tibia medially rotated; at about 30 degrees flexion, patient may have pain, stops flexion, and rotates tibia laterally.	Should have no pain with movements.	Pain with flexion and medial tibial rotation that disappears with lateral rotation indicates osteochondritis dissecans (loose body in knee).
Yeoman's	**Legs and knees:** With patient prone, examiner stabilizes pelvis and extends each of patient's hips in turn with knees extended.; then extends each leg with knee flexed.	No pain or discomfort should be noted.	Pain along lumbar spine may indicate pathologic process of discs or vertebrae.
Yergason	**Elbow and arm:** With patient's elbow flexed to 90 degrees, examiner cups elbow in hand, then externally rotates arm with other hand on wrist and pulls down on elbow.	No pain should be noted.	Pain may indicate that the biceps tendon has come out of its bicipital groove.

References

1. Altman RD: Osteoarthritis: pathogenesis, differential diagnosis, treatment, Orthop Rev 13(5):53-63, 1984.

2. American Nurses Association and National Association of Orthopaedic Nurses: Orthopaedic nursing practice, process, and outcome criteria for selected diagnoses, Orthop Nurs 6(2):10-16, 1987.

3. Andrews G and MacEwen GO: Idiopathic scoliosis, Orthopedics 12(6):809-816, 1989.

4. Avioli LV, editor: The osteoporotic syndrome, Orlando, Fla, 1987, Grune & Stratton, Inc.

5. Ball GV and Koopman WJ: Clinical rheumatology, Philadelphia, 1986, WB Saunders Co.

6. Batson E: Chemionucleolysis for herniated lumbar disk, JAMA 262(7):953-956, 1989.

7. Behrens F: General theory and principles of external fixation, Clin Orthop 241:15-23, 1989.

8. Benson DR: Idiopathic scoliosis: the last ten years and state of the art, Orthopedics 10(12):1691-1698, 1987.

9. Berg E and Moyle DD: Osteoporosis: an overview of causes, prevention, and therapy, J Musculoskel Med 5(1):64-81, 1988.

10. Betts K: Women should know risks of taking estrogen for osteoporosis, Oncol Times, 10(9):7, 27, 1988.

11. Bordelon RL: Evaluation and operative procedures for hallux valgus deformity, Orthopedics 10(1):38-44, 1987.

12. Brashear HR Jr and Raney RB Sr: Handbook of orthopaedic surgery, ed 10, St Louis, 1986, Mosby–Year Book, Inc.

13. Bray TJ and Templeman DC: Fractures of the femoral neck. In Chapman MW, editor: Operative orthopaedics, Philadelphia, 1988, JB Lippincott Co.

14. Broos PLO et al: Polytrauma in patients of 65 and over: injury patterns and outcomes, Int Surg 73:119-122, 1988.

15. Browner BD and Edwards CC: The science and practice of intramedullary nailing, Philadelphia, 1987, Lea & Febiger.

16. Buchanan WW: Managing arthritis in elderly patients, J Musculoskel Med (suppl) 4(3):S16-17, 1989.

17. Burke JF, Boyd RJ, and McCabe CJ: Trauma management: early management of visceral, nervous system and musculoskeletal injuries, St Louis, 1988, Mosby–Year Book, Inc.

18. Bynum TE: NSAID-induced gastropathy: a gastroenterologist's point of view, J Musculoskel Med (suppl), 4(3):S18-20, 1989.

19. Cooke TDV: Pathogenesis of osteoarthritis, Orthop Rev 17(5):527, 1988.

20. Corbett JV: Laboratory tests and diagnostic procedures with nursing diagnoses, East Norwalk, Conn, 1987, Appleton & Lange.

21. Crenshaw AH, editor: Campbell's operative orthopaedics, St Louis, 1987, Mosby–Year Book, Inc.

22. Crues J: Meniscal tears of the knee: accuracy of MR imaging, Radiology 164:445-448, 1987.

23. Dahlin DC and Unni KK: Bone tumors: general aspects and data on 8542 cases, ed 4, Springfield, Ill, 1986, Thomas Publishing Co.

23a. Darr KF et al: Giant cell tumor of bone, Orthop 11(1):209-221, 1988.

24. Deacon P and Dickson RA: Vertebral shape in the median sagittal plane is idiopathic thoracic scoliosis, Orthopedics 10(6):893-896, 1987.

25. Durning RP: Reflux of chymopapain, Surg Rds for Orthop 1(4):41-42, 1987.

26. Engler MB and Engler MM: The hazards of magnetic resonance imaging, AJN 86(6):650, 1986.

27. Enneking WF: A system of staging musculoskeletal neoplasms, Clin Orthop 204:9-24, 1986.

28. Enneking WF, editor: Limb salvage in musculoskeletal oncology, New York, 1987, Churchill Livingstone, Inc.

29. Epps CH, editor: Complications in orthopaedic surgery, ed 2, Philadelphia, 1986, JB Lippincott Co.

30. Esterhai JL et al: Treatment of chronic refractory osteomyelitis with adjunctive hyperbaric oxygen, Orthop Rev 17(8):809-815, 1988.

31. Firestone TP et al: Correction of hallux valgus using the Chevron osteotomy, Surg Rds for Orthop 8(9):24-32, 1988.

32. Gebhardt MC and Mankin HJ: Osteosarcomas: the treatment controversy. II, Surg Rds for Orthop 2(7):25-42, 1988.

33. Gentry LO: Overview of osteomyelitis, Orthop Rev 16(4):91-106, 1987.

33a. Gerstner DL and Omer Jr GE: Part II: Peripheral entrapment neuropathies in the upper extremity, J Musculoskel Med 5(4):37-49, 1988.

34. Good Morning, America: Lyme disease, July 5, 1989 (television broadcast).

35. Goldberg AL et al: The impact of magnetic resonance on the diagnostic evaluation of acute cervicothoracic spinal trauma, Skeletal Radiol 17:89, 1988.

36. Gossling HR: The cost of imaging technology, Complications in Orthopedics 3(2):31, 49, 1988.

37. Graham CE: Percutaneous posterolateral lumbar discectomy: an alternative to laminectomy in the treatment of backaches and sciatica. Proceedings of the Second Annual Meeting of the International Intradiscal Therapy Society, Inc, Orlando, FL. Mar 9-12, 1989, p. 23.

38. Green NE moderator, Alternatives in the treatment of idiopathic adolescent scoliosis, Cont Orthop 20(2):210-245, 1990 (symposium).

39. Green NE and Edwards K: Bone and joint infections in children, Orthop Clin North Am 18:1-22, 1987.

39a. Grimes DE: Infectious diseases, St. Louis, 1991, Mosby–Year Book, Inc.

40. Gulanick M, Klopp A, and Galenes S, editors: Nursing care plans, nursing diagnosis, and interventions, St Louis, 1986, Mosby–Year Book, Inc.

40a. Gustilo RB, Corpres V, and Sherman RE: Epidemiology, mortality and morbidity in multiple trauma patients, Orthopedics 8(12):1523-1528, 1985.

41. Guyton AC: Textbook of medical physiology, ed 7, Philadelphia, 1986, WB Saunders Co.

42. Hald RD and Mellion MB: Taping and wrapping of common sports injuries, J Musculosk Med 6(1):78-101, 1989.

43. Heaney RP: The role of calcium in prevention and treatment of osteoporosis, Phys & Spts Med 15(11):83-88, 1989.

44. Herbert MA and Bobechko WP: Paraspinal muscle stimulation for the treatment of idiopathic scoliosis in children, Orthopedics 10(8):1125-1132, 1987.

45. Hicks JE: Exercise for patients with inflammatory arthritis, J Musculoskel Med 6(10):40-56, 1989.

46. Hoaglund FT: Confirming the diagnosis of osteoarthritis, J Musculoskel Med 1(5):66-81, 1984.

46a. Hoare K and Donahue KM: Alterations in musculoskeletal function. In McCauce KL and Huether SE: Pathophysiology, St. Louis, 1990, Mosby–Year Book, Inc.

47. Hungerford DS: Response: the role of core decompression in the treatment of ischemic necrosis of the femoral head, Arthritis Rheum 32:801, 1989.

48. Ilizarov GA: The tension-stress on the genesis and growth of tissues, Clin Orthop 239:263-285, 1989.

49. Javernig PR: Organizing and implementing an Ilizarov program, Orthop Nurs 9(5):47-55, 1990.

50. Kaplan PE and Tanner ED: Musculoskeletal pain and disability, East Norwalk, Conn, 1989, Appleton & Lange.

51. Karpman RR and Baum J, editors: Aging and clinical practice: musculoskeletal disorders, Tokyo, 1988, Igaku-Shoin Medical Publishers, Inc.

52. Kengora JE: A rationale for the surgical treatment of bunions, Orthopedics 11(5):777-789, 1988.

53. Kim MJ et al: Pocket guide to nursing diagnosis, ed 2, St Louis, 1987, Mosby–Year Book, Inc.

54. Kostuik JP: Anterior Kostuik-Harrington distraction systems, Orthopedics 11(10):1379-1391, 1988.

55. Lane JM et al: Overview of geriatric osteopenic syndromes. II. Clinical presentation, diagnosis, and treatment, Orthop Rev 17(12):1231-1236, 1988.

56. Lawson JP and Steere AC: Lyme disease: radiographic findings, Radiology 154:37-43, 1985.

57. Legwold G: Lyme disease: diagnosis by observation, Cleve Clin J Med 56(3):230-231, 1989.

58. Legwold G: Tennis elbow: joint resolution by conservative treatment and improved technique, Phys & Spts Med 12(8):168-182, 1984.

59. Licata AO: Some thoughts on osteoporosis in women, Cleve Clin J Med 55(3):233-238, 1988.

60. Lonstein JE, moderator: Management of adult scoliosis (symposium), Contemp Orthop 12(1):71-93, 1986.

61. Luque ER and Rapp GF: A new semiridged method for interpedicular fixation of the spine, Orthopedics 11(10):1445-1450, 1988.

62. MacKenzie EJ, Shapiro S, and Siegel JH: The economic impact of traumatic injuries, JAMA 260(22):3290-3296, 1988.

63. Mader JT, Hicks CA, and Calhoun J: Bacterial osteomyelitis adjunctive hyperbaric oxygen therapy, Orthop Rev 18(5):581-585, 1989.

64. Magee DJ: Orthopedic physical assessment, Philadelphia, 1987, WB Saunders Co.

65. Mann RA: Treatment of the bunion deformity, Orthopedics 10(1):49-56, 1987.

66. Maquet PGJ: Biomechanics of the hip, New York, 1985, Springer-Verlag New York, Inc.

67. McCance KL and Huether SE: Pathophysiology, St Louis, 1990, Mosby–Year Book, Inc.

68. McGuire MH: The pathogenesis of adult osteomyelitis, Orthop Rev 18(5):564-570, 1989.

69. Mears DC and Rubash HE: Pelvic and acetabular fractures, Thorofare, NJ, 1986, Slack, Inc.

70. Melvin JL: Rheumatic disease in the adult and child: occupational therapy and rehabilitation, ed 3, Philadelphia, 1989, FA Davis Co.

71. Meyer HS: Trauma surgery (book review), JAMA 260(14):2127, 1988.

72. Moskowitz RW: An overview of osteoarthritis, J Musculoskel Med (suppl) 4(3):S13-15, 1989.

73. Mourad LA: Musculoskeletal system. In Thompson et al: Mosby's manual of clinical nursing, ed 2, St Louis, 1989, Mosby–Year Book, Inc.

74. Mozanec DJ and Grisanti JM: Drug-induced osteoporosis, Cleve Clin J Med 56(3):297-303, 1989.

75. Myers WJ and Small RA: A cost-efficient system for the irrigation of open fractures, Orthop Rev 17(5):520-521, 1988.

76. Niewoehner CB: Prevention of osteoporosis, J Musculosk Med 6(5):57-66, 1989.

77. Paley D: Bone transport: The Ilizarov treatment of bone defects, Surg Rds for Orthop 3(11):17-32, 1989.

78. Paulus HE, Furst DE, and Dromgoole SH: Drugs for rheumatic disease, New York, 1987, Churchill Livingstone, Inc.

79. Perdriolle R and Vidal J: Morphology of scoliosis: three-dimensional evolution, Orthopedics 10(6): 909-915, 1987.

80. Perry CR et al: Local antibiotic treatment of orthopaedic infections, Surg Rds for Orthop 2(4):32-42, 1988.

81. Post M: Physical examination of the musculoskeletal system, St Louis, 1987, Mosby–Year Book, Inc.

82. Potter PA and Perry AG: Fundamentals of nursing, ed 2, St Louis, 1991, Mosby–Year Book, Inc.

83. Rames RD et al: Lumbar discectomy: operative indications and technique, Surg Rds for Orthop 2(1):15-19, 1988.

84. Rang M et al: Management of displaced supracondylar fractures of the humerus (symposium), Contemp Orthop 18(4):497-535, 1989.

85. Renshaw TS: Pediatric orthopedics, Philadelphia, 1986, WB Saunders Co.

86. Sartoris DJ and Resnick D: Guide to the radiologic manifestations of osteoporosis. II. Most revealing changes in vertebra, femur, metacarpus, J Musculoskel Med 6(2):35-44, 1989.

87. Scherr L, reporter: Lyme disease, June 30, 1989 (television broadcast on 20/20).

88. Schumacher HR and Gall EP: Rheumatoid arthritis, Philadelphia, 1988, JB Lippincott Co.

89. Schwartsman V, McMurray MR, and Martin SN: The Ilizarov method—the basics, Contemp Orthop 19(6):628-638, 1989.

90. Sculco TP, editor: Orthopaedic care of the geriatric patient, St Louis, 1985, Mosby–Year Book, Inc.

91. Seidel HM et al: Mosby's guide to physical examination, ed 2, St Louis, 1991, Mosby–Year Book, Inc.

92. Simmons JV and Norwood SM: Calcitonin and osteoporosis: new mechanisms of pathophysiology, Orthop Rev 16(10):26-32, 1987.

93. Simon RR and Koenigsknecht SJ: Emergency orthopedics: the extremities, ed 2, East Norwalk, Conn, 1987, Appleton & Lange.

94. Simons GW, moderator: Current practices in the treatment of idiopathic clubfoot in the child between birth and five years of age. I., Contemp Orthop 17(1):63-98, 1988 (symposium).

95. Smyrnis T et al: Idiopathic scoliosis: characteristics and epidemiology, Orthopedics 10(6):921-930, 1987.

96. Stewart EL: Calcium intake and osteoporosis, Your Patient and Fitness 1(2):12-14, 1988.

97. Stulberg BN and Watson JT: Management of orthopedic complications of metabolic bone disease, Cleve Clin J Med 56(7):696-703, 1989.

98. Thibodeau GA: Anatomy and physiology, St Louis, 1987, Mosby–Year Book, Inc.

98a. Thompson JM et al: Mosby's manual of clinical nursing, ed 2, St Louis, 1989, Mosby–Year Book, Inc.

99. Tollison CD and Kriegel ML: Physical exercise in the treatment of low back pain. II. A practical regimen of stretching exercise, Orthop Rev 17(9):913-923, 1988.

100. Totty WG: Radiographic evaluation of osteomyelitis using magnetic resonance imaging, Orthop Rev 18(5):587-590, 1989.

101. Turek SL: Orthopaedics: principles and their applications, ed 4, vols 1 and 2, Philadelphia, 1984, JB Lippincott Co.

102. Vassar MJ et al: Early fluid requirements in trauma patients, Arch Surg 123(9):1149-1157, 1988.

103. Walker LG and Meals RA: Tendinitis: a practical approach to diagnosis and management, J Musculoskel Med 6(5):24-54, 1989.

104. Watts C: Chemonucleolysis: concerns. Proceedings of the Second Meeting of the International Intradiscal Society, Inc, Orlando, Fl, March 9-12, 1989.

105. Wiesel SW et al: The aging lumbar spine, Philadelphia, 1982, WB Saunders Co.

105a. Wilson SF and Thompson JM: Respiratory diseases, St Louis, 1990, Mosby–Year Book, Inc.

106. Wong AL and Weisbart RH: Rheumatoid arthritis: a review of current medical therapies, J Musculoskel Med 6(11):39-58, 1989.

107. Zaroukian MJ and Pera A: Diagnosing osteomyelitis, Surg Rds for Orthop 2(11):17-26, 1988.

108. Zwolski K: Lyme disease, Orthop Nurs 9(1):10-17, 1990.

109. Zinberg EM: Free-muscle transfer for chronic osteomyelitis, Surg Rds for Orthop 3(3):26-32, 1989.

Index

A

A band, 10, 11
Abdominal aorta, examination of, 34
Abdominal reflex, 35
Abduction, 15
Abduction pillow, 220, 221
Abduction splint, 174
Abscess, 128
    Brodie's, 121
Acetylsalicylic acid, 281
Achilles reflex, 35
Achilles tendon, 12
Acromioclavicular joint, examination of, 25
Actin, 10, 11
Adams test, 292
Adduction, 15
Adson test, 292
Advil; *see* Ibuprofen
A-hydroCort; *see* Hydrocortisone sodium succinate
Ak Dex; *see* Dexamethasone sodium phosphate
Alba Dex; *see* Dexamethasone sodium phosphate
Allen maneuver, 292
Allis sign, 292
Allopurinol, 287
Amcort; *see* Triamcinolone diacetate
A-methaPred; *see* Methylprednisolone sodium succinate
Amphiarthrotic joints, 14, 16
Amputation, 205-211
    contraindications and cautions, 206
    medical management, 206
    nursing care, 207-211
    patient teaching, 211
    preprocedural care, 206
    types of, 207
Anal reflex, 35
Anaprox; *see* Naproxen sodium

Anderson, Roger, external fixation apparatus, 204
Aneurysmal bone cyst, 160, 161-162
Angulated fracture, 52
Ankle(s)
    examination of, 33
    total joint replacement for, 225
Ankle jerk reflex, 35
Ankylosing spondylitis, 74-81
    complications, 75
    diagnostic studies and findings, 75-76
    medical management, 76
    nursing care, 77-81
    pathophysiology, 75
    patient teaching, 81
Ansaid; *see* Flurbiprofen
Antigout medications, 286-287
Antiinflammatory medications, 280-284
Antimalarial drugs, 287-288
Antirheumatic medications, 287-290
Antiulcer medications, 290
Anturane; *see* Sulfinpyrazone
Aorta, abdominal, examination of, 34
Apley test, 32, 292
Appendicular skeleton, 2
Aprazone; *see* Sulfinpyrazone
Aralen; *see* Chloroquine
Aristocort; *see* Triamcinolone
Aristospan; *see* Triamcinolone hexacetonide
Arm(s)
    bones of, 2
    carrying angle of, examination of, 25-26
    muscles of, 7
Arthritis
    Marie-Strümpell, 74
    patient teaching guide on, 261-262
    posttraumatic, 184
    rheumatoid; *see* Rheumatoid arthritis
Arthrodesis of vertebral column, 228
Arthrography, 42

Arthroscopy, 39
Articulations; *see* Joint(s)
Articulose; *see* Prednisolone acetate
AS; *see* Ankylosing spondylitis
ASA, 281
Aspirin, 280, 281
Assessment of musculoskeletal tissues, 17-35
Atolone; *see* Triamcinolone
Auranofin, 288
Aurothioglucose, 288
Avulsed fracture, 52
Avulsion, 12
Axial skeleton, 2
Axid; *see* Nizatidine
Azathioprine, 289
Azolid; *see* Phenylbutazone

B

Babinski sign, 35, 292
Back problems; *see also* Low back pain
    preventing, patient teaching guide on, 269
Baclofen, 285
Balanced suspension to femur, 193, 195-196
Ballottement examination of knee, 31
Ballottement sign, 292
"Bamboo spine," 75
Bands of muscle fibers, 10, 11
Banflex; *see* Orphenadrine citrate
Bankart procedure, 232
Barlow maneuver, 293
Barton's fracture, 55
Bechterew disease, 74
Benemid; *see* Probenecid
Bennett's fracture, 55
Betamethasone acetate, 284
Betamethasone sodium phosphate, 284
Biceps muscles, examination of, 24
Biceps reflex, 35

Biopsy of bone, muscle, and synovium, 43
Biosone; *see* Hydrocortisone sodium succinate
Blood serum values, 43-45
Blood supply to hip, 226, 227
Bone(s); *see also* specific types
  of arm, 2
  biopsy of, 43
  of body, 1
  cancellous, 5
  compact, 5
  diseases of; *see* specific diseases
  formation and resorption of, 5-6
  functions of, 2
  of leg, 2
  structure of, 4-6
  of trunk and pelvis, 3
  tumors of; *see* Musculoskeletal tumors
Bone cyst
  aneurysmal, 160, 161-162
  unicameral, 160, 162
Bone grafts, spinal fusion with, 228-229
Bone marrow, distribution of, 6
Bone scans, 38-39
Bone scintigraphy, 38-39
Boston brace, 265
Bouchard's nodes, 98
Braces for scoliosis, 265
Brachial plexus nerve entrapment, 104
Brachioradial reflex, 35
Bristow-Helfet-Latarjet procedure, 232
Brodie's abscess, 121
Brudzinski test, 293
Brush test, 293
Bryant traction, 193, 194
Bucket handle fracture, 46, 52
Buck's extension traction, 193, 194
Bulge sign of knee, 32
Bunnel-Littler test, 293
Bursae, 16
Bursitis, 87-91
  complications, 88
  diagnostic studies and findings, 88
  medical management, 88
  nursing care, 88-90
  pathophysiology, 87-88
  patient teaching, 91
Butazolidin; *see* Phenylbutazone
Butterfly fracture, 52

C

Cage test, 293
Calcium
  and bone formation, 5-6
  content of, in foods, 131
  and osteoporosis, 264
Calcium-troponin molecules, 10, 11

Camel sign, 293
Campylodactyly, 27
Canaliculi, 5
Cancellous bone, 4, 5
Carbuncle, 128
Carisoprodol, 285
Carpal tunnel syndrome, 104-109
  complications, 105
  diagnostic studies and findings, 105
  medical management, 106
  nursing care, 107-109
  pathophysiology, 105
  patient teaching, 109
Carrying angle of arm, 25-26
Cartilage, 4, 13
  tumors of; *see* Musculoskeletal tumors
Cast syndrome, 184
Casts, 179-192
  application of, 179-181
    care following, 181-182
  complications, 182-184
  for congenital talipes equinovarus, 176
  home care for, 272
  names of, 180
  nursing care, 185-191
  patient teaching, 192
  patient teaching guides on, 271, 272
  removal of, 184
  skin care and, 185
  types of, 180
Celestone Soluspan; *see* Betamethasone sodium phosphate
Cellulitis, 128
Cenocort A-40; *see* Triamcinolone acetonide
Cenocort Forte; *see* Triamcinolone diacetate
Cervical head halter, 193, 194
Cervical reflex, 35
Cervical spine, examination of, 21
Chaddock reflex, 35
CHD; *see* Congenital hip dysplasia
Chemonucleolysis, 243-248, 268
  contraindications and cautions, 244
  diagnostic studies and findings, 244
  medical management, 244
  nursing care, 245-248
  patient teaching, 248
  preprocedural care, 244
Chloroquine, 287-288
Chlorphenesin carbamate, 285
Chlorzoxazone, 285
Choline salicylate, 281
Chondroblastoma, 160, 161
Chondrocytes, 13
Chondroma, 160, 161
Chondromyxoma, 161

Chvostek sign, 293
Chymopapaine, 243, 268
Cimetidine, 290
Circulation checks, 260
Circumduction, 15
Clarke test, 293
Clavicles, examination of, 23, 24
Claw toe, 34
Clinoril; *see* Sulindac
Closed fracture, 52
Clubfoot; *see* Talipes equinovarus
Colchicine, 286
Cold, therapeutic uses of, 258
Collagen, 13
Colle's fracture, 55
Comminuted fracture, 46, 52
Compact bone, 4, 5
  cross-section of, 6
Compartment syndrome, 182-183
Compression fracture, 52
Computed tomography, 38
Condyles, 4
Congenital hip dysplasia, 173-175
  assessment, 173-175
  complications, 173
  diagnostic studies and findings, 174
  medical management, 174
  nursing care, 175, 176-178
  pathophysiology, 173
  patient teaching, 178
  signs of, 173
Congenital musculoskeletal conditions; *see* Congenital hip dysplasia; Talipes equinovarus
Contraction of muscle, 10-11
Contusion(s), 48, 49
Cortef; *see* Hydrocortisone
Corticosteroids, 283, 284
Corticotomy, 249
Cortisone, 283, 284
Cotrel-Dubousset instrumentation, 229, 230
Cotrel traction, 193, 195
Cotton's fracture, 55
Cozen test, 293
Cram test, 294
Cremasteric reflex, 35
Crutch walking, 188-189
  patient teaching guide on, 274
CT scans, 38
Cubital tunnel syndrome, 104
Cubitus valgus, 26
Cubitus varus, 26
Cullen sign, 294
Cuprimine; *see* Penicillamine
Curvatures of spine, 145-155
  kyphosis, 145-149
  lordosis, 155
  scoliosis, 150-154

Cyclobenzaprine, 285
Cyclophosphamide, 290
Cyst, bone
    aneurysmal, 160, 161-162
    unicameral, 160, 162
Cytotoxic drugs, 289-290
Cytoxan; *see* Cyclophosphamide

D

Dalalone; *see* Dexamethasone sodium
        phosphate
Dalalone LA; *see* Dexamethasone
        acetate
Dantrium; *see* Dantrolene
Dantrolene, 285
Decaject-LA; *see* Dexamethasone
        acetate
Degenerative musculoskeletal
        conditions; *see* Carpal tunnel
        syndrome; Hallux valgus;
        Osteoarthritis; Sciatic nerve
        injury
Delaxin; *see* Methocarbamol
Deltasone; *see* Prednisone
Deltoid muscles, examination of, 24
Depen; *see* Penicillamine
DepMedalone-40; *see*
        Methylprednisolone acetate
Depoject; *see* Methylprednisolone
        acetate
Depo-Medrol; *see* Methylprednisolone
        acetate
Dexamethasone acetate, 284
Dexamethasone sodium phosphate, 284
Dexoacen LA-8; *see* Dexamethasone
        acetate
Diagnostic procedures, 36-43
Diaphysis, 4
Diarthrotic joints, 14, 16
    range of motion of, 15
Diazepam, 285
Diclofenac, 282
Diflunisal, 280, 281
Discoraphy, 42
Disks, ruptured, 110-111
    patient teaching guide on, 268
Dislocation, 49
    congenital hip; *see* Congenital hip
        dysplasia
Dislocations, shoulder, recurrent, 232
Displaced fracture, 53
Dorsiflexion, 15
Dowager's hump, 146
Drainage system, suction, 220
Drawer test, 32, 294
Drugs; *see* specific drugs
Dunlop traction, 193, 195
Duralone; *see* Methylprednisolone
        acetate

E

Ectrodactyly, 27
Eden-Hybbinette procedure, 232
Elbow(s)
    examination of, 25
    total joint replacement for, 225
Electromyography, 40
Elevation of injured limbs, 182
Enchondroma, 161
Endomysium, 10
Endoprosthetic replacement of femoral
        head, 226-227
Enneking's system of lesions, 156-157,
        158, 159
Epicondyles, 5
Epicondylitis, 82-87
    complications, 83
    diagnostic studies and findings, 84
    medical management, 83
    nursing care, 84-87
    pathophysiology, 82-83
    patient teaching, 87
Epimysium, 10
Epiphyses, 4
Erb's palsy, 104
Eversion, 15
Ewing's sarcoma, 160, 162
Examination, physical, of
        musculoskeletal tissues, 19-35
Exercises
    after total hip replacement, 276
    after total knee replacement, 278
    for back problems, 269
    for low back pain, 267
    for osteoporosis, 264
Exercise programs for rehabilitation,
        258
Extension, 15
External fixation devices, 204
Extraarticular fracture, 53
Extremities; *see* Arm(s); Leg(s)

F

Faber test, 294
Face, examination of, 20
Famotidine, 290
Fasciculi, 10
Feet, examination of, 33-34
Feldene; *see* Piroxicam
Femoral head, endoprosthetic
        replacement of, 226-227
Femur, balanced suspension to, 193,
        195-196
Fenamate, 282
Fenoprofen, 282
Fibrosarcoma, 161, 162
Fibrous cartilage, 13
Finger flexor reflex, 35

Fingers, examination of, 26, 27-29
Finkelstein test, 294
Fixation devices
    external, 204
    internal; *see* Open reduction with
        internal fixation
Flat back, 146
Flexeril; *see* Cyclobenzapine
Flexion, 15
Flurbiprofen, 282
Folex; *see* Methotrexate
Foods
    calcium content of, 131
    high in iron, 74
    high in purines, 137
Fracture(s), 49, 50
    diagnosis of, 51
    healing of, 50-51
    nursing care, 52, 57-62
    patient teaching, 62
    proper names for specific
        (illustrated), 55-56
    treatments for, 51-52
    types and causes of (illustrated),
        52-54
Frejka pillow splint, 174
Froment test, 294
Frontal bone, 4
Fusion, spinal; *see* Spinal fusion

G

Gaenslen test, 294
Gag reflex, 35
Gait analysis laboratory, 257
Gait, examination of, 19, 20, 29
Galeazzi test, 292
Galeazzi's fracture, 55
Gastric acid inhibitors, 291
Giant cell tumor, 160, 161
Gibbus, 23, 146
Glenohumeral joint, examination of, 25
Glenoplasty, 232
Glucocorticoids, 283, 284
Gold compounds, 288
Gold sodium thiomalate, 288
Gold toxicity, 289
Golfer's elbow, 82
    assessment for, 294
Gomphoses, 16
Gordon reflex, 35
Gout, 136-140
    complications, 136
    diagnostic studies and findings, 136
    medical management, 137
    nursing care, 137-139
    pathophysiology, 136
    patient teaching, 140
Greenstick fracture, 53

H

H band, 10, 11
H₂ blockers, 290
Hallux valgus, 34, 115-119
  complications, 116
  diagnostic studies and findings, 116
  medical management, 116
  nursing care, 116-119
  pathophysiology, 115-116
  patient teaching, 119
Halo traction, 193, 196
Halo-femoral or halo-pelvic traction,
  193, 196
Hammer toe, 34
Hamstring reflex, 35
Hands, examination of, 26, 27-29
Harrington rods, 229
Haversian canal, 5, 6
Haversian system, 5
Head, examination of, 20
Head halter traction, 193, 194
Health history of musculoskeletal
  system, 18
Heat, therapeutic uses of, 258
Heberden's nodes, 98
Hematopoiesis (hemopoiesis), 6
Herniated disks; *see* Ruptured disks
Hip(s)
  blood supply to, 226, 227
  examination of, 29-31
Hip prostheses, 220, 275
Hip replacement, total; *see* Total hip
  replacement
Histamine H₂ antagonists, 290
History, health, of musculoskeletal
  system, 18
Hoffman external fixation apparatus,
  204
Homan sign, 294
Hubbard tank, 258
Hughston test, 295
Humpback, 146
Hyaline cartilage, 13
Hydeltrasol; *see* Prednisolone sodium
  phosphate
Hydrocortisone, 284
Hydrocortisone acetate, 284
Hydrocortisone cypionate, 284
Hydrocortisone sodium phosphate, 284
Hydrocortisone sodium succinate, 284
Hydrocortone Phosphate; *see*
  Hydrocortisone sodium
  phosphate
Hydroxychloroquine, 287-288
Hyndman test, 293
Hyperextension, 15
Hyperflexion, 15
Hyperlordosis, 155

I

I band, 10, 11
Ibuprofen, 282
Iliac crests, examination of, 29
Ilizarov method, 248-255
  nursing care, 250-254
  patient teaching, 255
  preprocedural nursing care, 249
Immunomodulating agents, 289
Impacted fracture, 53
Imuran; *see* Azathioprine
Indocin; *see* Indomethacin
Indole, 282
Indo-Lemmon; *see* Indomethacin
Indometh; *see* Indomethacin
Indomethacin, 282
Infectious musculoskeletal conditions;
  see Osteomyelitis; Wound
  infections
Inflammatory musculoskeletal
  conditions; *see* Ankylosing
  spondylitis; Bursitis;
  Epicondylitis; Lyme disease;
  Rheumatoid arthritis; Tendinitis
Injured limbs, elevation of, 182
Injury; *see* Trauma, musculoskeletal
Interphalangeal joint, examination of,
  26, 27, 29
Interstitial venous pressure,
  measurement of, 183
Intervertebral discs, ruptured, 110-111
  patient teaching guide on, 268
Intraarticular fracture, 53
Inversion, 15
Iron, foods high in, 74
Isotonic twitch, 12

J

Jaw jerk reflex, 35
Joint(s), 14-16; *see also* specific types
  movements of, 15, 16
  replacement of; *see* Total hip
    replacement; Total knee
    replacement; Total shoulder
    replacement
  structure of, 14-15
  synovial, structure of, 14
  temporomandibular, examination of,
    20-21
  types of, 14, 16
Joint capsule, 14
Joint play
  of ankles, 33
  of cervical spine, 21
  of feet, 34
  of hips, 31
  of knee, 33
  of shoulder muscles, 25

Joint play—cont'd
  of thoracic and lumbar spine, 23
  of wrists and fingers, 29

K

Kenacort; *see* Triamcinolone
Kenalog; *see* Triamcinolone acetonide
Kenoject; *see* Triamcinolone acetonide
Kernig sign, 295
Ketoprofen, 282
Key-Pred; *see* Prednisolone acetate
Key-Pred-SR; *see* Prednisolone sodium
  phosphate
K-Flex; *see* Orphenadrine citrate
Klumpke's paralysis, 104
Knee(s)
  examination of, 31-33
  ligaments and tendons of, 12
  meniscus of, 212
  structures of, 14
Knee prostheses, 223, 277
Knee replacement, total; *see* Total knee
  replacement
Kyphosis, 145-149
  complications, 146
  diagnostic studies and findings, 146
  medical management, 147
  nursing care, 147-149
  pathophysiology, 146
  patient teaching, 149
  x-ray of, 146

L

Laboratory values, normal, 43-45
Lachman test, 295
Lacunae, 5, 6
Laguere test, 295
Lamellae, 5, 6
Leg(s)
  bones of, 2
  examination of, 29, 33
  muscles of, 8
Leiomyoma, 161, 163
Leiomyosarcoma, 161, 163
Ligaments, 12
Linear fracture, 53
Lines and bands of muscle fibers, 10,
  11
Lioresal; *see* Baclofen
Liquid Pred; *see* Prednisone
Lopurin; *see* Allopurinol
Lordosis, 155
Low back pain, 110
  patient teaching guide on, 266-267
Lumbar puncture, 41
Lumbar spine, examination of, 22-23
Luque rods, 229
Lyme disease, 91-96
  complications, 91

Lyme disease—cont'd
  diagnostic studies and findings, 91
  medical management, 92
  nursing care, 92-96
  pathophysiology, 91
  patient teaching, 96

M

M line, 10
Macintosh test, 295
Magnuson-Stack procedure, 232
Magnesium salicylate, 281
Magnetic resonance imaging, 37
Malgaigne's fracture, 55
Maolate; *see* Chlorphenesin carbamate
Marbaxin; *see* Methocarbamol
Marflex; *see* Orphenadrine citrate
Marie-Strümpell arthritis, 74
McMurray test, 32, 295
Meclodium; *see* Meclofenamate
Meclofenamate, 282
Meclomen; *see* Meclofenamate
Median nerve entrapment, 104
Medications; *see* specific drugs
Medralone; *see* Methylprednisolone
    acetate
Medrol; *see* Methylprednisolone
Mefenamic acid, 282
Meniscectomy, 211-218
  contraindications and cautions, 212
  diagnostic studies and findings, 212
  medical management, 213
  nursing care, 214-218
  patient teaching, 218
  preprocedural care, 212
Meniscus, 14
Mepolone; *see* Methylprednisolone
Metabolic musculoskeletal conditions;
    see Gout; Osteomalacia;
    Osteoporosis
Metacarpophalangeal joint, examination
    of, 26, 27, 28
Metaphysis, 4
Metatarsus varus and valgus, 34
Metaxalone, 285
Methocarbamol, 285
Methotrexate, 290
Methylprednisolone, 284
Methylprednisolone acetate, 284
Methylprednisolone sodium succinate,
    284
Metiocorten; *see* Prednisone
Milgram test, 296
Milwaukee brace, 265
Monteggia's fracture, 56
Motor endplate, 10, 11
Motrin; *see* Ibuprofen
MRI, 37

Muscle(s), 7-12; *see also* specific types
  of arm, 7
  biopsy of, 43
  contraction and relaxation of, 10-11
  diseases of; *see* specific diseases
  fibers of, 10
  functions and types of, 7
  of leg, 8
  names of, 7
  of shoulder (rotator cuff), 231
  skeletal, structure of, 7-8
  striated, lines and bands in, 10, 11
  structure of, 7-10
  of trunk and pelvis, 9
  tumors of; *see* Musculoskeletal
      tumors
Muscle fibers, 10
Muscle spasm, 12
Muscle tone, 12
Muscle twitch, 12
Muscle-relaxant medications, 284-285
Musculoskeletal drugs, 280-291
  antigout, 286-287
  antiinflammatory, 280-284
  antirheumatic, 287-290
  antiulcer, 290
  muscle-relaxant, 284-285
Musculoskeletal system
  anatomy and physiology of, 1-16
  assessment of, 17-35
  disorders of; *see* specific disorders
Musculoskeletal trauma; *see* Trauma,
    Musculoskeletal
Musculoskeletal tumors, 156-171
  of bone and cartilage, 159-163
  classification of, with tissue of origin,
      157
  Enneking's system of, 158
  of muscles, 163-164
  nursing care, 164-171
  patient teaching, 171
  staging of, 157, 159
  surgical options for, 163-164
Myelography, 40-41
Myochrysine; *see* Gold sodium
    thiomalate
Myoglobin, 8
Myolin; *see* Orphenadrine citrate
Myosin, 10, 11

N

Naffsiger sign, 296
Nalfon; *see* Fenoprofen
Naprosyn; *see* Naproxen
Naproxen, 282
Naproxen sodium, 282
Neck, examination of, 21-22
Neer fracture, 56
Nerve entrapment syndromes, 104

Nerve injury, sciatic; *see* Sciatic nerve
    injury
Neurovascular checks, inside back
    cover
Nightstick fracture, 53
90-90 traction, 193, 196
Niscort; *see* Prednisolone acetate
Nizatidine, 290
Nodes
  Bouchard's, 98
  Heberden's, 98
Nodules, subcutaneous, 63
Nonangulated fracture, 53
Nondisplaced fracture, 53
Nonsteroidal antiinflammatory drugs,
    281-283
Norflex; *see* Orphenadrine citrate
Nor-Pred; *see* Prednisolone tebutate
NSAIDs; *see* Nonsteroidal
    antiinflammatory drugs
Nuprin; *see* Ibuprofen

O

OA; *see* Osteoarthritis
Oblique fracture, 54
Occult fracture, 54
Occupational therapists, 256
O-Flex; *see* Orphenadrine citrate
Open fracture, 54
Open reduction with internal fixation,
    218-219
  contraindications and cautions, 219
  medical management, 219
  nursing care, 233-243
  patient teaching, 243
  preprocedural care, 219
Oppenheim reflex, 35
Orasone; *see* Prednisone
ORIF: *see* Open reduction with
    internal fixation
Orphenadrine citrate, 285
Orthotist, 256
Ortolani click, 173
Ortolani maneuver, 296
Orudis; *see* Ketoprofen
Osteoarthritis, 97-103
  complications, 98
  diagnostic studies and findings,
      99-100
  medical management, 99
  nursing care, 100-103
  pathophysiology, 98
  patient teaching, 103
  patient teaching guide on, 261-262
  treatment of, 262
Osteoblasts, 6
Osteochondroma, 159-161
Osteoclastoma, 160
Osteoclasts, 6

Osteocytes, 5
Osteogenesis, 3
Osteoma, 159, 160
Osteomalacia, 140-144
  complications, 140
  diagnostic studies and findings, 140
  medical management, 141
  nursing care, 141-143
  pathophysiology, 140
  patient teaching, 144
Osteomyelitis, 120-127
  complications, 121
  diagnostic studies and findings, 122
  medical management, 123
  nursing care, 123-127
  pathophysiology, 121
  patient teaching, 127
  types of, 121
Osteophytes, 98
Osteoporosis, 129-136
  complications, 131
  diagnostic studies and findings, 130
  medical management, 132
  nursing care, 132-135
  pathophysiology, 130-131
  patient teaching, 136
  patient teaching guide on, 263-264
  treatment of, 264
  x-ray of, 130
Osteosarcoma, 160, 162
Osteotomy, 228
Oxicam, 282
Oxyphenbutazone, 282-283

P

Pain, low back; *see* Low back pain
Palsy, Erb's, 104
Pannus formation of synovium, 64
Pansol-S; *see* Prednisone
Paraflex; *see* Chlorzoxazone
Parafon Forte; *see* Chlorzoxazone
Parosteal osteosarcoma, 160, 162
Patellar reflex, 35
Pathologic fracture, 54
Patient teaching guides, 259-279
Pavlik harness, 174
Pectoralis major reflex, 35
Pediapred; *see* Prednisolone sodium
  phosphate
Pelvic belt, 193, 195
Pelvic sling, 193, 194-195
Pelvis
  bones of, 3
  examination of, 29
  muscles of, 9
Penicillamine, 288-289
Pepcid; *see* Famotidine
Perichondrium, 13
Perimysia, 10

Periosteum, 4
Peripheral nerve entrapment
  syndromes, 104
Peroneal nerve entrapment, 104
Pes cavus, 34
Pes planus, 34
Pes valgus, 34
Pes varus, 34
Phalen sign, 296
Phenylacetic acid, 282
Phenylbutazone, 282-283
Physical examination of musculoskeletal
  tissues, 19-35
Physical therapy, 256, 257, 258
Pins, transfixing, 204
Piroxicam, 282
Plantar flexion, 15
Plaquenil; *see* Hydroxychloroquine
Ponstel; *see* Mefenaminic acid
Posttraumatic arthritis, 184
Posture, examination of, 19-20
Pott's fracture, 56
Predaject; *see* Prednisolone acetate
Predalone; *see* Prednisolone tebutate
Predcor; *see* Prednisolone acetate
Predicort; *see* Prednisolone sodium
  phosphate
Prednicen-M; *see* Prednisone
Prednisolone acetate, 284
Prednisolone sodium phosphate, 284
Prednisolone tebutate, 284
Prednisone, 284
Probanlan; *see* Probenecid
Probenecid, 286
Pronation, 15
Propionic acid, 282
Prostheses
  ankle, 225
  elbow, 225
  of femoral head, 227
  hip, 220
  knee, 223
  wrist, 225
Prosthetist, 256
Prozalone derivatives, 282-283
Purines, foods high in, 137
Putti-Platt procedure, 232

Q

Q-pam; *see* Diazepam
Quick sign, 296
Quinacrine, 321, 324, 325
Quinine sulfate, 320-321

R

RA; *see* Rheumatoid arthritis
Radial nerve entrapment, 104
Radiocarpal groove, examination of, 26
Radiographic examination, 36

Range of motion
  of cervical spine, 21
  of diarthrotic joints, 15
  of elbow, 26
  of hip, 30, 31
  of knee, 32
  of lumbar spine, 23
  of shoulder, 24, 25
  of thoracic spine, 23
  of wrists, hands, and fingers, 27, 28
Ranitidine, 290
Reflexes, testing, 35
Rehabilitation, 255-258
  nursing considerations, 256-257
  team members and functions, 256
  various treatments used, 258
Rela; *see* Carisoprodol
Relaxation of muscle, 10-11
Rhabdomyoma, 161, 163
Rhabdomyosarcoma, 161, 163
Rheumatoid arthritis, 63-74
  complications, 64
  diagnostic studies and findings, 64
  medical management, 65
  nursing care, 65-74
  pathophysiology, 63-64
  patient teaching, 74
  patient teaching guide on, 261-262
  treatment of, 262
Rheumatrex; *see* Methotrexate
RICE, 260
Ridaura; *see* Auranofin
Robaxin; *see* Methocarbamol
Rods, metallic, spinal fusion with,
  228-230
Roentgenograms, 36
Roger Anderson external fixation
  apparatus, 204
Rotation, 15
Rotator cuff muscles, 231
  examination of, 24-25
Rotator cuff tears, surgery for, 230-231
  contraindications and cautions, 230
  medical management, 231
  nursing care, 233-243
  patient teaching, 243
  preprocedural care, 231
Round back, 146
Ruptured disks, 110-111
  patient teaching guide on, 268
Russell traction, 193, 194, 195

S

Salicylate toxicity, 281
Salicylates, 280-281
Salsalate, 281
Salter (Salter-Harris) fracture, 56
Sarcolemma, 10
Sarcoma, Ewing's, 160, 162

Sarcomere, 10
Sarcoplasm, 10
Scans, bone, 38-39
Scapula(e), examination of, 23, 24
Scheuermann's disease, 145, 146
Schober sign, 296
Sciatic nerve entrapment, 104
Sciatic nerve injury, 110-115
    anatomy of, 110
    complications, 111
    diagnostic studies and findings, 112
    medical management, 111
    nursing care, 112-114
    pathophysiology, 110-111
    patient teaching, 115
Scintigraphy, bone, 38-39
Scoliosis, 150-154
    complications, 150
    diagnostic studies and findings, 151
    medical management, 151
    nursing care, 151-154
    pathophysiology, 150
    patient teaching, 154
    patient teaching guide on, 265
Segmented fracture, 54
Sezone; *see* Dexamethasone sodium
        phosphate
Sharpey's fibers, 4
Shoulder(s)
    examination of, 23-25
    muscles of, 231
Shoulder dislocations, recurrent, 232
Shoulder replacement, total; *see* Total
        shoulder replacement
Skelaxin; *see* Metaxalone
Skeletal Dunlop traction, 193, 195
Skeletal muscles; *see* Muscles, skeletal
Skeletal traction; *see* Traction (skin and
        skeletal)
Skeleton, 1, 2-3; *see also* Bones
Skin care
    for braces with scoliosis, 265
    and casts, 185
Skin traction; *see* Traction (skin and
        skeletal)
Skull tongs, 193, 195
Sodol; *see* Carisoprodol
Solganal; *see* Aurothioglucose
Solu-Cortef; *see* Hydrocortisone sodium
        succinate
Solu-Medrol; *see* Methylprednisolone
        sodium succinate
Solurex; *see* Dexamethasone sodium
        phosphate
Soma; *see* Carisoprodol
Soprodol; *see* Carisoprodol
Spasm, muscle, 12
Speed sign, 296
Spinal fracture, 54

Spinal fusion, 228-230
    contraindications and cautions, 230
    medical management, 230
    nursing care, 233-243
    patient teaching, 243
    preprocedural care, 230
Spine
    cervical, examination of, 21
    curvatures of, 145-155
        kyphosis, 145-149
        lordosis, 155
        scoliosis, 150-154
    lumbar, examination of, 22-23
    thoracic, examination of, 22-23
Spondylitis, ankylosing; *see* Ankylosing
        spondylitis
Spondylolisthesis, 229
Sprains, 12
    classification of, 48, 50
    patient teaching guide on, 260
    symptoms of, 50
    treatment of, 49, 260
Staphylococcus aureus and
        osteomyelitis, 120
Stature, examination of, 19, 20
Stellate fracture, 54
Sterapred; *see* Prednisone
Sternoclavicular joint, examination of,
        25
Still's disease, 63
Straddle fracture, 54
Strain(s), 48, 49, 50
    classification of, 48, 50
    patient teaching guide on, 260
    symptoms of, 50
    treatment of, 48-49, 260
Stress fracture, 54
Striated muscle, lines and bands in, 10,
        11
Stroke test, 293
Stump wrapping, 210
Subcutaneous nodules, 63
Subluxation, 49
Suction drainage system, 220
Sulfinpyrazone, 287
Sulindac, 282
Supination, 15
Supraspinatus sign 296
Surgery; *see* specific types of surgery
Sutures, 16
Swayback, 155
Symphysis, 16
Synarthrotic joints, 14, 16
Syndesmoses, 16
Synovectomy, 232-233
    contraindications and cautions, 232
    medical management, 233
    nursing care, 233-243
    patient teaching, 243

Synovectomy—cont'd
    preprocedural care, 233
Synovial joint, structures of 14
Synovium, 14
    biopsy of, 43

T

Tac-D; *see* Triamcinolone diacetate
Tac-40; *see* Triamcinolone acetonide
Tagamet; *see* Cimetidine
Talipes equinovarus, 175-178
    casts for, 176
    complications, 175
    diagnostic studies and findings, 175
    medical management, 176
    nursing care, 176-178
    pathophysiology, 175
    patient teaching, 178
Tarsal tunnel syndrome, 104
Teardrop fracture, 56
Temporomandibular joint, examination
        of, 20-21
Tendinitis, 82-87
    complications, 83
    diagnostic studies and findings, 84
    medical management, 83
    nursing care, 84-87
    pathophysiology, 82-83
    patient teaching, 87
Tendons, 12
Tennis elbow, 82
Tenosynovitis; *see* Tendinitis
TENS, 270
Thighs, examination of, 33
Thomas test, 296
Thompson sign, 297
Thoracic outlet syndrome, 104
Thoracic spine, examination of, 22-23
THR; *see* Total hip replacement
Tibial nerve entrapment, 104
Tinel's sign, 106, 297
TKR; *see* Total knee replacement
TMJ; *see* Temporomandibular joint
Tolectin; *see* Tolmentin
Tolmentin, 282
Tomography, computed, 38
Tone, muscle, 12
Torticollis, 150
Torus fracture, 54
Total hip replacement, 220-222
    contraindications and cautions, 221
    medical management, 222
    nursing care, 233-243
    patient teaching, 243
    patient teaching guides on, 275, 276
    preprocedural care, 221
Total joint replacement for wrist,
        elbow, or ankle, 225

Total knee replacement, 222-223
  contraindications and cautions, 222
  medical management, 223
  nursing care, 233-243
  patient teaching, 243
  patient teaching guides on, 277, 278
  preprocedural care, 222
Total shoulder replacement, 224-225
  contraindications and cautions, 225
  medical management, 224
  nursing care, 233-243
  patient teaching, 243
  patient teaching guide on, 279
  preprocedural care, 225
Trabeculae, 5
Traction (skin and skeletal), 192-203
  complications, 192
  nursing care, 197-203
  patient teaching, 203
  patient teaching guide on, 273
  preparation before, 196
  principles of, 193
  types of, 193, 194-196
  uses of, 193
Transcutaneous electrical nerve
    stimulation (TENS), 270
Transfixing pins, 204
Transverse fracture, 54
Trapezius muscle(s), examination of,
    23, 24
Trauma, musculoskeletal, 46-62; *see
    also* Fracture(s)
  age-related injuries, 47

Trauma, musculoskeletal—cont'd
  nursing care, 57-62
  patient teaching, 62
  principles of management, 47, 48
  statistics, 46
  types of and care for, 48-52
Trendelenburg's sign, 31, 173, 297
Treppe, 11
Triamcinolone, 284
Triamcinolone acetonide, 284
Triamcinolone diacetate, 284
Triamcinolone hexacetonide, 284
Triceps muscles, examination of, 24
Triceps reflex, 35
Trochanters, 4
Trunk
  bones of, 3
  muscles of, 9
TSR; *see* Total shoulder
    replacement
Tubercles, 4
Tumors; *see* Musculoskeletal
    tumors
Twitch, muscle, 12

U

Ulnar drift, 63
Ulnar nerve entrapment, 104
Ulnohumeral joint, examination of,
    27-29
Unicameral bone cyst, 160, 162
Uricosuric drugs, 286-287
Urine laboratory values, 45

V

Valium; *see* Diazepam
Venous pressure, interstitial,
    measurement of, 183
Vitamin D
  and bone formation, 6
  and osteomalacia, 140, 141
  and osteoporosis, 264
Voltaren; *see* Diclofenac

W

Weber test, 297
Wipe test, 293
Wound infections, 128
Wrist(s)
  examination of, 26, 27-29
  total joint replacement for, 225
Wryneck, 150

X

X-ray examination, 36

Y

Yellow cartilage, 13
Yeoman's test, 297
Yergason test, 297

Z

Z line, 10, 11
Zantac; *see* Ranitidine
Zetran; *see* Diazepam
Zidovudine, 319, 320
Zurinol; *see* Allopurinol
Zyloprim; *see* Allopurinol

NEUROVASCULAR CHECKS

Parameter	Significance
Color of affected and surrounding tissues	Indicates adequacy of circulation; color should be pinkish, not pale or white. Injured tissues are usually paler than the contralateral tissues.
Temperature of affected tissue	Indicates circulatory adequacy or perfusion. Injured tissues are usually cooler than contralateral tissues.
Capillary refill of nails	Refill in 2-4 seconds indicates normal capillary perfusion. Initially, injured tissues may have normal refill, but gradual slowing may be noted with careful assessment; slowing to 4-6 seconds should be reported.
Edema	Presence indicates venous stasis. Injured tissues usually are noticeably more swollen than contralateral tissues.
Range of motion or movement of tissues	Indicates amount or degree of limitation(s) of movement. Injured tissues usually have decreased mobility (patient may hold the part to lessen pain).
Sensory functions (may not be diagnostic in newborn or very young baby)	Indicates pressure on nerves, noted by complaints of numbness, tingling, or "pins and needles" sensation.
Complaints of pain	Indicates injury, pressure, or trauma to tissues. Injured tissues usually are more painful than contralateral tissues.
Affected and unaffected tissues bilaterally	Indicates specific tissue involved when compared with other side.